JOSE JACOB
SENIOR I
PHYSIOTHERAPIST

D1352644

Dictionary of
Physiotherapy

For Elsevier:

Senior Commissioning Editor: Heidi Harrison
Development Editor: Siobhan Campbell
Production Manager: Caroline Horton
Design: Judith Wright
Illustration Manager: Bruce Hogarth
Cartoonist: David Banks

Dictionary of Physiotherapy

....

Stuart Porter
BSc (Hons), Grad Dip Phys, MCSP, SRP, CertMHS

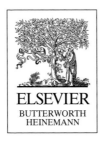

ELSEVIER
BUTTERWORTH
HEINEMANN

EDINBURGH LONDON NEW YORK OXFORD PHILADELPHIA
ST LOUIS SYDNEY TORONTO   2005

ELSEVIER
BUTTERWORTH
HEINEMANN

© 2005, Elsevier Ltd

The right of Stuart Porter to be identified as editor of this work has been asserted by them in accordance with the Copyright, Designs and Patents Act 1988.

No part of this publication may be reproduced, stored in a retrieval system, or transmitted in any form or by any means, electronic, mechanical, photocopying, recording or otherwise, without either the prior permission of the publishers or a licence permitting restricted copying in the United Kingdom issued by the Copyright Licensing Agency, 90 Tottenham Court Road, London W1T 4LP. Permissions may be sought directly from Elsevier's Health Sciences Rights Department in Philadelphia, USA: (+1) 215 239 3804, fax: (+1) 215 239 3805, e-mail: healthpermissions@elsevier.com. You may also complete your request on-line via the Elsevier Science homepage (http://www.elsevier.com), by selecting 'Support and contact' and then 'Copyright and Permission'.

First published 2005
  Reprinted 2007, 2009 (twice)

ISBN-13: 978 0 7506 8833 8

British Library Cataloguing in Publication Data
A catalogue record for this book is available from the British Library.

Library of Congress Cataloging in Publication Data
A catalog record for this book is available from the Library of Congress.

Note
Knowledge and best practice in this field are constantly changing. As new research and experience broaden our knowledge, changes in practice, treatment and drug therapy may become necessary or appropriate. Readers are advised to check the most current information provided (i) on procedures featured or (ii) by the manufacturer of each product to be administered, to verify the recommended dose or formula, the method and duration of administration and contraindications. It is the responsibility of the practitioner, relying on their own experience and knowledge of the patient, to make diagnoses, to determine dosages and the best treatment for each individual patient, and to take all appropriate safety precautions. To the fullest extent of the law, neither the publisher nor the editor assumes any liability for any injury and/or damage.

The Publisher

Contents

. . . .

For Kate and for Mary,
For bringing so many years of heartache to an end,
what you did was wonderful
– thank you.

Acknowledgements

No one writes a book alone and there are some people that I need to thank. Firstly to all the contributors who gave their precious time and effort to this project. Heidi Harrison and Robert Edwards at Elsevier Science for their continued faith in me; Sarah Wilkinson, Caroline Callister, Nichola Gale, Mark Clare, Richard Muir, David Wilkes – student physiotherapists; Ann Prescott, Niamh O'Sullivan and Peter Burley – The Health Professions Council, Park House, 184 Kennington Park Road, London; Brian R. Mulligan NZRP, Dip MT, FNZSP, MCTA and Jack Miller BSc (PT), Dip MT (NZ), FCAMT, MCTA; Stephen Ashmore, Leicester Primary Care Audit Group, Manager; Tracy Johnson, Leicester Primary Care Audit Group, Deputy Manager; Louise Fish, Senior Communications Manager, National Institute for Clinical Excellence; Dariel Terry MA BS, Assistant Professor of Information System Technology at Northern Virginia Community College, USA; Stephen May MCSP, Dip MDT, MSc Senior Lecturer in Physiotherapy Sheffield Hallam University; Robert Conlon and Chris Rees Evans and Alistair Dickson and Philip McCusker. As usual, my exceptional wife and children have been with me during the writing of this book.

This is the third book to bear my name – a fact that I still cannot quite believe. I hope that fact is some inspiration to those students who feel that they will not make it past graduation. If I can do it, so can you.

Contributors

Stuart B. Porter BSc (Hons) Grad Dip Phys MCSP SRP Cert MHS
Lecturer in Physiotherapy
University of Salford Manchester UK
Hon Research Fellow Wrightington Wigan and Leigh NHS Trust
UK

Sue Porter RGN, DPSN
Field Manager
Innovex (UK) Ltd.
UK

Nigel Palastanga MA BA FCSP DMS DipTP ILTM
Pro Vice-Chancellor
Dept Physiotherapy Education
School of Healthcare Studies
University of Wales College of Medicine
UK

Heather A. Thornton MBA PGCE MCSP SRP ILTM
Senior Lecturer
Department of Allied Health Professions – Physiotherapy
University of Hertfordshire
UK

Sally French
Freelance Researcher and Writer
Associate Lecturer at the Open University
UK

Jackie Hindle Grad Dip Phys MMACP MCSP SRP
Department of Physiotherapy
Manchester Metropolitan University
UK

Ruth Anderson BSc (Hons) MCSP SRP MMACP
Department of Physiotherapy
Manchester Metropolitan University
UK

Kay Fitton BSc (Hons) MCSP SRP
Department of Physiotherapy
Manchester Metropolitan University
UK

John Swain
Professor of Disability and Inclusion
Faculty of Health, Social Work and Education
University of Northumbria
Newcastle-upon-Tyne
UK

Val J. Robertson PhD BAppSci (Physio) BA (Hons)
Professor of Allied Health
University of Newcastle and Central Coast Health
Gosford
Australia

Susan Pieri-Davies MSc MCSP SRP DipRGRT
Project Manager & Senior Respiratory Lecturer
Respiratory Education and Training Centres
Aintree University Hospital
Liverpool
UK

Ralph Hammond MSc MCSP
Professional Advisor
The Chartered Society of Physiotherapy
London
UK

Cherry Kilbride MSc MCSP SRP
Deputy Head of Therapy Services
Royal Free Hampstead NHS Trust
London
UK

Tim Watson
Professor of Physiotherapy
Department of Allied Health Professions
University of Hertfordshire
UK

Prefixes

Commonly encountered Prefixes and their meanings

an-	absence of, e.g. atrophy = absence of growth
ab-	away from
acro-	extremity
acou-, acu-	hear
adeno-	gland
alg-	pain, e.g. arthralgia = joint pain
an-	without
andro-	man androgens are male hormones
ankylo-	crooked, curved, e.g. ankylosing spondylitis
angio-	vessel, e.g. angiogram is a test to examine the arteries
ant-	against
ante-, antero-	before, e.g. antenatal classes occur before birth
anteri-	front, forward
anti-	against, e.g. anti-gravity muscles work against gravity
arterio-	artery, e.g. arteriogram
arthro-	joint, e.g. arthritis means inflammation of a joint
articul-	joint
athero-	fatty
audio-	hearing
aut-	self, e.g. auto-assisted exercises are assisted by the patient themselves
bi-	two or twice
bili-	bile
bi-, bis-	double, twice, two
brady-	slow, e.g. bradykinesia = slowness of movement, bradycardia = slow heart rate
carcin-	cancer
cardio-	heart
cephalo-	head
cerebro-	brain
cervic-	neck
chemo-	chemico

chole-	bile, or referring to gall bladder
cholecysto-	gall bladder
chondro-	cartilage
circum-	around, about
contra-	against, counter
corpor-	body
costo-	rib
cranio-	skull
cut-	skin
cryo-	cold
cyano-	blue
cysto-	bladder
cyto-	cell
dactyl-	finger
deca-	ten
deci-	one-tenth
dent-	tooth
dermato-	skin
diplo-	double
dors-	back
dys-	abnormal
ecto-	outside
electro-	electricity
encephalo-	brain
endo-	within
entero-	intestine
erythro-	red
extra-	outside
ferro-	iron
gastro-	stomach
gen-	originate
gynae-	female
haemato-	blood, e.g. haematologist
hemi -	half, e.g. hemiarthroplasty
hepato-	liver, e.g. hepatitis
hetero-	dissimilar
homo-	same
hydro-	water

hyper-	excessive, high, e.g. hypertension is high blood pressure
hypo-	deficient, low, e.g. hypotension is low blood pressure
hystero-	uterus, e.g. hysterectomy
iatro-	doctor, e.g. if a condition has been caused by the medical profession is iatrogenic
infra-	beneath, e.g. infra patellar fat pad
inter-	among, between, e.g. an inter muscular haematoma lies between two muscles
intra-	inside, e.g. the anterior cruciate ligament is an intra articular ligament
iso-	the same
laparo-	flank, abdomen
latero-	side
leuko-	white leukocyte – white blood cell
linguo-	tongue, e.g. a medicine which is given sub lingually is under the tongue
lipo-	fat, e.g. liposuction
lympho-	lymphatic
macro-	large
mal-	bad, abnormal, e.g. malabsorption
mammo-	breast, e.g. mammography
masto-	breast
meningo-	membranes, e.g. meningitis is inflammation of the meninges, membranes that surround the brain
micro-	small
milli-	one-thousandth
mono-	one
multi-	many
myo-	muscle, e.g. myometer measures muscle strength
myelo-	marrow, e.g. myeloma
naso-	nose
necro-	death, e.g. avascular necrosis means death of tissue due to lack of blood supply
nephro-	kidney, e.g. nephrectomy is removal of a kidney
neuro-	nerve, e.g. neurology
oophoro-	ovaries, e.g. oophrectomy means removal of the ovaries
osseo-	bone
osteo-	bone
oto-	ear

ovari-	ovary
paed-	child
para-	beside
patho-	disease
peri-	around
phago-	eat, destroy
pharm-	drug
pharyngo-	throat
phlebo-	vein
pleuro-	pleura
pneum-	breath, air
pneumono-	lung
poly-	much, many
post-	after
posteri-	back, behind
procto-	anus
pseudo-	false
psycho-	mind
pulmono-	lung
pyelo-	kidney
pyo-	fever
quad-	four
reno-	kidneys, e.g. renal failure
retro-	behind
rhino-	nose, e.g. rhinoplasty
sacro-	sacrum
salping-	fallopian tube
sclero-	hard, e.g. scleroderma
scope-	instrument, e.g. arthroscope or bronchoscope
scopy-	examination
semi-	half
socio-	sociology
spleno-	spleen
spondylo-	vertebra, e.g. spondylosis
sub-	beneath
supra-	above, e.g. supraspinatus comes from above the spine of the scapula
syn-	united with

tachy-	fast, quick, e.g. tachycardia is a rapid heart rate
therap-	treatment, e.g. exercise therapy
thoraco-	chest
thrombo-	clot, lump, e.g. thrombosis
tomy-	incision (operation by cutting), e.g. laparotomy
tracheo-	trachea
trans-	across
uro-	urine
utero-	uterus
vaso-	vessel, e.g. vasoconstriction referring to blood vessels
veno-	vein, e.g. venogram

Suffixes

Commonly used suffixes

-able	capable
-aemia	blood
-aesthesia	sense perception
-algia	pain
-blast	cell
-centesis	to puncture
-ectomy	removal by cutting
-emia	blood
-epi	outer, superficial,
-graph	measuring instrument
-itis	inflammation, e.g. tendinitis
-kinesis, -kinetic	movement
-lysis, -lytic	to break down
-malacia	softening
-morph	form or shape
-odynia	pain
-ogen	a precursor
-oid	resemblance
-ology	study of
-oma	tumour
-opsy	examine
-ostomy	to form an opening
-otomy	to make a cut
-pathy	disease
-penia	lack of
-peps, -pept	digest
-phagia	swallowing
-phasia	speech
-philia	love of
-phobia	fear of
-plasty	reconstruction
-pleg(ia)	paralysis

-pnea	breathing
-pod(o)	foot
-poie	make, produce
-ptosis	falling
-rhage	burst forth
-rhythmia	rhythm
-scope	to examine with a probe
-stasis	cessation of movement
-tome	surgical cutting tool
-trophy	growth
-uria	urine

Abbreviations

AAA	Abdominal aortic aneurysm
ABGs	Arterial blood gases
ACBT	Active cycle breathing technique
ACL	Anterior cruciate ligament
ADL	Activities of daily living
AE	Air entry
AFO	Ankle foot orthosis
AIDS	Aquired immunodeficiency syndrome
AP	Antero posterior
ARDS	Acute respiratory distress syndrome
ARF	Acute renal failure
AF	Atrial fibrillation
AS	Ankylosing spondylitis
AVR	Aortic valve replacement
BCG	Bacille Calmette–Guérin
BID	Twice a day (medication)
BiPAP	Bi-level positive airway pressure
BM	Blood glucose monitoring
BP	Blood pressure
BPM	Beats per minute
BS (x2)	Breath or bowel sounds
B/slab	Back slab
Ca	Carcinoma
CABG	Coronary artery bypass graft
CAD	Coronary artery disease
CAPD	Continuous ambulatory peritoneal dialysis
CBC	Complete blood cell count
CCF	Congestive cardiac failure
CDH	Congenital dislocation of hip
CI	Chest infection
CK	Creatine kinase
CPK	Creatine phosphokinase
CT	Computerised tomography
C/O	Complains of
COP	Completion or change of plaster
COPD	Chronic obstructive pulmonary disease
CPAP	Continuous positive airway pressure
CPM	Continuous passive motion
CRP	C-reactive protein
Crash team	Cardiac arrest team
C-section	Caesarean section

CTEV	Congenital talipes equinovarus
CVA(IN)	Cerebro vascular accident (incident)
CVS	Cardio vascular system
c/w	Consistent with
CXR	Chest X-ray
D&C	Dilation & curettage
DBE	Deep breathing exercises
DDD	Degenerative disc disease
DH	Drug history
DISH	Diffuse idiopathic skeletal hyperostosis
DOA (x2)	Dead on arrival or date of admission
DMARD	Disease modifying anti-rheumatic drug
DNA (x2)	Deoxyribonucleic acid or did not attend
DM	Diabetes mellitus
DTs	Delirium tremens
DU	Duodenal ulcer
DVT	Deep vein thrombosis
DW	Discussed with
ECG	Electrocardiogram
EIA	Exercise induced asthma
EMG	Electromyogram
EPAP	Expiratory positive airway pressure
EPP	Equal pressure point
ERV	Expiratory reserve volume
ESR	Erythrocyte sedimentation rate
ESRF	End stage renal failure
ET	Endotracheal tube
EUA	Examination under anaesthesia
FBC	Full blood count
FET	Forced expiratory technique
FEV1	Forced expiratory volume in one second
FFD	Fixed flexion deformity
FH	Family history
F(A)ROM	Full (active) range of motion
FRC	Functional residual capacity
FVC	Forced vital capacity
FWB	Full weight bearing
GA	General anaesthetic
GH	Gleno-humeral
GI(t)	Gastro intestinal (tract)
GOR	Gastro oesophageal reflux
GTN	Glyceryol trinitrate
Hb	Haemoglobin
HDL	High density lipoprotein
HDU	High-dependency unit
HIV	Human immunodeficiency virus
HLA	Human leucocyte antigen

HPC	History of present condition
IABP	Intra aortic balloon pump
IBS	Irritable bowel syndrome
ICD	Intercostal drain
ICP	Intracranial pressure
IDC	Indwelling catheter
IF	Interferential therapy
IgG	Immunoglobulin G
IM (x2)	Intramuscular or intra-medullary
INH	Inhalation
INR	International normalized ratio
IRQ	Inner range quadriceps
IPPV	Intermittent positive pressure ventilation
IPS	Inspiratory pressure support
IRV	Inspiratory reserve volume
IS	Incentive spirometry
ITU	Intensive therapy unit
IV	Intravenous
IVI	Intravenous infusion
°JACCOL	No jaundice, anaemia, clubbing, cyanosis, oedema, lymphadenopathy
LA	Local anaesthetic
°LKKS	No liver, kidney, kidney, spleen
LBP	Low back pain
LCL	Lateral collateral ligament
LDL	Low density lipoprotein
LFA	Low friction arthroplasty
LFT (x2)	Lung or liver function tests
LL	Lower lobe or limb
LP	Lumbar puncture
LSCS	Lower segment caesarean section
MAOI	Monoamine oxidase inhibitors
MCL	Medial collateral ligament
MDT	Multi-disciplinary team
ME	Myalgic encephalomyopathy
MI	Myocardial infarction
MMR	Measles-mumps-rubella (vaccine)
MUA	Manipulation under anaesthesia
MRI	Magnetic resonance imaging
MSU	Mid-stream urine
MWM	Mobilizations with movement
MVR	Mitral valve replacement
NAD	No abnormality detected
NAG	Natural apophyseal glide
NAI	Non-accidental injury
NBI	No bony injury

NBM	Nil by mouth
NCPAP	Nasal continuous positive airway pressure
NG	Nasogastric
NOF	Neck of femur
NSAID	Non-steroidal anti inflammatory drug
NIDDM	Non-insulin dependent diabetes mellitus
NIPPV	Non-invasive intermittent positive pressure ventilation
NWB	Non-weight bearing
OA	Osteoarthritis
Occ	Occasional
OE (x2)	Objective examination or on examination
OPD	Out-patient department
ORIF	Open reduction internal fixation
PA	Postero anterior
PCIRV	Pressure controlled inverse ratio ventilation
PCL	Posterior cruciate ligament
PE	Pulmonary embolism
PERLA	Pupils equal reacting to light and accommodating
PEME	Pulsed electromagnetic energy
PFTs	Pulmonary function tests
PFJ	Patello femoral joint
PIFR	Peak inspiratory flow rate
PIP	Peak inspiratory pressure
PMH	Past medical history
PMR	Polymyalgia rheumatica
PID (x2)	Pelvic inflammatory disease or prolapsed inter vertebral disc
PAIVM	Passive accessory inter vertebral movement
PPIVM	Passive physiological inter vertebral movement
POMR	Problem oriented medical records
POP	Plaster of Paris
PU	Passed urine
PR	Per rectum
PRN	As needed (pro re nata)
PVD	Peripheral vascular disease
PWB	Partial weight bearing
Px	Prescribing
QD	Every day
QID	Four times per day
QOD	Every other day
RA	Rheumatoid arthritis
RBC	Red blood cell
RIP	Rest in peace
RR	Respiratory rate
RS	Respiratory system
RSD	Reflex sympathetic dystrophy
RSI	Repetitive strain injury

RTA	Road traffic accident
Rx	Treatment
SAB	Sub acromial bursa
SC	Sub cuticular
SCI	Spinal cord injury
SFL/SFR	Side flex left/right
SH	Social history
SIJ	Sacro iliac joint
SL	Sub lingual
SLE	Systemic lupus erythematosus
SLAP	Superior labrum anterior and posterior
SLE	Systemic lupus erythematosus
SLR	Straight leg raise
SUF(c)E	Slipped upper femoral (capital) epiphysis
SNAG	Sustained natural apophyseal glide
SOB(OE)	Short of breath (on exertion)
SVD	Spontaneous vaginal delivery
SVT	Supra ventricular tachycardia
TA	Tendo Achilles
TAA	Thoracic aortic aneurysm
TATT	Tired all the time
TAR	Total ankle replacement
TDS	Three times a day
TED stocking	Thromboembolic deterrent stocking
TEE	Thoracic expansion exercises
TFCC	Triangular fibrocartilaginous complex (at the wrist)
TFT	Thyroid function tests
THR	Total hip replacement
TIA	Transient ischaemic attack
TKR	Total knee replacement
TTO	To take out (medication)
TURP	Trans urethral resection of prostate
TV	Tidal volume
U&E	Urea and electrolytes
URTI	Upper respiratory tract infection
US	Ultrasound
UTI	Urinary tract infection
VAS	Visual analogue scale
VER	Visual evoked response
VF	Ventricular fibrillation
VMO	Vastus medialis obliquus
VSD	Ventricular septal defect
WBC	White blood cell
X-ray	X-ray

Other symbols seen in medicine

<	Less than
>	More than
°	No (absence of)
#	Fracture
△	Diagnosis

Diagram of abdomen

. . . .

A band The cross striations in the myofibrils of muscle where thick myosin and thin actin filaments overlap.

    See *Muscle structure*

Abdomen The portion of the body between the thorax and the pelvis. This cavity contains the abdominal viscera and is enclosed by a wall formed by the abdominal muscles, vertebral column and the iliac bones.

Abdominal aorta The portion of the aorta below the diaphragm that splits into the right and left common iliac arteries.

Abdominal hernia A hernia protruding through a defect or weakness in the abdominal wall, e.g. an umbilical hernia is a type of abdominal hernia.

Abdominoplasty A surgical operation to remove fatty tissue or excess skin from the lower to middle portions of the abdomen.

Abduction Anatomical term meaning movement of a limb away from the midline of the body. The opposite of adduction.

Abortion Removal or loss of a foetus from the uterine cavity.

Abscess A localized collection of pus in tissues, organs or confined spaces, which is usually caused by some infective organism.

Absolute risk reduction Research term – the difference in the event rate between two groups in a comparative study; the control group (CER) and treated group (EER):

$$ARR = CER - EER$$

Absorption Electrotherapy term – varies with the type, intensity and properties of the energy as well as the types and distribution of tissues through which it passes. Absorption is the inverse of penetration, therefore, higher frequency ultrasound (e.g. 3 MHz) with its shorter wavelength is absorbed more readily than lower frequency ultrasound (e.g. 1 MHz or less).

Abstract Research term – a succinct summary of a research paper. A good abstract should accurately summarize the article.

    ➲ Student tip You should read the article and not just the abstract when you are studying a topic.

Abuse Harm caused to or perpetrated on by one person on another. Abuse may be physical, verbal, sexual, psychological, emotional, financial or through neglect. It is often committed by those who have power over people who are relatively powerless and includes criminal offences. Abuse may also be ingrained within the structure and ethos of institutions where it is referred to as 'systems abuse'. In addressing abuse the wishes of the victim should be paramount.

Academic title The title of an academic member of staff, e.g. from most junior upwards – lecturer, senior (principal) lecturer, professor, dean, pro vice chancellor, provost, vice chancellor, chancellor.

Academic unit The term used to describe a distinct academic part of a university, e.g. in progressive order of size – section, department, division, school, faculty, college.

Acceleration Acceleration is the rate of change of velocity, i.e. the change in velocity over a given time:

$$\text{Acceleration} = \text{Change in Velocity} \div \text{Time}$$

Accessory movement A movement that cannot be performed voluntarily by the patient, e.g. rotation of the MCP joint, but that is necessary for normal joint function. Includes movements such as spin, roll and glide.

Accessory nerve The nerve that supplies the sternocleidomastoid and the trapezius muscles.

Accommodation Property of nerve. If stimulus increases too slowly the sodium pump adjusts and there will be no action potential. The nerve has accommodated.

Accountability The provision of explanations and justifications and being responsible for actions. Physiotherapists are accountable to their patients and clients, the organizations in which they work and their professional body. The interests of these groups may conflict making accountability difficult to achieve.

ACE inhibitors Drugs used to treat high blood pressure and congestive heart failure.

Acetabular labrum A fibrocartilaginous ring attached around the margin of the acetabulum in the pelvis, it serves to deepen the socket and aids joint stability. The glenoid of the shoulder also possesses a labrum.

Acetylcholine Also known as ACh, acetylcholine serves as a neurotransmitter at many synapses in the peripheral nervous system and central nervous system including neuromuscular junctions.

Achilles tendinitis Inflammation of the Achilles tendon.

Achilles tendon The tendon that attaches the gastrocnemius and soleus muscles to the calcaneus or heel bone.

○ Clinical point The test that diagnoses a ruptured Achilles tendon is the Thompson test (not to be confused with Thomas test, which tests for a hip flexion contracture).

See *Thompson test*

Acid–base balance The normal balance between acid and base in blood plasma, measured in terms of hydrogen ion concentration or pH. Normal acid–base values for humans are shown in the table below.

Normal acid–base values for adults

Units	Mean	Range
pH	7.4	7.36–7.44
[H^+] mmol/l	39.8	35.8–43.8
$PaCO_2$ kPa	5.47	4.97–6.00
$PaCO_2$ kPa @ 40 years	12.6	10.5–14.7
[HCO_3^-] mmol/l	24.8	22.6–27.0
SaO_2 %		94.0–97.5

See *Metabolic and respiratory acidosis/alkalosis*

Acidosis A condition resulting from the accumulation of too much acid or loss of base. If caused by the respiratory system it is known as a respiratory acidosis, if another factor is the cause then it is called a metabolic acidosis.

Acne rosacea A skin disorder that results from chronic inflammation of the cheeks, nose, chin, forehead and or eyelids. It is treated with antibiotics.

Acoustic impedence The term to describe the resistance of tissues to the passage of ultrasound.

Acoustic neuroma This is schwannoma of the eighth cranial nerve. It is a benign tumour and usually presents with hearing loss in the side affected. Other symptoms can occur especially as it grows and presses on the trigeminal nerve, including dizziness, poor balance, facial pain and tinnitus. It is usually successfully removed by surgery, but in many cases the hearing loss is permanent. The main complication of surgery is damage to the facial nerve for which the patient may be referred to physiotherapy.

Acoustic streaming The unidirectional movement of fluid in an ultrasound field. It is thought to stimulate cell activity if it occurs at boundaries such as between the cell membrane and surrounding tissue fluid. It may alter cell membrane permeability resulting in:

- increased protein synthesis
- increased secretion from mast cells
- increased mobility of fibroblasts
- release of growth factors by macrophages.

Acquired immunodeficiency syndrome (AIDS) The syndrome caused by infection with the human immunodeficiency virus (HIV).

Acrodynia Pain in the extremities.

Acromegaly A metabolic disorder caused by an excess of growth hormone. Body tissues enlarge including the bones of the face, jaw, hands, feet and skull. It may also affect the heart, leading to its enlargement.

Acromio-clavicular joint (ACJ) The joint between the acromion process of the scapula and the medial end of the clavicle.

Actin A protein involved in muscle contraction.
See *Myosin, sliding filament theory*
Actin and myosin slide past in such a way as to cause shortening of a muscle.
See *Sliding filament theory*

Actinotherapy Electrotherapy term – an alternative name for ultraviolet radiations (UVR) used therapeutically in certain skin disorders.

Action potential (AP) Name given the electrical impulse transmitted along a nerve axon. Initiated by a receptor (e.g. pain receptors in the skin, afferent nerve) or centrally (e.g. at spinal level if motor nerve, efferent nerve). Impulse is an electrochemical change, an action potential, that can travel proximally or distally along the axon. Action potential has five distinct phases: normal state (potential difference of approximately $-70\,mV$ inside axon with respect to outside); depolarization (if increasing level of sodium ions inside axon membrane and proportionately fewer potassium ions is sufficient, nerve reaches 'threshold' and action potential is inevitable – 'All or none law'); peak (overshoot of charge – to same level irrespective of strength of stimulus); absolute refractory period (stimulation not possible as ion balance starts to revert to normal state); relative refractory period (stimulation possible but requires high intensity stimulus); normal state (stable ion balance level).

Action research A form of applied social research that involves the systematic implementation and review of change within the situation being researched. Following the investigation of an issue, a course of action is implemented that is then subjected to evaluation through further research. Action research can, therefore, be a continuous process of investigation and evaluation.

Active assisted exercise An exercise in which part of the activity is undertaken by the patient and part by the therapist or other equipment. For example, shoulder-assisted flexion in lying using a pole.

Active cycle of breathing technique (ACBT) A method of facilitating the clearance of excessive pulmonary secretions.
The whole cycle should be repeated two to three times or until the patient becomes non-productive. In early post-operative patients, fatigue may be an issue and treatment should be terminated at this point. The thoracic expansions should be slow deep breaths, in through the nose and sigh out through the mouth. The end inspiratory hold can improve airflow to poorly ventilated regions (Hough 2001), the breath hold should be encouraged at the height of the inspiratory effort for 2–3 s.

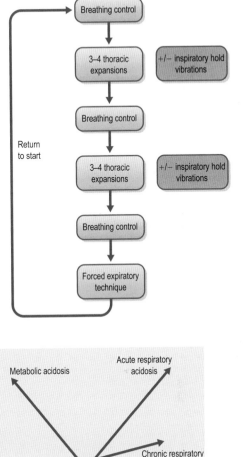

A

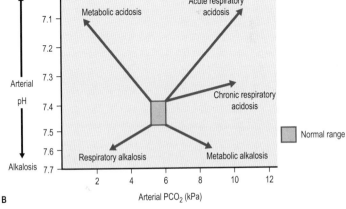

B

(**A**) Breathing control. Adapted from Physiotherapy for respiratory and cardiac problems Pryor & Prasad 2002 ISBN 0443 07075 x Churchill Livingstone; (**B**) Acid–base relationships

Active insufficiency This affects muscles that span two joints, it occurs when the muscle cannot contract maximally across both joints at the same time. An example would be the finger flexors. When you make a strong fist, you may notice that the wrist is in a neutral or an extended position. Now, if you attempt to actively flex your wrist joint whilst keeping your fingers flexed, you will

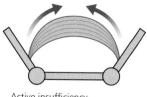

Active insufficiency

find that the strength of the grip is greatly diminished. This is because the wrist and finger flexors are unable to shorten any further and, therefore, the fingers begin to extend or lose grip strength.

Compare with passive insufficiency, which is the inability of a muscle to stretch maximally across two joints at the same time.

Active movement Movement performed by a person, unaided by any external factor or influence.

See *Passive movements, Active assisted movement* and *Resisted movement*

Activities of daily living (ADL) The things we normally do during the course of our daily living, e.g. putting on clothes. The person's ability to perform these can be used as an outcome measure. Physiotherapists need to be aware that what constitutes normal daily living for one individual is not the same as another.

Acupuncture The traditional Chinese practice of therapy and pain relief using needles.

Acute Having severe symptoms and/or a short course.

Acute bacterial endocarditis A condition caused by pyogenic organisms such as streptococci or staphylococci.

See *Self-advocacy*

Acute-phase protein Chemical mediators that are released in response to tissue damage.

Acute respiratory distress syndrome (ARDS) ARDS is a severe and acute form of respiratory failure precipitated by a wide range of catastrophic events including shock, septicaemia, major trauma, aspiration or inhalation of noxious substances (Barnard et al. 1994).

Adaptation To modify in response to a stimulus, can be permanent (e.g. change limb dominance following severe trauma to previously dominant limb) or temporary change.

Addison's crisis An acute life-threatening state of profound adrenocortical insufficiency.

Addison's disease An endocrine disorder that results from failure of the adrenal glands to produce correct amounts of aldosterone and cortisol.

Symptoms include weakness, low blood pressure, anaemia, low blood sugar and problems with electrolyte balance.

❶ Point of interest US president John F. Kennedy had this disease.

Adduction Anatomical term meaning movement towards the midline of the body.

Adenoidectomy Surgical removal of the adenoid glands.

Adenopathy This term refers to enlargement of a gland, used especially in relation to lymph nodes.

Adenosine triphosphate (ATP) A nucleotide present in all living cells that serves as an energy source.

Adjustment Psychological accommodation, behavioural or emotional, to a particular set of circumstances or events.

ADL Common medical abbreviation – Activities of daily living.

Adrenal cortex This is the outer segment of the adrenal gland and releases cortisol when stimulated by the pituitary hormone adrenocorticotropin (ACTH).

Adrenal gland Two glands that sit on top of the kidneys, they have a cortex and a medulla, each with separate functions.

Adrenocorticotrophic hormone (ACTH) A hormone produced by the anterior pituitary gland. It stimulates the adrenal cortex to secrete glucocorticoid hormones.

Adverse neural tension (ANT) The term that refers to restricted movement of the nervous system, such as is seen with a case of nerve root tethering following a prolapsed intervertebral disc.

Adverse reaction Undesirable effects of medication or other therapy, e.g. a person who develops a rash after being given antibiotics has suffered an adverse reaction.

Advocacy Takes a variety of forms with the emphasis on ensuring the effective representation of the views of a client, patient or service user. This may be through direct participation of the person him or herself (self-advocacy) or by an advocate who presents and safeguards the interests of an individual. Advocates can be professional (paid) or voluntary.
See *Self-advocacy*

AE Common medical abbreviation – Air entry.

A&E Abbreviation – Accident and emergency.

Aerobic Metabolic processes that require the presence of oxygen.

AF Common medical abbreviation – Atrial fibrillation.

Afferent This means approaching the central nervous system and so is used to describe nerve fibres carrying impulses into the spinal cord and the rest of the central nervous system (CNS) from the rest of the body. For example, sensory information from the hand would travel along afferent fibres to the CNS.
See *Efferent*

Affirmative action Policies or practices that favourably support disadvantaged groups (including women, ethnic minorities and disabled people) who have experienced institutionalized discrimination. It is also referred to as positive discrimination.

The concept is complex and the practice of affirmative action can, in some circumstances, be illegal.

A fibres See *Nerve fibre types*

Afterload Refers to position of a muscle when the elastic tissue 'in series' is slack – less than resting length. During contraction, the slack has to be taken up.

After pain The pain that typically comes on the day after treatment.

Ageism Stereotyped, negative beliefs about old people which may lead to discrimination. Ageism frequently leads to the denial of appropriate services to old people and to a lack of equal opportunities in comparison with other citizens.

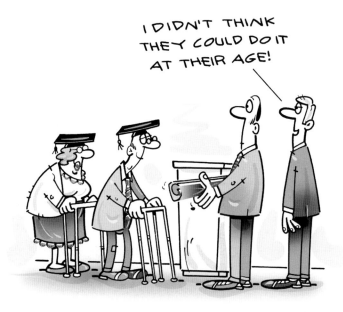

Agglutination test A blood test that is used to demonstrate the presence of blood antibodies. It is dependent on the clumping of cells or particles when they are mixed with a specific antiserum.

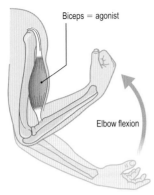

Biceps = agonist

Elbow flexion

Elbow flexion

Agonist A prime mover, e.g. when raising a cup to the mouth, the biceps and brachialis muscles are agonists, triceps would be the antagonist in this example.

Agnosia This is where the individual is unable to attach meaning or recognize something despite receiving sensory information. For example, a patient might be able to feel a hairbrush but not recognize that it was a hairbrush. This is associated with damage to the posterior parietal areas of the brain.

Agree instrument Tool developed by the AGREE collaboration that facilitates systematic evaluation of the quality of a clinical guideline. The AGREE Collaboration is an international group of researchers and policy makers whose aim is to improve the quality and effectiveness of clinical practice guidelines. Go to http://www.agreecollaboration.org

AIMS2 A useful measuring tool in arthritic conditions (Meenan et al. 1992).

Airway conductance This is the ease with which gas flows along the airways and is calculated by flow/pressure. This is the reciprocal of airway resistance.

Airways These are passages to the lungs consisting of upper (URT) and lower (LRT) respiratory tracts. The URT consists of the nose, pharynx and larynx and warms, filters and moistens the inhaled air prior to its passage down the LRT. The URT is also important for the functions of speech, taste and smell. The LRT comprises the conducting system and begins at the trachea, which bifurcates to the point of the terminal bronchioles before the formation of the gas exchange unit of the lung (alveolar sacs).

Airways resistance (Raw) This is the pressure required to elicit airflow between the mouth and the alveolus. Airway resistance increases as the calibre of the airway is reduced, e.g. through inflammation, bronchial smooth muscle contraction or thickening of the airway walls through remodelling in various disease processes. Raw is calculated by the change in pressure along a tube, divided by the flow.

A-K amputation Abbreviation for above-the-knee amputation.

Akinesia Inability to initiate or a delay in initiating movement, often seen in Parkinson's disease.

Alar ligaments A ligament in the upper cervical spine that extends from the side of the dens of the axis to the medial occipital condyle, may be ruptured following certain disorders, such as rheumatoid arthritis.

Aldosterone A steroid produced by the adrenal cortex, that controls salt and water balance via the kidney.

Alendronate (Fosamax) A bisphosphonate drug used specifically for the prevention and treatment of osteoporosis.

Algesic Painful or causing pain. Analgesia means pain relief.

Algodystrophy See *Complex regional pain syndrome*

Alignment Refers to the postural inter-relationship of body segments, in different planes. Physiotherapists assess alignment in different positions, e.g. standing, sitting, as normal alignment is integral to efficient movement. There is considerable variability of alignment and so individual assessment and clinical judgement is important.

Alkalosis A pathological condition caused by an accumulation of base or loss of acid with respiratory (hyperventilation) or metabolic primary causes.

Allergic reaction The body's response to an allergic stimulus. It may be localized or generalized and may include: rash, itching and swelling, or the reaction may be much more severe.

Allocation concealment Research term – the process used to prevent advance knowledge of group assignment in a Randomized controlled trial (RCT). The allocation process should be impervious to any influence by the individual making the allocation, by being administered by someone who is not responsible for recruiting participants (NICE 2004).

Alopecia Absence of the hair from skin areas where it normally is present.

Alpha 1 antitrypsin deficiency (AAT) This is an inherited form of destructive emphysema resulting from the absence or inadequate levels of the chemical alpha 1 antitrypsin that inhibits trypsin (a proteolytic enzyme. Neutrophil elastase may go unchecked in this deficiency resulting in the destruction of elastin and subsequent dissolution of the alveolar walls). This should be suspected in patients around the age of 40 years or less, who present with COPD (a disease usually associated with later years).

Alpha motor neurone This is the nerve that innervates the extra fusal fibres of the skeletal muscle.

Alternating current Electrotherapy term – one of three recognized categories of therapeutic currents (pulsed, direct and alternating currents). A continuous series (train) of biphasic pulses. Continuous pulses can be interrupted (bursts).

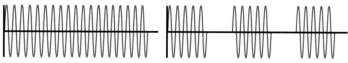

A Continuous series of pulses

B Trains of pulses (bursts) separated by interburst intervals

See *Pulse* for more characteristics

Alternative medicine Medical treatment and practice that lies outside ortho-dox medical and paramedical services. Alternative medical practices may, however, become orthodox, for example physiotherapists now practice acupuncture within the NHS and general practitioners may provide coun-selling services. Alternative medicine can, therefore, be defined as practice that is not endorsed by orthodox medicine.

Alveolar cell Cell of the air sac of the lung.

Alveolar-arterial difference for oxygen (P_AO_2-PaO_2 gradient) This is a measure of lung efficiency for gaseous exchange. Ideally, the two values would be the same but in the normal lung, the alveolar arterial oxygen difference equates to 0.5–2 kPa. In hypoventilation states, the difference will be small since both are reduced. However, where V/Q mismatch is present or diffusion problems experienced, the PaO_2 will be relatively normal, but the P_AO_2 will be reduced, so resulting in a greater $_{A-a}PO_2$ difference.

Alveolar cell A cell of the alveolus (the air sac of the lung in which gas exchange occurs).

Alveolitis Inflammation of the alveoli.

Alveolus This is the gas exchange unit of the lung (an air sac). It is particularly suited to its function of exchanging gases since it has a large cross sectional area, an abundant blood supply and is only a single cell thick, thus facilitat-ing diffusion across the alveolar capillary membrane.

Alzheimer's disease This is the most common cause of dementia in the eld-erly. It results in progressive dementia ultimately leading to loss of functioning in all ADL. Alzheimer's disease is defined pathologically by a presence of an excess number of neurofibrillary tangles and senile plaques seen in the cortex.

Amenorrhoea Cessation of menstruation.

Amino acid Substances that contain an amino group and can combine to form proteins in living beings.

Amitriptyline A drug that is used to treat depression.

Amnesia A severe loss of memory. This can be further categorized as:
- anterograde amnesia – unable to form new memories
- retrograde amnesia – loss of memory of events prior to injury
- transient global amnesia – a short period of both of the above usually only lasting hours or days.

  The physiotherapist will come across this most commonly when treating head-injured patients, although it can occur in other brain disorders.

Amnion The thin membrane that lines the chorion and contains the foetus and the amniotic fluid.

Amortisation phase The term to describe the time period between eccentric and concentric muscle contractions.

Amplitude Electrotherapy term – the intensity of a current, clinically meas-ured in mA or µA. Represented in illustrations of a pulse by the height.
  See *Pulse*

Amplitude modulated frequency (AMF) – also known as beat frequency This occurs when using interferential therapy, two medium frequency currents 'interfere' or cancel each other out in a predictable fashion to produce a desired frequency.

Amputee A person with an amputated limb or part of limb.

Amygdala This nucleus is situated in the anterior temporal lobe and is associated with emotion learning and memory.

Amyloidosis The deposition of amyloid, this is a common complication of several diseases, such as rheumatoid arthritis, the deposits may cause kidney and other systemic problems.

Amyotrophic lateral sclerosis (ALS) The most common form of motor neurone disease. Characterized by wasting fasiculated muscles especially in the thenar eminences and brisk reflexes are present indicating involvement of cortico-spinal tract. This is a deteriorating disease with no proven treatment and so provision of care and management of symptoms by a multidisciplinary team is important. There is a very active support group the Motor Neurone Disease Association. Go to http://www.mndassociation.org

Anabolic steroids Testosterone derivatives used as performance-enhancing drugs, to increase muscle bulk and strength. May be taken orally or as an injection.

Anaemia Too few red blood cells in the bloodstream. There are many types of anaemia including:

- aplastic anaemia; results from failure of the bone marrow
- haemolytic anaemia; an anaemia resulting from destruction of erythrocytes
- hypoplastic anaemia; anaemia resulting from inadequately functioning bone marrow
- iron deficiency anaemia; a form of anaemia due to lack of iron in the diet or to iron loss as a result of chronic bleeding
- macrocytic anaemia; when the average size of erythrocytes is larger than normal
- microcytic anaemia; when the average size of erythrocytes is smaller than normal
- refractory anaemia; any anaemic condition that is not successfully treated by any means other than blood transfusions.

Anaerobic Metabolic processes that require an absence or low levels of oxygen.

Anaesthesia The complete loss of feeling or sensation. May be induced deliberately prior to surgery to permit performance of surgery or other painful procedures or may be used to describe loss of sensation following, for example, severance of a nerve.

Anakinra A relatively new and potentially very successful biologic therapy for use in rheumatological conditions.

Analgesia Pain relief.

Analysis by intention to treat Research term – a data analysis method in which the primary calculations of outcome data are by assigned treatment, regardless of future adherence to treatment.

Anaphylactic shock – also known as anaphylaxis A severe, potentially fatal systemic reaction to a sensitizing substance such as a drug, vaccine, food, serum, venom or chemical. Symptoms include increased anxiety, sweating, weakness and shortness of breath. As shock progresses, symptoms can include hypotension (fall in blood pressure), nausea and diarrhea.

Anatomical position The upright position of the body, the head facing forwards with arms by the sides palms forwards and feet together. This is used as the land map to describe all anatomical directions and structures.

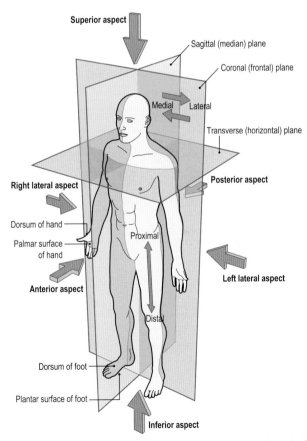

The anatomical position showing the cardinal planes and directional terminology

Aneurysm This is where there is a weakness in the wall of a blood vessel and so a bulge occurs. There are many causes of aneurysm. Inter-cranial aneurysms are found in approximately 1% of the population. They do not cause any symptoms usually, but if they rupture then they cause a sub-arachnoid haemorrhage. Treatment usually requires neurosurgery. In some cases patients have neurological deficits that require treatment and management.

Angina (Pectoris) An angina attack is characterized by severe pain and heaviness or tightness behind the sternum. Pain radiating to the arms, neck, jaw, back or stomach is also common. A cause of angina may be physical activity, particularly after a large meal. However, sufferers can also get an attack during other forms of stress, or whilst resting or even asleep.

Angiography A contrast medium opaque to X-ray is injected into the blood vessels leading to the brain. Computerized tomography (CT) scans can then be taken and digitally enhanced so that the blood vessels can clearly be seen. This is used for assisting in the diagnosis of aneurysms and AVMs and in assessing the relationship of blood vessels with tumours. Recent developments have resulted in magnetic resonance imaging (MRI) being used. Previously, this procedure often had major side effects including death due

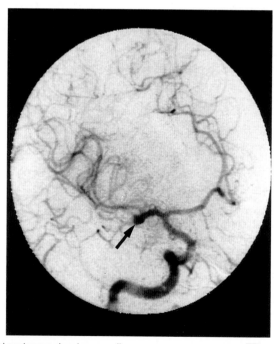

Cerebral angiogram showing a small aneurysm

to arterial spasm, but due to improving techniques and contrast mediums this is now a much safer procedure.

Angioplasty-balloon Balloon angioplasty of the coronary artery, is a non-surgical procedure that relieves narrowing and obstruction of the coronary arteries. This allows more blood and oxygen to reach the heart muscle.

Angiotensin-converting enzyme (ACE) This enzyme changes angiotensin I (biologically inactive) to angiotensin II.

Angiotensin II causes contraction of vascular smooth muscle and thus raises blood pressure.

Angular Work

$$= \text{Force} \times \text{Distance moved}$$

Angular Power

$$\frac{\text{Work done}}{\text{Time taken}}$$

Ankle foot orthosis (AFO) This is a splint for the ankle foot complex, usually designed to enable function. They are useful in patients with insufficient dorsiflexion to clear the floor on swing through when walking or with unstable ankle and subtalar joints. The orthosis usually allows for some dorsiflexion, but prevents plantarflexion beyond plantargrade. This means that the patient can walk without tripping up. The stability provided by the orthosis can often enable patents to walk more safely and quicker and have greater confidence when walking outside. They are usually made of plastic material. As with all external devices care needs to be taken to ensure correct fitting to prevent skin damage.

Ankle sprain Overstretch of the ligaments of the ankle joint, most commonly from an inversion injury, resulting in injury to the anterior talofibular ligament (ATF).

➲ Student tip Sprain = Ligament
           Strain = Muscle or tendon

Ankylosed Stiffened: bound by adhesions or fused.

Ankylosing spondylitis A sero negative polyarthritis involving predominantly the spine, which is characterized by inflammation at the site or attachment of ligament or tendon to bone (enthesopathy) resulting in progressive, painful stiffening of the joints and ligaments. It almost exclusively commences in early adulthood and typically affects males to females in a 3:1 ratio.

It is closely associated with HLA B27, 90% of sufferers are HLA B27 positive, however, a proportion of the population are B27 positive and do not have ankylosing spondylitis.

Ankylosis A fibrous or bony fusion of a joint.

Annular ligament The ligament at the elbow that holds the radial head in place, it is rather like the cuff on an elbow crutch.

Annulus fibrosis The outer portion of the intervertebral disc, consisting of collagen fibres arranged in lamellae or sheets each with a slightly different orientation. The posterior aspect of the annulus fibrosis is thinner than the rest of the annulus, therefore, more likely to rupture.

See *Disc prolapse*

The annulus and nucleus interact with each other providing a resilient hydrodynamic complex.

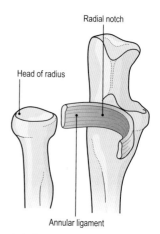

Articular surfaces of the superior radioulnar joint exposed

Nucleus pulposus

- Type 11 collagen
- Hydrophilic (water loving)
- Kept in check by the annulus
- No nerve endings.

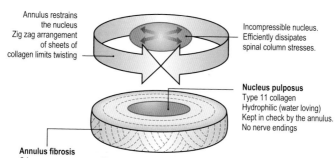

Annulus restrains the nucleus
Zig zag arrangement of sheets of collagen limits twisting

Incompressible nucleus. Efficiently dissipates spinal column stresses.

Nucleus pulposus
Type 11 collagen
Hydrophilic (water loving)
Kept in check by the annulus.
No nerve endings

Annulus fibrosis
Criss cross arrangement of lamellae or sheets. Each layer has a slightly different orientation of fibres, this makes the disc resistant to torsional movements.
The annulus permits a small amount of disc bulging.
Type I collagen (typical of tendon) provides the disc with tensile strength.
Type II collagen (typical of cartilage) provides the disc with compressive strength.
Nerve endings in outer portion.

Annulus and nucleus interaction

Annulus fibrosus

- Criss-cross arrangement of lamellae or sheets
- Each layer has a slightly different orientation of fibres, this makes the disc resistant to torsional movements
- The annulus permits a small amount of disc bulging
- Type 1 collagen (typical of tendon) provides the disc with tensile strength

- Type 11 collagen (typical of cartilage) provides the disc with compressive strength
- Nerve endings in outer portion.

Anode Electrotherapy term – a conductor with a positive charge, attracting negatively charged atoms or groups of atoms (anions). Usually has a red lead and is used as the indifferent electrode for motor stimulation with a monophasic or an unbalanced pulse. Anodal block – if used distally, the anode may block an action potential as it moves distally down an axon (i.e. positively charged ions at the anode may be sufficient to block the ionic changes that comprise the action potential by creating a local hyper-polarization).

Anoxia This means lack of oxygen. Patients can be described as having anoxic brain damage, where their brain has been starved of oxygen for a sufficient period to cause brain damage. Examples of how this could occur are in head injury where ventilation is not maintained, or in partial strangulation or carbon-monoxide poisoning in attempted cases of suicide.

Antalgia Away from pain, e.g. an antalgic gait is the gait adopted by a person in an attempt to produce the minimum amount of pain when walking.

○ Clinical point An antalgic posture is often adopted by someone with acute neck or back pain in an attempt to find the least painful position.

Anterior Anatomical term meaning nearer the front of the body.

Anterior cruciate ligament (ACL) One of the main stabilizing ligaments of the knee, it lies inside the joint and also plays a large part in providing

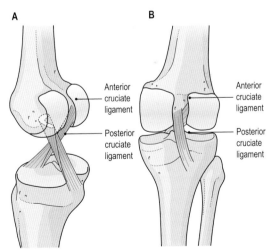

The anterior and posterior cruciate ligaments (**A**) oblique view showing twisting of fibres; (**B**) posterior view showing them crossing in space

proprioception. It attaches on the anterior portion of the tibial plateau, extends upwards and posteriorly and inserts to the medial aspect of the lateral femoral condyle. Commonly injured during twisting type sports or those involving rapid deceleration. The cruciates play a very important role in proprioception, which is so important for knee joint control.

Anterior (PA) draw test A test to detect rupture of the anterior cruciate ligament.

The patient lies supine. The therapist sits on the patient's foot to stabilize the leg and grasps around the proximal tibia and tibial tuberosity and pulls the tibia forwards.

A positive sign is elicited by excessive translation of the tibia anteriorly.

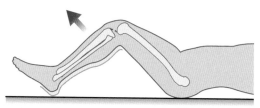

Illustration – A positive PA draw

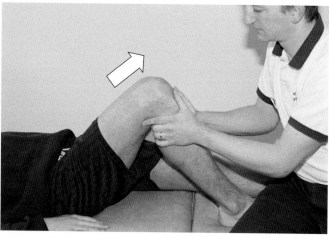

PA draw test. Normal finding – normal translation is approximately 6 mm. Abnormal finding translation of 1.5 cm confirms rupture. Compare this to the other side

Anterior fontanel The diamond-shaped membranous interval at the junction of the skull sutures in a newborn baby.

Anterior horns These are the projections of grey matter that lie anteriorly in the grey matter in the spinal cord. The anterior horns size reflects that amount of skeletal muscle innervated at that level. So they are larger in the cervical and lumbar regions due to the innervation of the limb musculature.

Anterior talofibular ligament (ATF) The most anterior of the three lateral collateral ankle ligaments and the most commonly injured following inversion injuries.

The three ligaments in the complex are:

1. posterior talofibular ligament
2. calcaneofibular ligament
3. anterior talofibular ligament

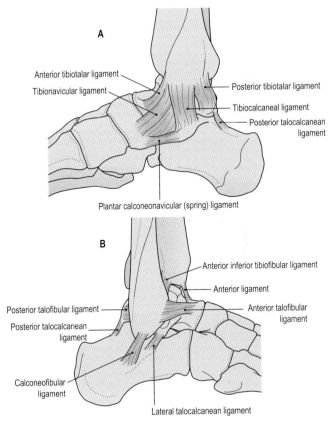

The deltoid (**A**) and the lateral collateral (**B**) ligaments of the ankle

Anthropometric Concerned with measurement of the body.

Antibiotic A substance that kills or inhibits the growth of bacteria.

Anticholinergic Pertains to the blockade of acetylcholine receptors, thus inhibiting parasympathetic nervous activity. Anticholinergic drugs, therefore, reduce spasm in smooth muscle most notably the bladder, bronchi (causing bronchodilation) and intestines. They also decrease gastric, bronchial and salivary secretions. Certain types of these drugs are used in the treatment of such conditions as Parkinson's disease and dystonia.

Anticipatory postural adjustments These are part of the overall balance mechanism. They occur in postural muscles prior to movement or movement of a body part. For example, prior to moving the arm there would be anticipatory postural adjustments in the trunk. These small changes, which may be invisible to the naked eye, are essential in maintaining equilibrium.

Anticoagulant A substance that reverses the tendency of the blood to clot, examples include heparin and warfarin.

> **✪ Clinical point** Anticoagulant therapy has systemic effects, so physiotherapists need to be aware if a person is undergoing anticoagulant therapy, for example, manipulation may be contraindicated.

Anti-discriminatory practice Professional policy, practice and provision that actively seeks to reduce institutional discrimination experienced by individuals and groups, particularly on the grounds of age, race, gender, disability, social class and sexual orientation. Anti-discriminatory practice can utilize particular legislation, such as the Sex Discrimination Act (1975) and the Disability Discrimination Act (1995), to challenge discrimination.

Antigen Any substance that stimulates the immune system to produce antibodies. Antigens are commonly foreign substances or objects such as bacteria or viruses that invade the body.

Anti-inflammatory drugs There is a broad selection of drugs that have an anti-inflammatory effect, most work by blocking the conversion of arachidonic acid to prostanoids. The commonest type of anti-inflammatory drugs are non-steroidal anti-inflammatory drugs (NSAIDs) such as ibuprofen, naprosyn and voltarol. They often have side effects, including damage to the lining of the gastric mucosa.

Anti-nuclear antibody (ANA) These are found in persons whose immune system may be predisposed to cause inflammation against their own body tissues.

Anti-oppressive practice A term often used interchangeably with 'anti-discriminatory practice'. Anti-oppressive practice emphasizes the need to change power relations by minimizing power differences in society. This demands fundamental challenges and changes to social values and within relationships and institutions.

Anxiety A state of unease or apprehension. The object of anxiety (for example future prospects or inability to control events) is often unspecific.
   See *Stress*

Aortic coarctation A heart abnormality that is a common cause of congestive heart failure.

AP Common medical abbreviation – Antero posterior.

Apgar score A method of recording of the physical health of a newborn infant, determined after examination of respiration, heart action, muscle tone, skin colour and reflexes. The total numerical score is 10.

Aphasia This is an impairment caused by brain damage leading to the inability to comprehend written or spoken language or express oneself.

Apical Pertaining to the apex, e.g. apical fibrosis in the lung.

Aplasia A lack of development of an organ or tissue – the opposite of hyperplasia.

Aplastic anaemia The form of anaemia where bone marrow fails to provide sufficient numbers of peripheral blood elements.

Apley's test (AKA grind test) This tests the menisci of the knee. The test comprises of compression of the knee (in 90° of flexion, with patient lying prone) and then performing both medial and lateral rotation of tibia on femur.

Apneustic centre The part of the respiratory control centre responsible for the cessation of inspiration to enable expiration.

Apnoea Cessation of breathing.

> ○ Clinical point Apnoea alarms are encountered in clinical practice, especially in paediatric units.

Apnoea hypopnoea index (AHI) This is the hourly frequency of apnoeas and hypopnoeas during sleep. The AHI is a measure commonly used to diagnose/ assess the severity of sleep apnoea. The index is calculated by measuring the number of apnoeic (episodes of no airflow) or hypopnoeic (episodes of reduced airflow) events per hour of sleep. An index of <5 is considered normal while an index >40 is reflective of moderate to severe sleep apnoea (there is no clear agreement as to the exact number of events) (SIGN OSA Guidelines 2003).

Apophyseal joint See *Zygapophyseal joint*

Apparent leg length See *Leg length*

Appeal The process whereby a student can challenge a decision by offering (mitigating) circumstances or reasons for poor performance. Students are not allowed to challenge the academic judgement of staff.

Apprehension test A test that places a joint in a position that would simulate subluxation or dislocation, visible 'apprehension' on the patient's face is a positive result.

Apraxia The inability to carry out familiar movements in the absence of motor or sensory impairment. Possibly caused by disconnection between the area of the brain that formulates the idea of movement and the area that is supposed to receive it (Stokes 1998).

APTA American Physical Therapy Association representing over 63 000 members.

Aquanatal classes   Classes undertaken in a pool specifically for women who are pregnant or those women in the postnatal period.

Arachnoid   The inner surface of the dura of the brain is lined with the arachnoid membrane. There is a space between the arachnoid membrane and the pia mater, this space, which is called the sub-arachnoid space, is filled with cerebro-spinal fluid.

See *Sub-arachnoid haemorrhages*

Arnold chiari malformation   This neural tube defect is where a herniation of the brainstem and part of the cerebellum occurs through the hole at the base of the skull known as the foramen magnum.

Arrhythmia   Any variation from the normal rhythm of the heart beat, it may include sinus arrhythmia, heart block, atrial fibrillation or atrial flutter. The most clinically significant arrythmias to recognize are SVT (supraventricular tachycardia), VT (ventricular tachycardia) and VF (ventricular fibrillation).

Arterial blood gases (ABGs)   Arterial blood gases (performed by sampling the arterial blood either from an artery or a capillary) measure the acid–base status (the pH, i.e. levels of acidosis or alkalosis) of an individual. The results obtained will determine the primary cause (respiratory or metabolic) of an imbalance and detect the presence/absence of compensatory mechanisms. They measure the pH (plasma hydrogen ion levels), partial pressures of oxygen (PaO_2) and carbon dioxide ($PaCO_2$) and bicarbonate (SBC) levels and are diagnostic of respiratory failure.

The four primary acid–base disturbances

Primary disturbances	Primary alteration	Secondary response	Mechanism of secondary response
Respiratory acidosis A transient increase in acid excretion occurs coupled with sustained enhancement of HCO_3^- reabsorption by the kidney	Increase in $PaCO_2$	Increase in plasma $[HCO_3^-]$	Acid titration of the tissue buffers
Respiratory alkalosis A transient suppression in acid excretion occurs coupled with sustained reduction of HCO_3^- reabsorption by the kidney	Decrease in $PaCO_2$	Decrease in plasma $[HCO_3^-]$	Alkaline titration of the tissue buffers
Metabolic acidosis	Decrease in plasma $[HCO_3^-]$	Decrease in $PaCO_2$	Alveolar hyperventilation
Metabolic alkalosis	Increase in plasma $[HCO_3^-]$	Increase in $PaCO_2$	Alveolar hypoventilation

The arterial values obtained should lie within the normal ranges of:

pH (H^+): 7.35–7.45 (<7.35 represents acidosis; >7.45 represents alkalosis).

$PaCO_2$: 4.5–6.0 kiloPascals (kPa)

PaO_2: 11–15 kPa

SBC: 22–28 mmol/l

It should be remembered that CO_2 is an acid gas; bicarbonate is a base and, therefore, alkaline. Hence, either an elevated CO_2 or a depleted bicarbonate level would cause an acidosis (or fall in pH below 7.35). A lowered CO_2 or elevated bicarbonate would cause an alkalosis (or rise in pH to above 7.45). While the PaO_2 is an important measure (and needed for the diagnosis of respiratory failure and to ascertain the oxygenation status of a patient) it is not helpful when interpreting the acid–base status of the patient. The main considerations for this purpose are the pH; $PaCO_2$ and SBC. To interpret the data, the following steps can be used:

1. Determine the pH (low = acidosis; high = alkalosis)
2. Determine the respiratory status (is the CO_2 within normal parameters and does this account for the pH?)
3. Determine the metabolic involvement (is the bicarbonate {SBC} within normal parameters and does this account for the pH?)
4. Consider compensatory mechanisms, for example:
   a. pH 7.25; $PaCO_2$ 9.6; SBC 24 would indicate a respiratory acidosis (pH is low; CO_2 raised and bicarbonate is normal)
   b. pH 7.46; $PaCO_2$ 5.4; SBC 35 would indicate a metabolic alkalosis (pH is raised and SBC is elevated)

Determining compensatory mechanisms

Where an acid–base imbalance occurs, the lungs can compensate rapidly for metabolic disturbances, but it takes the kidneys longer to alter the bicarbonate levels in response to respiratory disturbances. When the pH is maintained within normal limits there is 'full compensation' occurring.

Is the compensation full or partial?

Where compensation has occurred (through homeostatic mechanisms), it is unlikely that the pH will be returned beyond the centre point of 7.4. Hence, a fully compensated respiratory acidosis will be reflected by a pH between 7.35 and 7.4; a raised CO_2 (as the primary cause of the original acidosis) and raised bicarbonate levels (renal compensation to bring the pH back to within normal levels). Alternately, a fully compensated metabolic acidosis will be reflected by a low side of normal pH, low CO_2 (compensatory hyperventilation) and a low SBC (the cause of a reduced pH). For example: 3. pH 7.36; $PaCO_2$ 9.6; SBC 32 would indicate a fully compensated (pH is within the normal range so is fully compensated – the bicarbonate level is raised), respiratory acidosis (a raised CO_2 would cause the acidosis). This could not be a metabolic cause, as to make a patient acidotic; the bicarbonate level must be lowered. If the pH is not maintained within normal limits, but the other parameters are deranged, then only partial compensation of the problem has occurred. For example: 4. pH 7.3; $PaCO_2$ 9.6; SBC 30 represents a partially compensated respiratory acidosis (since the pH is still acidotic, despite the elevated bicarbonate). The primary cause of the acidosis is the elevated CO_2 level.

Test your comprehension

1. pH 7.4; $PaCO_2$ 5.8; SBC 26 (normal)
2. pH 7.18; $PaCO_2$ 10.8; SBC 35 (partially compensated respiratory acidosis)
3. pH 7.49; $PaCO_2$ 5.1; SBC 33 (metabolic alkalosis)
4. pH 7.3; $PaCO_2$ 7.1; SBC 30 (partially compensated respiratory acidosis)
5. pH 7.36; $PaCO_2$ 6.6; SBC 30 (fully compensated respiratory acidosis)
6. pH 7.21; $PaCO_2$ 3.4; SBC 16 (partially compensated metabolic acidosis).

Arteriovenous malformations (AVMs) Developmental abnormalities of vasculature. These can be asymptomatic. When they occur in the brain or spinal cord they may cause neurological deficits and if they leak or burst they can lead to sub-arachnoid haemorrhage.

Arthritis A general term to describe inflammation within a joint.

Arthritis impact measurement scale (AIMS) A useful measuring tool in arthritic conditions (Meenan et al. 1982).

Arthritis self-efficacy scale (ASES) A useful measuring tool in arthritic conditions (Lorig et al. 1989).

Arthrodesis A surgical operation to produce bony fusion across a joint, still occasionally preferred to joint replacement (arthroplasty) commonly done to correct such deformities as hammer toes or following certain complex fractures.

Arthroplasty Any operation to fashion a new joint:

- Excision arthroplasty: removal of a joint to allow fibrous union instead
- Low friction arthroplasty: hip replacement.

Arthroscope/Arthroscopy Use of a probe or camera, this procedure is minimally invasive and it allows the surgeon to assess, examine, diagnose, repair or reconstruct tissues both within and around joints. It results in less trauma than open surgical techniques, therefore, facilitating rehabilitation.

Articular Pertaining to a joint.

Articular cartilage The soft specialized tissue that covers the ends of bones and allows the distribution of compressive loads over the cross section of bones, as well as providing an almost frictionless surface for joint movement.

Structure of articular hyaline cartilage

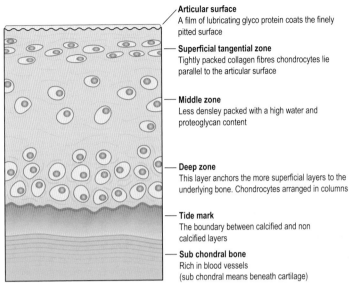

Articular surface
A film of lubricating glyco protein coats the finely pitted surface

Superficial tangential zone
Tightly packed collagen fibres chondrocytes lie parallel to the articular surface

Middle zone
Less densley packed with a high water and proteoglycan content

Deep zone
This layer anchors the more superficial layers to the underlying bone. Chondrocytes arranged in columns

Tide mark
The boundary between calcified and non calcified layers

Sub chondral bone
Rich in blood vessels
(sub chondral means beneath cartilage)

Articular disc An anatomical term used to describe a plate of fibrocartilage attached to the joint capsule and separating the articular surfaces of the bones for a varying distance, it improves joint congruency (fit).

Asbestosis This respiratory disease is a member of the occupational interstitial lung disease group and is one of the three most common (the others being silicosis and pneumoconiosis). Patients with asbestosis will report exposure to asbestos (which may be many years prior to presentation) and demonstrate parenchymal scarring with various symptoms, including dyspnoea on exertion, crackles on auscultation with reduced spirometric values of a restrictive nature, reduced gas diffusing capacity and radiological changes of reticulonodular infiltrates affecting both lung bases, pleural effusion or pleural plaques.

Ascites Is a collection of excess fluid in the space between the membranes lining the abdomen and abdominal organs known as the peritoneal cavity.

Aseptic necrosis See *Avascular necrosis*

Ashworth scale The Ashworth Scale is a scale to measure tone. It has two versions, a standard and a modified version. It is easy to use in the clinical setting and consists of a five-point graded scale. It has been used extensively in research, although there is considerable debate in the literature as to if it really measures tone or simply the resistance to movement, which could be due to contracture or other factors. It has been modified and more recent research tends to favour the newer Modified Ashworth Scale.

Modified Ashworth Scale

0 = No increase in muscle tone

1 = Slight increase in muscle tone, manifested by a catch and release or by minimal resistance at the end range of motion when the part is moved in flexion or extension/abduction or adduction, etc.

1+ = Slight increase in muscle tone, manifested by a catch, followed by minimal resistance throughout the remainder (less than half) of the ROM

2 = More marked increase in muscle tone through most of the ROM, but the affected part is easily moved

3 = Considerable increase in muscle tone, passive movement is difficult

4 = Affected part is rigid in flexion or extension (abduction or adduction, etc.)

Aspergillosis A fungal infection. This infection may affect the lungs, ear canal, skin or the mucous membranes of the eye, nose or urethra. It is found especially in people who are immunocompromised.

Aspiration The use of a sterile needle and syringe to drain fluid. The term can also mean accidental inhalation of a substance into the lungs, e.g. aspiration of vomit, which causes aspiration pneumonia. Typically, the aspiration involves the right lung due to its anatomical features, i.e. the right main bronchus leaves the trachea at a straighter angle than the left main bronchus.

Aspirin An analgesic (pain relieving) antipyretic (fever relieving) and anti-inflammatory drug that also has anticoagulant effects.

Assisted movement These are movements that are either assisted by the therapist or by equipment. Auto-assisted movements are where the person helps himself or herself in moving the body part. For example, where a person helps to lift up their injured/affected arm using the non-affected arm.

Associated movements There are a variety of uses of this term in the literature (Stephenson et al. 1998). Bobath (1985) describes these as normal co-ordinated movements, which often accompany movements made with considerable effort such as when learning a new task. Other authors use the term to describe both normal and pathological movements.
  See *Associated reactions*

Associated reactions This term was used by Walshe (1923) to describe postural reactions in muscles released from normal neurological control. They appear as involuntary stereotyped movement patterns, e.g. the arm flexes, adducts and internally rotates. Usually seen when a patient is using effort for a task or is finding it difficult to maintain their balance, however, they may also occur when a patient sneezes or yawns.

Association of chartered physiotherapists in respiratory care (ACPRC) Go to http://www.csp.org.uk/membergroups/clinicalinterestgroups/microsites/apcp.cfm
  See *Clinical interest groups*

Association of physiotherapists interested in neurology (ACPIN) ACPIN is a special interest group of physiotherapists. They have regional groups that hold regular meetings that both members and non-members can attend. Go to http://www.acpin.net

See *Clinical interest groups*

Asthma A clinical syndrome characterized by episodic attacks of cough, wheezing, chest tightness and breathlessness owing to narrowing of the intrapulmonary airways. These symptoms are usually variable, but nocturnal symptoms are characteristic of asthma. Onset of the disease is most common in childhood, but asthma can occur at any age. The severity of the narrowing varies over short periods of time and is reversible either spontaneously or as a result of treatment. Various trigger factors are known to exist. These include exercise, house and dust mites, pollen and animals.

The pathological process underpinning is that of airway inflammation (largely eosinophilic in nature), causing mucosal oedema and increased mucus secretion. Management of this condition takes a step-wise plan consisting of bronchodilators and inflammatory agents, in addition to patient education and guidance with self-management (BTS Asthma Guidelines 2003).

Astrocytoma An intrinsic malignant tumour of the astrocytes in the brain. These can occur in any age group, although most common from 40 to 60 years. They are graded 1–4 depending on the malignancy, with the lowest grade being 1. Management options include neurosurgery, chemotherapy and radiotherapy, with ongoing management of neurological deficits by the multidisciplinary team. Astrocytomas grow more slowly than more malignant tumours such as glioblastomas.

Asymptomatic There are no symptoms.

✚ Clinical point For example a loose body in the knee joint can be asymptomatic until it moves and causes joint locking.

Asystole Cardiac arrest or the absence of a heartbeat.

Ataxia Failure of muscular co-ordination, varieties include sensory, labyrinthine and cerebellar:

- Sensory ataxia is caused when there is a loss of sensation from the peripheral nerves, causing wide-based gait and compensation by the eyes (Edwards 2002) neurological physiotherapy a problem solving approach.
- Vestibular ataxia may occur with either peripheral or central disorders and may include vertigo and visual problems.
- Cerebellar ataxia results from disorders of the cerebellum.
- Conditions in which ataxia may be seen are multiple sclerosis, Friedrich's ataxia, alcohol abuse and posterior fossa damage.

Ataxic gait Walking that is clumsy and uncoordinated, typically with a wide base.

Atelectasis Collapse of the airways due to hypoventilation. Varying degrees of atelectasis may occur from that which is undetectable clinically, to plate/band or lobar atelectasis. White opacities may be seen on chest X-ray, while a total lung collapse is referred to as a 'white out'.

Atheroma/Atherosclerosis A term used to describe the deposits of plaques on the arterial walls characterized by thickening and fatty degeneration of the inner coat of the arteries.

○ Clinical point Lay people often refer to this as hardening of the arteries.

Athetosis This is a term used to describe random movements that move from one area of the body to another in a writhing movement. It is seen in some children with cerebral palsy, although can be present in other conditions. The term chorea is often used to describe a similar movement pattern in adults.

Atopy An inherited immediate allergic reaction such as with asthma or dermatitis.

Atrial fibrillation (AF) Cardiac arrhythmia in which the atria beat in a chaotic manner. Atrial fibrillation (AF) may be transient or persistent and may contribute to ineffective pumping of blood by the heart.

Atrial flutter The term that describes regular atrial activity that is so rapid that the conduction of impulses to the ventricles may be impaired so that only every other or every third impulse excites ventricular activity and a detectable pulse.

Atrial septal defect (ASD) An inherited condition where the foramen ovale at birth does not close and results in congenital heart disease.

Atrioventricular block A heart conduction disturbance that results in delay or block of an electrical impulse, between atria and ventricles.

Atrophy Shrinking in size, usually following a period of disuse, disease or immobility. The opposite of hypertrophy.

○ Clinical point Muscle atrophy is commonly encountered by physiotherapists in clinical practice, it can develop rapidly, but do not forget that function is more important than the outward appearance of a muscle.

Attention This is the ability to concentrate, an essential cognitive ability for all activities. Patients who have attention deficits are likely to find learning how to manage their disability difficult and will be at greater risk of injury.

Attitude An orientation towards people, situations and ideas that has behavioural, cognitive and emotional dimensions. It involves a readiness to respond in a predetermined way.

Audit-clinical With kind permission from Stephen Ashmore, Leicester Primary Care Audit Group, Manager Tracy Johnson, Leicester Primary Care Audit Group, Deputy Manager

An initiative that strives to improve patient care outcomes through structured peer review. It involves clinicians examining own practice and comparing and contracting these results against a set of standards of guidelines.

Florence Nightingale, during the Crimean War, reputedly undertook the first clinical audit in the mid-19th century. From the time of Florence

Nightingale in 1850 to 1988, audit activity in the NHS remained very fragmented. Although a number of healthcare professionals within the NHS were interested in the quality of service they delivered to patients, very few systematically audited their work. In effect, during this time period, enthusiasts only carried out audit activity.

From 1989 to 1998 audit evolved considerably. The main reason why audit started to gather momentum in 1989 was because the Conservative government of the day decided to place greater emphasis on evaluating the quality of care delivered in the NHS. The government's 1989 white paper '*Working for Patients*' established hospital audit departments and Medical Audit Advisory Group (MAAGs) to assist general practitioners (GPs) in auditing their own work. Both MAAGs and hospital audit teams were involved in assisting healthcare staff to participate in audit work. Initially, at the start of the 1990s, the focus was on medical audit, but by the mid-1990s audit involved many disciplines and hence the name was changed to clinical audit. Since 1998, audit has gained considerable momentum and it is now firmly embedded in the NHS, largely owing to the fact that it is a central component of clinical governance. Unlike in the 1990s, when audit work was very much voluntary, there is now an expectation that healthcare professionals will conduct regular clinical audits. For example, the Coronary Heart Disease National Service Framework formally states that practices must have audit data that are no more than 12 months' old by April 2003. Moreover, recent developments within the NHS, such as the Shipman and Bristol enquiries, have heightened the profile of audit.

Definitions of clinical audit
Leicestershire Primary Care Audit Group have defined clinical audit as follows:

Clinical Audit is a structured process which ensures we are carrying out best practice by reviewing what we are doing, compared with what we should be doing.

Stages of the audit cycle
Selecting an appropriate audit topic
The first stage of any audit is to select an appropriate topic to be audited. However, selecting an appropriate audit topic is not as straightforward as it may appear. It is important that your audit topic focuses on a real problem and that it is also measurable and relevant to your field of work/practice.

Choosing appropriate criteria and standards
Criteria and standards are two audit terms, which often confuse people. This is unfortunate, as criteria and standards are not difficult to understand. In essence, if we refer back to our definition of audit, criteria and standards relate to 'what we should be doing'.

A criterion is essentially an item of care or an aspect of practice that we can use to assess quality. Each criterion should be recorded as a succinct statement. Therefore, an example of a criterion would be: 'The records show that patients with coronary heart disease are reviewed annually'.

A standard is a statement of the proportion of occasions or patients, which must fulfil each criterion. Standards are expressed as percentages. For example, we may set a standard stating that 100% of coronary heart disease (CHD) patients should have an annual review recorded in their records.

Criteria and standards should be based on the latest available research and evidence. If evidence is not available, it is acceptable to base criteria and standards on a consensus agreement by members of the team.

Collecting data

Once you have set the criteria and standards for your audit (i.e. decided what you are going to measure against) you will need to collect audit data. There are a number of factors to consider at this point. Audit data must be representative and, therefore, you will need to ensure that enough patients are included in the audit to make sure that the data collected is valid and representative. Second, it is important to make sure that any data collection form used is understandable, consistent and robust. If two people using the same audit data collection form interpret the questions and data differently, the audit will be prone to failure. Therefore, in order to make sure the data collection form is valid, it is advisable that teams pilot their data-collection tools.

In recent times, NHS staff have started to move from manual collection of audit data to the electronic capture of data. This is preferable as electronic capture of data is likely to be much quicker and more accurate. However, it is important that electronic audit tools are thoroughly checked, as problems can still emerge.

Analyzing data

Once audit data have been collected they need to be analyzed.

In most instances, analysis of audit data simply involves calculating basic percentages. For instance, using our earlier example, the team would firstly focus on the actual percentage of CHD patients who had no record of an annual review in their notes. This calculation would inform the practice if they were meeting the expected standard or not.

Audit data should also be analyzed to identify particular trends and problems. For example, using our CHD example once again, analysis of the audit data might reveal that a particular group of patients is not being reviewed annually (e.g. housebound patients) or that recently diagnosed CHD patients are not being invited back for a review after 1 year.

Implementing changes

The penultimate stage of the audit cycle is one of the most crucial and often also one of the most difficult.

Once all audit data have been analyzed and the audit results calculated, the audit team needs to decide what changes need to be implemented. Obviously, changes should be designed to rectify any major problems that the audit has identified.

Implementing changes that will be effective and lead to improvements is complex. In some cases, subtle changes will lead to considerable improvements. However, in other instances, major changes will need to be set in place.

Whatever changes result from an audit, it is vital that the change process is not left to chance. In other words, a detailed audit action plan should be made stating exactly who, when, what and how changes are to be implemented. Further, all members of the team should be informed of the proposed changes and someone should take a lead role in overseeing that the changes take place.

Re-audit

The final phase of the audit cycle is to undertake a re-audit, i.e. recollect audit data and analyze this. The main purpose of the re-audit phase is to find out if the changes that were implemented have led to an improvement.

Auscultation This is the art of using a stethoscope to listen to the effects of sound transmission through the lung tissue. These sounds must be taken into consideration with other findings and should not be used in isolation to arrive at a differential or absolute diagnosis. The phase of breathing at which the sound occurs, the loudness and the pitch of the sound, should all be considered. Sounds occur due to the turbulent flow of air through the upper and central airways and constitute high- and low-pitched components.

Normally aerated lungs filter out the high-pitched but transmit the low-pitched sounds well. Where disease is present, these sounds may change, e.g. transmission is reduced over areas of pleural effusion, while consolidated lung tissue transmits high-pitched sounds. Semantics are often confusing and the following terminology may be used (some of which is 'old-hat', but still in use) to describe sounds: bronchial breathing, vesicular breath sounds, creps (crepitations), rhonchi and rhales.

Autism A complex developmental disorder. It affects normal development of social and communication skills. Autism encompasses a broad spectrum of behaviours.

Autogenic drainage A variable breathing technique, which has been designed to facilitate the clearance of pulmonary secretions, maintains optimal chest-wall movement and improves ventilation.

This technique originated from Belgium and involves the use of breathing control to alter the rate, depth and location of respiration with the aim of providing a more effective method while allowing the patient more independence (the technique can be performed without the aid of others). The Belgian technique (incorporating three phases) has been slightly modified by the Germans (involves only a single phase), but the aims of both are to obtain the greatest possible airflow through the bronchi and facilitate sputum clearance through means of controlled breathing in patients with an abnormal nature or quantity of pulmonary secretions.

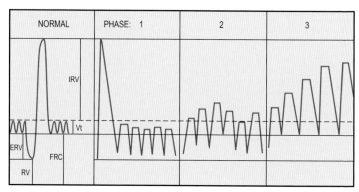

Autogenic drainage: Belgian method. Phases of autogenic drainage shown on a spirogram of a normal person. Phase 1: unstick; Phase 2: collect; Phase 3: evacute. (Vt = tidal volume, ERV = expiratory reserve volume, RV = reserve volume, FRC = functional residual capacity, IRV = inspiratory reserve volume, IRV + Vt + ERV = vital capacity) Reproduced with permission from Schoni MH 1989.

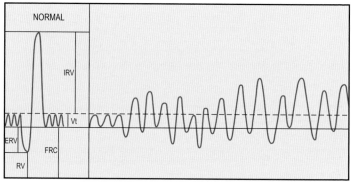

Autogenic drainage: German method. Autogenic drainage shown on a spirogram of a normal person. The method is not divided into separate phases. (Vt = tidal volume, ERV = expiratory reserve volume, RV = reserve volume, FRC = functional residual capacity, IRV = inspiratory reserve volume, IRV + Vt + ERV = vital capacity) Autogenic drainage: a modern approach to physiotherapy in cystic fibrosis. Journal of the Royal Society of Medicine, 82 (suppl. 16): 32–37.

Autoimmune disease Any disease that involves the production of host antibodies to host tissue.

Autonomic dysfunction The abnormal reaction of the autonomic nervous system following disease or injury or chemical imbalance. More often seen within the sympathetic system as a response to a noxious stimulus, for example, redness swelling and sweatiness of the hand.

Autonomic nervous system Neurones that are not under voluntary control, comprising the sympathetic and parasympathetic nervous systems. The autonomic nervous system has two divisions, their effects on body systems are listed below.

The effect of sympathetic and parasympathetic nerve stimulation on various tissues

Organ	Receptor type	Sympathetic	Parasympathetic
Heart			
SA node	β_1	Rate ↑	Rate ↓
Atrial muscle	β_1	Force ↑	Force ↓
AV node	β_1	Automaticity ↑	Conduction velocity ↓ AV block
Ventricular muscle	β_1	Automaticity ↑ Force ↑	No effect
Blood vessels			
Arterioles			
Coronary	α	Constriction	
Muscle	β_2	Dilatation	No effect
Viscera Skin Brain	α	Constriction	No effect
Erectile tissue Salivary gland	α	Constriction	Dilatation
Veins	α β_2	Constriction Dilatation	No effect
Viscera			
Bronchi			
Smooth muscle	β_2	No sympathetic innervation, but dilated by circulating adrenaline	Constriction
Glands		No effect	Secretion
Gastrointestinal tract			
Smooth muscle	α_2, β_2	Motility ↓	Motility ↑
Sphincters	α_2, β_2	Constriction	Dilatation
Glands		No effect	Secretion
Uterus			
Pregnant	α	Contraction	Variable
Non-pregnant	β_2	Relaxation	
Male sex organs	α	Ejaculation	Erection

(*Continued*)

Organ	Receptor type	Sympathetic	Parasympathetic
Eye			
Pupil	α	Dilatation	Constriction
Ciliary muscle	β	Relaxation (slight)	Contraction
Skin			
Sweat glands	α	Secretion (mainly cholinergic)	No effect
Pilomotor	α	Piloerection	No effect
Salivary glands	α, β	Secretion	Secretion
Lacrimal glands		No effect	Secretion
Kidney	β_2	Renin secretion	No effect
Liver	α, β_2	Glycogenolysis	No effect
		Gluconeogenesis	No effect

Adapted from Rang HP, Dale MM, Ritter JM 1999 Pharmacology, 4th edn. Churchill Livingstone, Edinburgh

Autopsy (Post mortem) A surgical procedure, which involves the examination of body organs often used as a means to determine cause of death.

Avascular necrosis – also known as aseptic necrosis Death of tissue due to depletion of blood supply.

✚ Clinical point Common following scaphoid and navicular fractures and with fractures of the femoral neck, leading to death of the head of the femur. For this reason it may be necessary to remove the femoral head and perform a replacement arthroplasty.

Avulsion fracture Where the insertion of a ligament, muscle or tendon may pull a fragment of bone off when it is damaged.

✚ Clinical point Examples seen in clinical practice include avulsion of the tip of the medial malleolus following an eversion injury owing to the strength of the deltoid ligament at the ankle.

Axillary nerve A nerve that arises from the posterior cord of the brachial plexus passes through quadrangular space with the winds round the surgical neck of the humerus and supplies the deltoid and teres minor muscles.

Axon The main outgrowth of a neurone along which impulses travel.

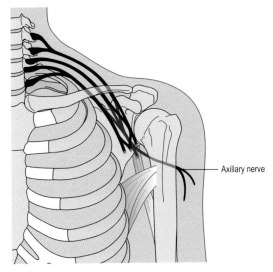

The axillary nerve

Axonotmesis Nerve injury characterized by disruption of the axon and myelin sheath, but preservation of the connective tissue fragments. The result is degeneration of the axon distal to the injury. Good-quality spontaneous regeneration usually occurs.

Axoplasmic transport The process of transporting materials down an axon.

Babinski reflex – also known as plantar response It is an abnormal response that occurs when a blunt object is drawn up the lateral aspect of the sole of the foot:

- Normal finding the big toe flexes
- Abnormal finding the big toe extends – this indicates upper motor neurone damage.

✚ Clinical point This primitive reflex is seen in newborn babies but disappears in time.

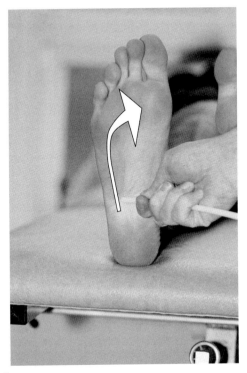

Babinski reflex

Back-slab   A back-slab is a splint made to fit the posterior surface of a limb. It is put on using bandages or straps and so immobilizes a joint. With new materials it is possible to make a back-slab that encases the limb with the front portion flexible and the back part firm. It is commonly used for the lower limb with the slab extending from the ankle to the hip, hence immobilizing the knee. It can be used to prevent contractures by maintaining positioning, as well as an adjunct to treatment. For example, a patient could be stood with a back-slab on the weaker leg, to allow them to weight bear through the leg.

Baclofen   Baclofen is a drug that is given to reduce spasms and hypertonicity. It can be given orally or intrathecally by a subcutaneous pump. Normally it is given orally, in increasing doses until the desired effect is achieved. It does have significant side effects including muscle weakness, drowsiness and fatigue. It should, therefore, be used with caution and following discussion between the patient and the multidisciplinary team.

Bacteraemia   The presence of bacteria in the blood.

Baker's cyst – also known as popliteal cyst   Bursitis of the semimembranosus or the medial gastrocnemius bursa. Often presents as a soft mass in the posterior knee area.

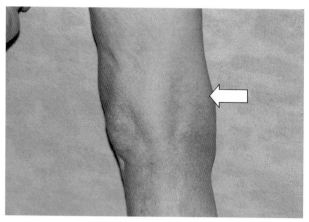

Bakers cyst. With thanks to Harry Clifford Arlow

Balance   The ability to attain and maintain the body's centre of gravity over the base of support in a given sensory environment for function. Balance reactions are complex responses based on prior experiential learning on a foundation of normal nervous system functioning. The two most commonly described responses are:

- righting reactions – these are automatic reactions that serve to bring the head and trunk back into midline

- equilibrium reactions – these are small often unperceivable reactions that help to maintain posture and position during movement.

Ballism The pathological condition where there are uncontrolled ballistic movements and is associated with damage to the sub-thalamus.

Ballismus Abnormal large involuntary movements of the limbs or one limb (hemiballismus).

Ballistic movement These are high-speed, large-amplitude movements requiring reciprocal activity between agonists and antagonist muscle groups, they may normally occur during fast movements such as serving a tennis ball.

Bamboo spine The term for the X-ray appearance in advanced ankylosing spondylitis, fusion of adjacent vertebrae makes the spine look like a piece of bamboo.

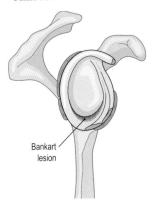

Bankart lesion

Bankart lesion A deformity that can occur following anterior shoulder dislocations, it leaves a deficit in the anterior restraining mechanisms of the shoulder. A Bankart lesion consists of avulsion of the inferior glenohumeral ligaments, the labrum and the capsular attachment of the glenoid.

Barium enema An X-ray test in which barium is placed into the rectum and colon through the anus to enhance X-ray pictures of the large bowel (colon). These X-rays are used to diagnose normal and abnormal anatomy of the colon and rectum.

Baroreceptor A pressure receptor. These are found in the heart, vena cava, aortic arch and carotid sinus and play a part in the homeostatic mechanisms of cardiorespiratory function.

Barotrauma This is damage caused by the application of excessive positive pressure. Such has been reported on the lung with the application of positive pressure mechanical ventilation, e.g. pneumothorax.

Barrel chest A term used to describe the shape of the thorax in states of hyperinflation. Most marked is the increased antero-posterior diameter of the chest. A change in the shape of the chest cage that may occur in certain lung diseases.

Barthel index The Barthel Index is an outcome measure that contains 10 items. It assesses the ability to undertake activities of daily living and mobility. The items include feeding, moving from wheelchair to bed and return, grooming, transferring to and from a toilet, bathing, walking on level surface, going up and down stairs, dressing, continence of bowels and bladder. It is easily applied with good reliability, but has limitations. It has limited responsiveness to change and a low ceiling affect, i.e. you can achieve the maximum score, but still be dependent, as it does not assess the effect of cognition.

Bartholin's abscess An abscess of the vulvovaginal gland.

Basal Pertaining to the lower portion, e.g. basal segment of upper lobe.

Basal ganglia A collection of five nuclei at the base of the cerebral cortex. It includes the caudate nucleus, the putamen, globus pallidus, substantia nigra and sub-thalamic nucleus. Degeneration or damage in this area can cause Parkinson's disease, Huntington's disease and hemiballism.

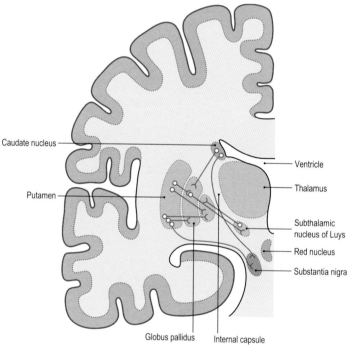

Location of the nuclei comprising the basal ganglia

Basal metabolic rate (BMR) The amount of energy needed to maintain body functioning at rest. Metabolic rates increase with exercise, stress, fear and/or illness.

Baseline data The set of data collected on a specific patient or set of patients prior to it being randomized.

Base of support The area between the body parts and the surface on which they rest. A large base of support generally leads to a lowering of muscular activity. For example, if you lay down on a bed you tend to relax as you have a large base of support, whereas if you stand on one leg you will have considerable activity to maintain your balance over the small base of support. In patients with neurological deficits normal postural reactions to taking up the base of support may not be present. For example, a patient with a head injury who demonstrates marked extensor tone may arch off the bed if placed in supine such that only his head and heels are in contact with the bed's surface.

Basfi bath ankylosing spondylitis functional index A useful measure of function in ankylosing spondylitis (Calin et al. 1994).

Basilar artery The artery that supplies the pons and gives rise to the vertebral arteries.
See *VBI*

Basophil A blood cell with large basophilic granules that contain histamine.

BCG Common medical abbreviation – Bacille Calmette-Guérin used for immunization against tuberculosis.

Behaviour The activities of one person that can be observed and possibly measured by another person.

Behaviour modification This describes an approach to change behaviour. It is used where patients are exhibiting behaviours that are inappropriate, e.g. hitting their carers or being sexually uninhibited, following brain damage. Desired behaviour is rewarded and undesired behaviour is either ignored or punished. Star charts and token economies can be used, amongst other methods. A psychologist usually devises programmes, but require the whole team's support to make them effective.

Bell's palsy A disorder caused by damage to cranial nerve VII, involving sudden facial drooping and decreased ability to move the face.
Clinical features may include:

- pain behind or in front of the ear
- loss of taste
- sensitivity to sound on the affected side
- headaches
- face feels pulled to one side
- problems eating and drinking
- facial droop
- difficulty with some facial expressions
- paralysis of one side of the face
- difficulty closing one eye
- difficulty with fine facial movements
- drooling due to inability to control facial muscles
- dry eye secondary to being unable to close eye properly because of facial weakness.

Beneficence An ethical principle that dictates that we should strive to do good to others and promote their welfare.

Benign The term that tends to be used with reference to cancer, it means not dangerous to health or progressive.

Compare with malignant (characterized by progressive and uncontrolled growth).

Benign proximal positional vertigo (BPPV) Transient attacks of dizziness (vertigo) associated with a change in head position. This condition may respond to the Brandt Daroff technique.

Bennetts fracture This is a fracture dislocation affecting the carpo metacarpal joint of the thumb.

Bereavement To be deprived of something or somebody that is valued and cherished, usually a close relative or friend through death. During the early stages of bereavement people are more prone to illness and disease.

See *Grief*

Berg scale This measures balance during 14 tasks and includes sitting, sit to stand, picking up objects from the floor and turning through 360°. It has good reliability and is easy to undertake in the clinical environment.

Beta-blockers These are anti-arrhythmic drugs that work by altering the conduction rates of the cardiac action potential through the heart muscle.

Bias Research term – deviation of the results from their true values.

Confounding bias

Occurs when two factors are closely associated and the effects of one confuses or distorts the effects of the other factor. The distorting factor is called a confounding variable.

Measurement bias

The act of being studied or measured can affect the outcome.

Recall bias

The recall of events may differ in cases and controls. Questions may be asked more times and more intensively in cases compared to controls.

Referral bias

Healthcare referrers may attract individuals with specific disorders or exposures.

Spectrum bias

The sample population chosen is not representative of the population, e.g. an appropriate spectrum of students were not included in the study of their exam results.

Volunteer bias

Volunteers may exhibit outcomes that may differ from non-volunteers (e.g. volunteers tend to be healthier).

Withdrawal bias
Patients who withdraw from studies may differ systematically from those who remain.

Bibliography A list of material used in constructing a piece of written work, but which is not directly cited in the reference list.

Biccinosis An interstitial lung disease of occupational nature, e.g. as experienced by those working in the cotton industry.

Bicondylar joint A joint in which two distinct, rounded surfaces of one bone articulate with shallow channels on the corresponding bone. The knee joint is a modified bicondylar joint.

BID Common medical abbreviation – Twice a day (medication).

Bile Is a thick digestive fluid secreted by the liver and stored in the gallbladder. It aids digestion by breaking down fats into fatty acids, which can then be absorbed by the digestive tract. The main bile pigment is bilirubin, which is formed from the breakdown of haem.

Bi-level positive airway pressure (B₁PAP®) See *NIV*

Biliary atresia A rare condition that is caused by the abnormal development of the bile ducts.

Bilobectomy This is the surgical removal of two pulmonary lobes.

Biofeedback The use of some form of instrument to bring physiological processes to the conscious awareness of the individual, using visual or auditory signals.

Biological therapy Treatment with substances that can stimulate the immune system to fight disease more effectively. Particularly successful in rheumatological conditions.

Biomedical model A model of health and disease that conceptualizes the body as a machine. The model is grounded in an understanding of anatomy and physiology and does not take into account psychological, sociological, cultural and spiritual influences.

Biopsy A diagnostic technique that involving the surgical removal of a small portion of tissue for microscopic examination and/or culture.

Biopsychosocial model A therapeutic model that recognizes that psychological and social factors must be included along with the biological in understanding a person's medical illness.

> ⊕ Clinical point This model is particularly important when dealing with people with chronic pain.

Biphasic Electrotherapy term – a pulse with two oppositely charged phases. See *Phase, Pulsed* and *Alternating currents*
The two phases may be balanced (equal charges in the positive- and negative-going phases) or unbalanced (level of charge in each phase not equal). If balanced there is no ion buildup over time on skin, if unbalanced the skin will become more alkaline under the cathode and more acidic under the

anode. These changes will manifest as skin irritation, typically, itchiness initially.

Bipolar Electrotherapy term – two equal-sized electrodes usually placed at either end of a muscle or muscle group to be stimulated. For example, to stimulate quadriceps femoris: two large, equal sized, electrodes are placed on the line running from the superomedial pole of the patella to the ASIS. The proximal electrode is placed approximately 30% of the distance from the ASIS (over vastus lateralis and rectus femoris) and the distal 90% (over vastus medialis and rectus femoris).

Bipolar electrodes

Bird See *IPPB*

Bisphosphonates A family of drugs specifically for the prevention and treatment of osteoporosis. The three most commonly used drugs within this family are alendronate (Fosamax), risedronate (Actonel) and etidronate (Didronel).

Bladder calculi Stones of the urinary bladder.

Blind or blinding (Masking) A research process for keeping study participants, caregivers, researchers and outcome assessors unaware of the interventions to which the participants have been allocated in a study.

○ Clinical point Physiotherapy is open to bias just like any other profession, always make efforts to minimize bias in any research project that you undertake.

Blood–brain barrier (BBB) The selective barrier between brain blood vessels and the brain. It restricts what may pass from the blood into the brain. Certain compounds and drugs can readily cross the blood–brain barrier, others cannot.

Blood gas values See *Arterial blood gases*

Blood pressure A measurement of the force applied to the walls of the arteries as the heart pumps blood through the body. The pressure is determined by the force and the amount of blood pumped and the size and flexibility of one's arteries. In clinical practice, blood pressure is presented as two numbers: for example, 120 over 80 (written as 120/80). The first number is the systolic blood pressure (the pressure exerted when the heart contracts), the second number is the diastolic blood pressure (the pressure in the arteries when the heart is at rest).

Blow-out fracture A fracture of the floor of the orbit or eye socket.

Bobath approach A form of neurological rehabilitation based on an approach pioneered by Berta and Karel Bobath. It aims to achieve the re-education of movement and function via the graded facilitation of movement through the use of proprioceptive input. Assessment is guided by the person's reaction to being handled by the therapist (Stokes 1998).

Body chart A body chart is a useful tool to help visualize and record a person's symptoms or problems, see below for a typical example.

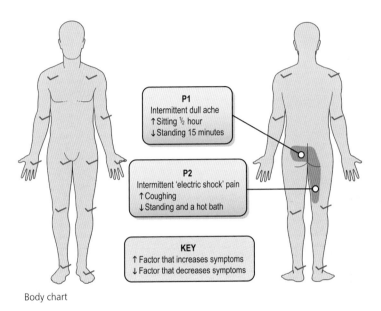

Body chart

Body mass index (BMI) This is a simple measurement tool for broadly assessing the nutritional status of a patient. It is calculated by:

$$\text{weight (kg)} \div (\text{height})^2 \text{ (m)}$$

The normal range for BMI is 21–25. A BMI <16 is indicative of severe malnourishment, with a BMI >30 indicative of severe obesity.

Body protected areas (BF) Electrotherapy term – level of electrical safety required when patients have contact with electromedical equipment. Less stringent than type **CF**, used when direct connection to the heart may occur.

Bohr effect This is the effect of the H^+ concentration (pH) on the position of the oxyhaemoglobin dissociation curve. In states of acidosis, the curve is shifted to the right and to the left in alkalotic states. These changes occur in response to the changes in shape of the Hb molecule as pH alters. Right shifts, reduces Hb affinity for O_2 (so better unloading of O_2 at the tissues occurs), while a shift to the left (with a raised pH) increases Hb affinity for O_2 (and therefore increases its uptake at the alveolus).

Other factors may also cause a shift in the curve, e.g. body temperature changes and abnormal Hbs (changes in amino acid sequences within the Hb will alter its shape and therefore its affinity for O_2).

Bone density   See *Bone mineral density*

A description of bone mass, this is diminished in osteoporosis.

Bone mineral density (BMD)   A measure used to assess density of bone in an individual, typically follows the pattern below in normal individuals and is altered in osteoporosis.

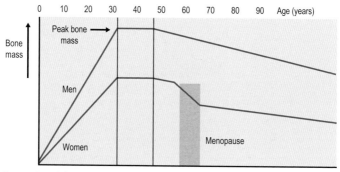

Bone mineral density throughout life in males and females

Bone scan   A radiographic technique that often involves giving an injection of a mildly radioactive substance that attaches itself to white blood cells, waiting for a period, then performing a scan to ascertain where areas of active inflammation or infection are. Also useful for identifying sites of tumours.

Borg dyspnoea scale   A validated measurement scale for patients, used to quantify the severity of perceived dyspnoea.

Botulinum toxin   A neurotoxin produced by the bacterium Clostridium botulinum; it produces weakness in targeted muscles by blocking the release of acetylcholine at the neuromuscular junction. It is used in the treatment and management of focal plasticity. The effects lasts for up to 3 months and it should only be given as an adjunct to treatment.

Bouchards nodes   Bony swellings of the intermediate interphalangeal joints seen in primary osteoarthritis.

See *Heberdens nodes*

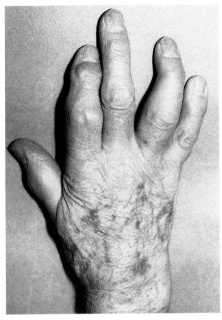

Heberden and Bouchard's nodes (bony swellings of the distal and intermediate interphalangeal joints respectively) in primary ostreoarthritis. Reproduced with permission from Dandy DJ, Edwards DJ 2003 Essential orthopaedics and trauma. Edinburgh, Churchill Livingstone

Boutonnière deformity A common finger deformity seen in rheumatoid arthritis.

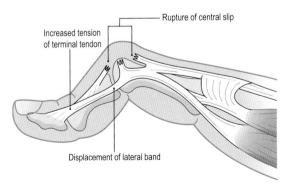

Boutonnière deformity. Reproduced from Eddington 1993 Boutonnière Deformity. In: Clark et al. Hand Rehabilitation, a practical guide. Churchill Livingstone

Bow legs See *Varus deformity*

BP Common medical abbreviation – Blood pressure.

Brachial plexus The collection of nerves in the neck that give rise to the nerves of the upper limb.

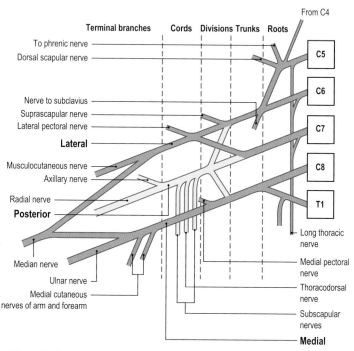

Schematic diagram of the brachial prexus

Bradycardia An abnormally slow heart rate (<60 beats/min).

Bradyglossia Abnormal slowness or deliberation in speech.

Bradykinesia An abnormal slowness of movement or initiating movement, seen in Parkinson's disease for example.

Bradykinin Is a substance produced in the plasma from kininogen. It has many pro-inflammatory reactions and also stimulates nociceptors (Davies et al. 2001).

Bradypnoea An abnormally slow respiratory rate, i.e. slow breathing.

Brain The part of the central nervous system situated within the skull. Includes the cerebrum, cerebellum, brain stem and retina.

Brain death Brain-stem reflexes are tested to ascertain brain death. The tests include pupil response to light, corneal reflex, gag reflex, motor response in muscles supplied by the cranial nerves, breathing and vestibular-occular reflex. These tests have to be undertaken by two senior clinicians and repeated following a set period of time for the patient to be declared brain dead. This procedure is required if patients are on life support machines, prior to the machine being switched off.

Brain stem The term used to describe the mid brain, pons and medulla.

Braxton hicks contraction Rhythmic uterine muscle contractions that occur during pregnancy.

Breast augmentation A surgical procedure, often involving the use of a prosthetic implant, to increase the size or alter the shape of the breast. A breast reconstruction may be carried out post mastectomy.

Breathing exercises The training of patients to take maximal inspirations achieves increases in lung volumes and promotes airflow through collateral channels (Menkes & Britt 1980), so facilitating ventilation and clearing pulmonary secretions. Positioning has an important influence on the distribution of ventilation so should be used in conjunction with the above.
    See *Active cycle breathing technique*

Breathlessness This is one of the four cardinal symptoms of respiratory disease. Breathlessness has been described as the perceived intensity of stimuli produced with breathing (Altose 1989). It is a subjective perception, related to life experience and is, therefore, a symptom reported and detailed by the patient. The clinician cannot fully appreciate nor judge the level of dyspnoea, as with other similar sensations, e.g. pain, fear, hunger, grief. It should not be confused with tachypnoea (a rapid respiratory rate). The sensation becomes distressing when the breathlessness perceived is greater than that expected for the activity undertaken. This symptom is thought to play a significant role in the deconditioning, which occurs through avoidance measures undertaken by patients suffering from chronic lung disease.

Breath sounds
Normal breath sounds
These represent filtering of the bronchial breath sounds generated in larger airways. They can be heard all over the chest wall during inspiration and for a limited time during expiration.

Bronchial breath sounds
The normal sounds that are transmitted though airless lung that does not attenuate the higher frequencies.

Diminished breath sounds
These happen when there is a reduction in the generation of sound or increased attenuation of the sound.

Wheeze – also known as rhonchi
Any condition that causes airway narrowing can cause a wheeze.

Crackles – also known as crepitations

Clicking sounds heard during inspiration, they may be early, late, coarse fine, localized or widespread.

Pleural rub

A creaking sound that occurs when the pleura are inflamed (Pryor & Prasad 2002).

Breech delivery The extraction of the baby that occurs when the baby emerges buttocks or feet first.

Bricanyl A drug used to relieve bronchospasm. It works by stimulating beta$_2$-receptors, which are widespread throughout the respiratory system.

Brittle bone disease (Osteogenesis imperfecta) A genetic disease that results in brittle and frail bones that break with minimal trauma.

   This is not the same condition as osteoporosis. For more information about osteogenesis impefecta contact: The Brittle Bone Society at www. brittlebone.org

Broca's aphasia A disturbance of language where the person has difficulty speaking or repeating words, but has a good understanding. Named after the area of the brain that is damaged in this disorder: the Broca's area that is in the Frontal lobe.

Bronchi The larger airways of the lungs, which divide to form smaller branches to the lung lobes and segments.

Bronchial Pertaining to the airways.

Bronchiectasis This is a chronic, suppurative lung disease characterized by the abnormal and irreversible dilatation of the bronchi through destructive and inflammatory changes in the airway walls. The classical feature is the production of excessive quantities of purulent sputum with the disease being either localized or diffuse. Cystic bronchiectasis results in sac-like dilatations of the distal airways and may be easily visible on the plain chest radiograph. The management includes bronchial hygiene and antibiotics, sometimes requiring sputum culture for the most appropriate prescription.

Bronchioles These are smaller divisions of the bronchi (commencing five to 14 divisions below the segmental bronchi), usually 2 mm or less in diameter, containing no cartilage within their muscarinic walls. The presence of bronchial smooth muscle enables changes in the diameter of the airways, with contraction resulting in bronchoconstriction (airway narrowing) and changes in airway resistance. The respiratory bronchioles are smaller subdivisions and these terminate at the terminal bronchioles prior to the alveoli. The bronchioles are held open by the outward traction pull of adjacent alveoli.

Bronchiolitis Inflammation and obstruction of the bronchioles resulting usually from an acute lower-respiratory-tract infection caused by the respiratory syncytial virus (RSV). This is a common respiratory infection in children under the age of 2 years with symptoms including breathlessness, wheeze and respiratory distress.

Bronchitis Inflammation (acute or chronic in nature) of the mucus membranes of the tracheobronchial tree. Symptoms include wheezing, dyspnoea and increased mucus production.

Bronchoconstriction This is narrowing of the bronchi due to contraction of the smooth muscle. This can occur through irritation of the respiratory tract in response to the inhalation of noxious substances, e.g. post aspiration, cigarette smoking, smoke inhalation and trauma. Symptoms include wheeze and dyspnoea.

Bronchodilation This is a widening of the tracheobronchial tree through relaxation of the smooth muscle contained within the airway walls. This may result from stimulation of the sympathetic nervous system, but can also occur as a result of pharmacological blockade of anticholinergic receptors thus causing relaxation of smooth muscle.

Bronchophony A modification of the voice sounds, by which they are intensified and heightened in pitch; observed in auscultation of the chest in certain cases of intra-thoracic disease.

Bronchopleural fistula (BPF) This is communication between the lung and the pleura and occurs as a thoracic surgical complication, most commonly, post pneumonectomy (spillage of the space contents occurs into the opposite lung via the stump of the surgically removed lung). BPF is more likely to occur when resections have been performed for tuberculosis or fungal infections and the severity of patient presentation varies with the size of the fistula.

Bronchopulmonary segment These are subdivisions of the lobes of the lungs, each containing its own segmental bronchus.
See *Lobes*

Bronchoscopy A procedure during which an examiner uses a tube to evaluate a patient's airways including the voice box and vocal cord, and trachea.

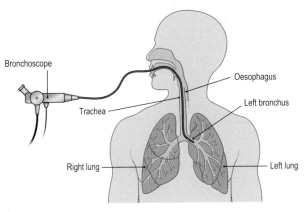

Bronchoscopy

Bronchus The first division of the airways. The bronchi (left and right) arise from the trachea. The left bronchus is longer and more angled than the right, so that accidental inhalation of material enters the right lung more readily than the left. The bronchi contain cartilaginous walls providing upper-airway stability during respiration. There are around 10 divisions of bronchi from the trachea.

Brown-sequard syndrome A type of spinal cord lesion in which damage to one side of the spinal cord distributes thermal and pain sensations from the opposite side of the body and positional sense from the same side below the level of the lesion. This injury is classically caused by a stabbing injury.

Brunnstrom approach A technique developed by Brunnstrom for maximizing recovery after stroke. It is based on the idea that reflex activity and movement synergies are used as the basis for voluntary movement and a progression from gross proximal movement towards distal fine movement.

Brushing A technique used in an attempt to facilitate muscle, controversy persists about its benefits (Stokes 1998).

Bruxism Grinding of the teeth.

BS (X2) Common medical abbreviation – Breath or bowel sounds.

B/Slab Common medical abbreviation – Back slab.

Bucket handle tear A type of tear of the meniscus in the knee joint. It extends along the length of the meniscus, within the body of the meniscus. This tear allows for the internal portion of the torn meniscus to slip into the joint. This commonly causes a 'locked' knee.

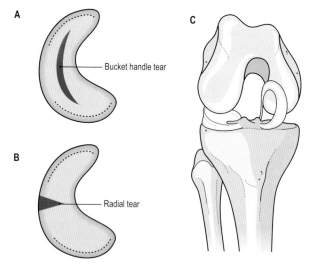

(**A**) Bucket handle tear; (**B**) Radial tear; (**C**) Complete detachment

Bulbar Pertaining to or involving the medulla oblongata, e.g. bulbar palsy.

Bullae The thin walled air sacs that develop in emphysema.

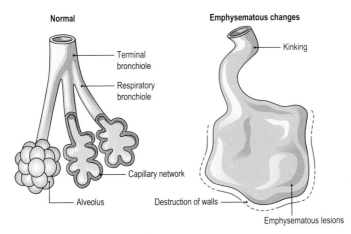

Normal

Emphysematous changes

Terminal bronchiole

Kinking

Respiratory bronchiole

Capillary network

Alveolus

Destruction of walls

Emphysematous lesions

Emphysematous changes in the lung

Bundle of his A bundle of modified myocardial fibres in the interventricular septum, responsible for the transmission of the cardiac impulse from the atrioventricular node to the ventricles.

Burnout An anxiety or stress response sometimes categorized as a disorder, resulting from overwork. It involves feelings of exhaustion, anxiety, cynicism and depression.

Burns An injury to body tissue that is caused by exposure to electricity, chemicals, fire, radiation or hot gases, they are classified as follows:

- A first degree burn is superficial and has similar characteristics to a typical sunburn; the skin is red in colour and sensation is intact.
- Second degree burns look similar to the first degree burns, however, there is blistering of the skin and the pain is usually more intense.
- Third degree burns involve damage that has progressed to the point of skin death. The skin is white and without sensation.

A method for gauging the Total Body Surface Area is 'the rule of nines'. This divides the body surface into 11 areas, each constituting 9% of the total. The perineum is counted as 1%. Other charts may be used for example the Lund and Browder chart.

See *TBSA*

Bursa A tissue space lined with synovial membrane that contains a small quantity of synovial fluid. They facilitate friction-free movement.

Bursitis Inflammation of a bursa, usually caused by overuse, infection or direct trauma.

Burst Electrotherapy term – a continuous series of biphasic pulses (train) followed by no pulses (i.e. an interburst interval) and then more bursts of pulses, depending on the burst frequency. Burst frequency is the number of bursts per second, if Russian current is 50 bursts per second (i.e. each burst typically has a 10 ms duration) followed by a 10 ms interburst interval. The burst and interburst intervals can be changed. For example, reducing the burst duration to 5 ms and increasing the interburst interval to 15 ms will reduce the rate of muscle fibre fatigue during motor stimulation.

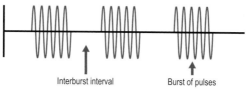

Interburst interval   Burst of pulses

Burst frequency

C

Cachexia The term used to describe general ill health and malnutrition marked by weakness and emaciation. Usually associated with terminal illness.

Cadence The cadence is the number of steps taken in a given time. This is often used as an outcome measure. The most common test used is the 10 m-walking test.

Caecum The first portion of the large intestine.

Caesarean section Surgical procedure in which the abdomen and uterus are incised and the baby is delivered transabdominally. Usually performed when conditions arise that would make a vaginal delivery of the baby hazardous.

Calcaneal spur The formation of a bony spur, extending from the calcaneum into the plantar fascia.

Calcitonin A hormone produced by the thyroid that causes a reduction of calcium ions in the blood.

Calcium channel antagonist A class of drugs that act by selective inhibition of calcium ion influx through or across cell membranes and they are used primarily in the treatment of certain heart conditions and stroke.

Calcium pump The ion pump that maintains a higher concentration of calcium ions outside the cell than inside the cell. Ion channels control the movement of ions in and out of the cells, along with the ions such as sodium and potassium, this gradient created an electrical potential difference (PD). This is of importance to physiotherapists since there is evidence that certain electrotherapy modalities such as pulsed electromagnetic energy (Tsong 1989) and ultrasound (Dyson 1985) can alter an abnormal potential difference in an injured cell or cells and restore it back to normal thus promoting healing and restoration of function.

See *Sodium pump* and *Potassium pump*

Calf squeeze test See *Thompson test*

Calipers External orthosis that are used to assist patients to walk, by mechanically stabilizing joints and providing support for the intrinsic weight of the limb. They are commonly used by paraplegic patients.

Callus The first bone laid down in the process of fracture healing.

Canals of lambert These are collateral channels of ventilation between the terminal bronchioles and alveoli. They remain in an open state even during bronchial smooth muscle contraction and are around 30 μm in size.

Candidiasis A fungal infection commonly found in the mucus membrane and skin. When restricted to the mouth, the infection is referred to as thrush. This infection can spread systemically in the immunocompromised individual.

Canaliculi In bone are channels that run through the calcified matrix between lacunae containing osteocytes. In the liver are small channels through which bile flows to the bile duct.

Cancellous bone Bone consisting of mineralized regularly ordered parallel collagen fibres more loosely organized than the lamellar bone found in the shaft of adult long bones. Found in the ends of the long bones such as the femur.

Capacitance Electrotherapy term – the ability of a capacitor to store electrical charge (C), measured in farads. Capacitance is increased by having larger capacitor plates, a higher dielectric of the material between them (e.g. water, kidney and fatty tissue all have a higher dielectric than bone marrow) and inversely reduced with increasing distance between the plates.

> See *Impedance*

Skin resistance is a combination of the capacitive reactance (mainly provided by the outer drier thicker skin layers) and resistance.

Capsular patterns The capsule of a joint affected by arthritis over a prolonged period behaves in a predictable way. Movements are lost in a classical pattern as the joint capsule contracts. Knowledge of capsular patterns can provide useful diagnostic clues for the presence of some form of arthritis (capsular pathology).

Joint	Capsular pattern (largest restriction listed first)
Shoulder (glenohumeral)	Lateral rotation more than abduction more than medial rotation
Elbow	Flexion more than extension
Wrist	Flexion and extension equally
Fingers	Flexion most of all
Trapeziometacarpal	Abduction extension
Hip	Flexion more than abduction then medial rotation
Knee	Flexion more than extension
Ankle	Plantarflexion more than dorsiflexion
Subtalar	Loss of varus

Carboxyhaemoglobin The substance created when carbon monoxide binds itself to the haemoglobin in the blood. Carbon monoxide has a great affinity for haemoglobin.

Cardiac cycle In a resting individual with a heart rate of around 70 beats/min each cardiac cycle lasts approximately 0.8 s. The contraction phase, known as systole, lasts around 0.3 s. The relaxation phase, known as diastole, lasts longer (around 0.5 s), during this period the heart chambers fill with

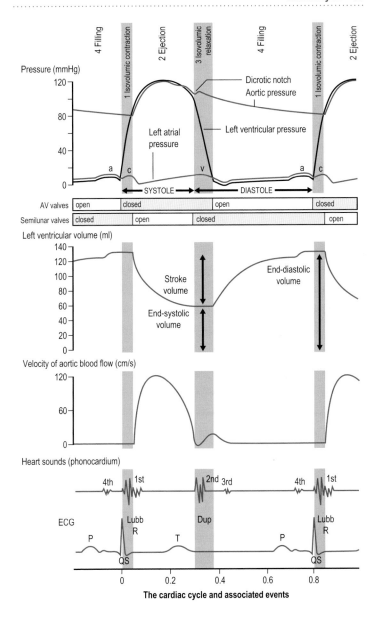

The cardiac cycle and associated events

returning blood. Each cycle is initiated by spontaneous generation of an action potential in the sinoatrial node. The figure shows the relation between the electrical events and mechanical events during the cardiac cycle.

Cardiac enzymes Damaged cardiac muscle cells release these; they can, therefore, be used as a diagnostic indicator of a myocardial infarction.

Cardiac output Defined as stroke volume multiplied by heart rate. It is measured in l/min.

The factors that determine cardiac output are: heart rate, preload, myocardial contractility and after load.

Cardiac rehabilitation A widely used form of management for people with cardiac disease. It aims to restore full physical, psychological and social status and to promote and undertake secondary prevention for optimum long-term prognosis (Pryor & Prasad 2002).

Cardiac tamponade The name given to the condition involving compression of the heart caused by blood or other fluid that accumulates in the space between the myocardium and the pericardium.

Cardiomyopathy (myo relates to muscles and pathy refers to damage).

Reproduced with permission from Porter S 2003 Tidy's physiotherapy, 13th edn. Elsevier Ltd, Edinburgh.

Cardiomyopathy describes a syndrome of non-inflammatory heart muscle damage or changes that affect the heart's pumping performance. Although other forms of heart disease, e.g. coronary heart disease can eventually lead to cardiomyopathy, the term is generally reserved for myocardial changes that are independent of other forms of heart disease; some clinicians use the terms primary and secondary to distinguish between the causes.

They may be divided into three main classes: dilated, hypertrophic obstructive and restrictive.

Dilated cardiomyopathy (DCM)

Also known as congestive cardiomyopathy, DCM is most notable for an enlarged heart that contracts poorly. Stretching, or dilatation, of the heart walls causes them to become thin and flabby so that the heart becomes weak and is unable to pump as well as it should. This is indicated by a reduction in ejection fraction.

Hypertrophic cardiomyopathy (HCM)

The most notable sign of hyperthrophic cardiomyopathy, also known as hypertrophic obstructive cardiomyopathy (HOCM), is an excessive thickening of the heart muscle. This wall thickening, or hypertrophy, can result in problems with obstruction to outward flow and problems with relaxation of the ventricles and can thereby affect the ability of the heart to fill. The distribution of hypertrophy is variable; the left ventricle is almost always affected and in some individuals the muscle of the right ventricle also thickens.

Restrictive cardiomyopathy (RCM)

The hallmark feature of RCM is ventricles with normal or near normal ventricular pumping function, but abnormal filling due to fibrosis or scarring of the myocardium. Because a stiff rigid ventricle has difficulty in filling, damming of blood behind one or both AV valves ensues and the atria become distended and enlarged. The ventricles remain normal or near normal in size. RCM is notable for increased work of breathing, often associated with a respiratory illness such as colds, bronchitis and pneumonia. Other symptoms are those of left and right heart failure, including systemic and pulmonary congestion. RCM is a very rare form of cardiomyopathy, accounting for around 5% of patients with cardiomyopathy. It may be idiopathic or may be secondary to other systemic diseases.

Care A multi-faceted concept suggesting concern and consideration for others. Care can be expressed in many ways including giving practical assistance, emotional support, social support, advice, physical intimacy and prayer. Care can be stifling and oppressive if the recipients have little control over the amount of care they receive, who provides it and the ways in which it is given. Care, in this situation, can be closely linked to control.

Care management A process whereby a professional person (usually a social worker) assesses the needs of individuals in order to cost, plan and monitor 'care packages'. The system of care management was introduced with the NHS and Community Care Act (1990).

Carer (caregiver) Someone other than a health professional who is involved in caring for a person with a medical condition.

Carpal bones The bones of the hand.

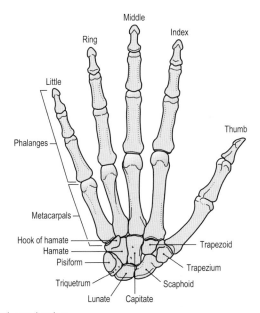

Right hand, anterior view

Carpal tunnel The 'tunnel' formed at the wrist, by the flexor retinaculum and the carpal bones.

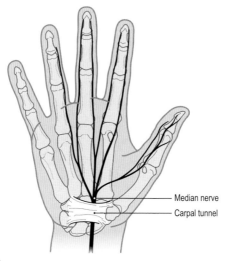

Carpal tunnel

Carpal tunnel syndrome Compression of the median nerve in the carpal tunnel, resulting in sensory and motor disturbances of the hand.
See *Phalen's test*

Case series A report of a number of cases of a given disease or with an outcome of interest, usually covering the course of the disease and the response to treatment. No control group is involved.

Casting See *Plaster of Paris*
Cast is the term usually applied to a splint made from either plaster of Paris or polyurethane resin or fibreglass, they are individually made for the patient. In addition to musculoskeletal and orthopaedic disorders, casts are used in the treatment of neurological patients as an adjunct to:

- increase or maintain range of movement
- correct muscle imbalance
- enable function.

Catchlike current Electrotherapy term – the first few pulses in each on-time have a higher frequency, typically 80 Hz, than the later pulses, often 40 Hz. The aim is to reduce the muscle fatigue associated with using pulsed current.

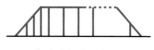

'On time' showing pulses
at different frequencies

Catchlike current

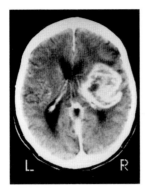

CAT scan

CAT scan – also known as a CT scan A computerized axial tomography scan. It is an X-ray procedure that combines many X-ray images with a computer to generate cross-sectional views or 3-dimensional images of the internal organs and structures of the body.

Catheter A venous line used to inject fluids into the body, or to drain fluids out.

Cathode Electrotherapy term – a conductor with a negative charge, attracting positively charged atoms or groups of atoms (cations). Usually is the black (or white) lead, attached to the distal electrode. Usually used as the stimulating electrode for motor stimulation with a monophasic or unbalanced pulse.
See *Anode* and *Anodal block*

Cauda equina The collection of spinal roots that emerge from the lower end of the spinal cord.

Caudate nucleus This is part of the basal ganglia and involved in motor control.

Causalgia An autonomic nervous system pain characterized by intense burning and hyperaesthesia throughout the distribution of an incompletely damaged peripheral nerve.
See *Algodystrophy, Complex regional pain syndromes* and *CRPS*

Cavitation Electrotherapy term – formation of bubbles of a gas previously absorbed in a liquid. Can be stable (remain relatively unchanged) or unstable (tend to form and burst rapidly leading to release of heat). Can be produced by ultrasound. Unlikely with therapeutic ultrasound applied to a living human body if the output is in the frequency range 0.8 to 3 MHz and the intensity 0 to 3 W/cm^2. Often described in explanations of how therapeutic ultrasound works but relevance to outcome is not clarified.

CBC Common medical abbreviation – Complete blood cell count.

CDH Common medical abbreviation – Congenital dislocation of hip.

Cell-mediated immunity (CMI) The portion of the immune system responsible for the reaction to foreign material by specific defense cells (T-lymphocytes, killer cells, macrophage and other white blood cells) rather than antibodies.

Cellular streaming See *Microstreaming*

Central line Special intravenous (IV) line placed in a large vein that goes to the heart. Can be used to give high levels of nutrition.

Central nervous system The term that refers to the brain, spinal cord and spinal nerves.

Central pattern generators A network of neurones that can generate repetitive rhythmic output, e.g. stepping and breathing without sensory feedback. They are found in the spinal cord.

Central tendency Research term – The middle of a distribution.

Central venous pressure (CVP) The blood pressure in the large veins of the body, distinguished from the peripheral veins in the arms and legs. A catheter inserted into the patient's vena cava can measure the pressure.

Centre of pressure (COP) Biomechanical term referring to the forces acting beneath the foot.

Cerebellar cortex The grey matter that lies under the pial surface of the cerebellum.

Cerebellum A structure of the brain located in the posterior fossa. It is attached to the brain stem at the pons and is important in the control of movement.

Cerebral aqueduct The canal filled with cerebro-spinal fluid within the mid brain. If blocked this leads to hydrocephalous.

Cerebral haemorrhage The term used to describe a haemorrhage from a blood vessel in the brain. They are usually described on the basis of location; sub-arachnoid, extradural, subdural and inter-cerebral within the brain matter itself. Can result in neurological damage.

Cerebral hemispheres The two side of the cerebrum in the brain.

Cerebral palsy A motor function disorder caused by a permanent non-progressive brain defect or lesion present at birth or shortly after. The neurological deficit may result in spastic hemiplegia, monoplegia, diplegia or quadraplegia, athetosis or ataxia seizures, parathesia, along with varying degrees of learning disabilities, impaired speech, vision and hearing.

Cerebrospinal fluid (CSF) Fluid produced by the choroid plexus in the brain, which flows through the ventricular system into the subarachnoid space. Where too much fluid is produced or blockage to the flow of the fluid occurs hydrocephalus can result.
   See *Lumbar puncture*

Cerebro-vascular accident (CVA) A term given to a sudden interruption of the blood supply to the brain leading to neurological deficit lasting more than 24 h. This is commonly used interchangeably with the term stroke. It can either be caused by a haemorrhage or an infarct.

Cerebrum The brain.

Cervical lordodsis See *Lumbar lordosis*

Cervical smear Secretions and superficial cells of the cervix are removed with a sterile applicator from the external uterine wall. The specimen is spread on a slide and sent for examination.

Cervical spine Seven vertebrae – C1–C7. Articulates with the occiput superiorly and the T1 vertebra inferiorly. Commonly known as the neck.

Cervical spondylosis Degenerative arthritis that affects the cervical spine.
   See *Lumbar spondylosis* and *Vertebro basilar insufficiency*

C fibres See *Nerve fibre types*
These are nerve fibres that are postganglionic and autonomic in nature, with temperature and pain sensation capabilities.

Challenging behaviour A term most often applied to the behaviour of people with learning difficulties judged to be unacceptable by the social standards relevant to age and cultural background. It may involve self-injurious behaviour, sexual behaviour or verbal or physical violence. Challenging behaviour may, however, be considered in terms of the impact it has on the life of the individual and others and as challenging the adequacy of service provision. 'Challenging behaviour' is thus a broader term than 'difficult' or 'problem' behaviour that takes the environment into account.

Chance Research term – Random variation. Statistical methods are used to estimate the probability that chance alone has accounted for the difference in outcome.

Charge Electrotherapy term – a fundamental property of matter, measured in coulombs (C). For example, an electron has a negative charge and a particle or body that loses sufficient electrons (1 or more depending on the initial state) will become positively charged. Current is flow of charge per unit time:

$$I = Q/t$$

where

$$I = \text{current [A], } Q = \text{charge [C] and } t = \text{time [sec]}$$

Charnley, Sir John Early pioneer of the hip replacement that now bears his name – Charnley low-friction arthroplasty, much of his work was at Wrightington Hospital in Lancashire, UK.

Chemoreceptor A sensory receptor that responds to a chemical substance.

Chemotaxis The process through which phagocytic cells are attracted to a substance and then follow the concentration gradient from an area of low concentration moving towards a high concentration. A number of chemical factors are known to stimulate leukocyte chemotaxis, for example the anaphylatoxin C5a platelet-activating factor (PAF) and leukotriene B_4 (LTB_4).

Chemotherapy The treatment of disease by chemical agents; usually refers to cancer treatment.

Chest drain/chest tube A tube inserted into the chest to drain off excess fluid or air, they usually incorporate a strip that is visible on X-ray.
See *Underwater seal drainage*

Chest percussion A respiratory assessment technique used in clinical examination of the patient. This technique enables the location of some key structures (e.g. the liver and heart) and enables evaluation of the transmission of air through the lungs. Percussion sounds should be compared on either side throughout the full length of the lungs. 'Dullness' of sounds is associated with poor aeration, e.g. pleural effusion, lung collapse, consolidation and, less commonly, an elevated diaphragm, tumour and thickened pleura.

However, abnormalities, which lie deeper, may not be detected by changes in percussion resonance so its use is limited.

This phrase also refers to the technique of clapping/cupping – a physio-therapeutic technique used to facilitate the clearance of excessive bronchial secretions. It has been demonstrated that the technique raises intrathoracic pressure. However, its efficacy has yet to be scientifically proven. The technique should be performed using a cupped hand (in order to trap air) that is struck over the chest wall (thus, causing a vibratory shock wave to pass through the chest wall and loosen secretions), but avoiding contact with bony structures.

Where the patient is thin, emaciated or frail, the technique can be made more comfortable by placing a folded towel across the chest wall prior to percussion of the area and should not be performed over rib fractures. This technique should be applied with care and can be single or double handed and performed quickly or slowly. When performed by an experienced practitioner, at a slower pace with one hand, it can be used to reduce muscular tension and promote relaxation in an anxious, distressed patient.

Chest X-ray

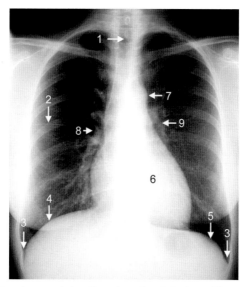

Interpretation of a normal chest X-ray. 1: trachea; 2: horizontal fissure; 3: costophrenic angle; 4: right hemidiaphragm; 5: left hemidiaphragm; 6: heart shadow; 7: aortic arch; 8: right hilum; 9: left hilum

Cheyne–Stokes respiration An abnormal pattern of respiration characterized by alternating patterns of apnoea followed by deep, rapid breathing. The respiratory cycle begins with slow, shallow breaths and gradually increases to abnormal depth and rapidity.

Chlamydia pneumoniae An atypical pneumonia pathogen.

Chondroma A tumour of cartilage.

Chondromalacia patellae (CMP) Common name given to a collection of syndromes that result in softening of the cartilage on articular surface of the patella. Commonly seen in adolescents, young women and commonly associated with functional and biomechanical deficiencies of the patello-femoral joint such as an abnormal Q angle.

> See *Q angle*

> It is common in adolescents and it may be related to overuse, trauma and/or abnormal forces on the knee. It is more common in females.

> Symptoms include:

- knee tenderness
- recurrent effusions and increased joint temperature
- anterior knee pain that worsens after prolonged sitting
- a grating or grinding sensation under the patella on knee extension.

Cholecystectomy Surgical removal of the gallbladder.

Cholesterol Cholesterol is a fat-like compound. It is found in many foods, in the bloodstream and in all cells. Cholesterol is essential for:

- formation and maintenance of cell membranes
- formation of sex hormones
- production of bile salts, which help to digest food
- conversion into vitamin D in the skin when exposed to sunlight.

There are two types of cholesterol, commonly considered to be good and bad types. 'Bad' cholesterol is the low-density lipoprotein (LDL), the major cholesterol carrier in the blood. High levels of these LDLs are associated with atherosclerosis. 'Good' cholesterol is the high-density lipoprotein (HDL); a greater level of HDL – think of this as the drain cleaner you put in the sink – is thought to provide some protection against artery blockage.

Chorea A neurological term that refers to irregular spontaneous movements, often abrupt, it may vary in appearance from restlessness to fidgeting to a flow of violent movements (Stokes 1998).

Chronaxie Electrotherapy term – a measure applied to a strength-duration graph to evaluate peripheral nerve function. Calculation based on the rheobase as is defined as the duration required for a minimally perceptible response (motor or sensory, depending on the test) at twice rheobasic intensity using a monophasic pulse and a frequency of approximately 1 Hz. Normal values vary whether constant current or constant voltage stimulator used. Go to electrotherapy textbooks for normal values.

Chronic Ongoing for a long time, typified by a stage of stasis within the tissues.

Chronic bronchitis A lung disease characterized by the presence of cough and sputum production every day for at least 3 months in each of 2 consecutive years (GOLD Guidelines 2001).

Chronic obstructive pulmonary disease (COPD) This disease is characterized by progressive and largely irreversible airflow limitation associated with abnormal inflammatory responses of the lung to noxious agents. The airway damage affects both the small airways and parenchymal walls. Chronic inflammation results in the remodelling and narrowing of the small airways, while ingestion of elastase by lung proteases, destroys the elastic supporting structures and alveolar attachments, resulting in air trapping.

Diagnosis is obtained through the detection of airflow limitation on spirometric testing in conjunction with details of a full patient history and clinical findings (NICE COPD Guidelines 2004). The severity of airflow limitation is categorized through evaluation of the FEV1 (Forced expiratory volume in the first second) and clinical examination.

Tobacco smoking is a major cause of COPD (approximately 90% of COPD sufferers carry a smoking history). COPD is a major cause of chronic mortality and morbidity around the world and poses a significant burden both personally, socially, economically and psychologically. The disease course is variable but inevitably irreversible. A multi professional team of experts should lead the holistic management strategies including pharmacological support, oxygen therapy, pulmonary rehabilitation, smoking cessation and nutrition (see GOLD guidelines (2001) and NICE guidelines (2004) for more detailed information).

Chylothorax The accumulation of chyle in the thorax following damage to the thoracic duct.

Cilia These are fine hair-like structures present within the airways from the nose to the terminal bronchioles. The cilia are an important component of the body's defence mechanism. There are approximately 200 cilia on each epithelial cell, each beating in a wave-like motion (mitochronial wave) with a frequency of 10–20 times/s, in order to move inhaled debris towards the pharynx for expectoration (or to be swallowed).

Cinahl Cumulative Index to Nursing and Allied Health is an electronic database, which has authoritative coverage of literature related to nursing and allied health.

Circle of Willis A vascular structure located on the floor of the cranial cavity. The circle of Willis loops around the brainstem, above the pons, giving off the major vessels supplying the brain.

Circumduction Movement of a limb in a circular motion so that the limb traces out a cone shape.

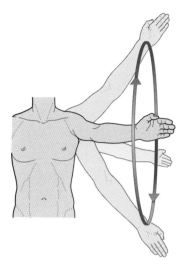

Circumduction

Citizenship The range of human and civil rights and obligations expected in a democratic society. These include the right of participation in the selection of a legitimate government, the right of free speech and the right of religious freedom. Obligations include obeying the law and taking the needs of others into consideration.

CK Common medical abbreviation – Creatine kinase.

Clarke's test Compression of the patella with simultaneous resisted knee extension. It is commonly used as a test of chondromalacia patellae.

Clasp knife phenomenon A type of spasticity seen upon passive movement of a limb with resistance to the movement (the catch), which disappears upon further attempts to passively move the joint.

Classification of recommendations A code (such as A, B, C, D) given to a guideline recommendation, indicating the strength of the evidence supporting that recommendation (NICE 2004).

Claudication Disorder characterized by cramp-like pains in the calves, caused by poor circulation of the blood to the leg muscles. The condition is most commonly associated with atherosclerosis. Intermittent claudication is a form of the disorder that is conspicuous only at certain times usually after prolonged periods of walking and relieved by rest.

Climbing fibres The axon of an inferior olive neuron that innervates a Purkinje cell of the cerebellum.

Clinical audit See *Audit*

Clinical effectiveness The extent to which an intervention produces an overall health benefit in routine clinical practice.

Clinical efficacy The extent to which an intervention achieves its desired effect when studied under controlled research conditions.

Clinical governance A legal duty placed upon NHS establishments to improve their services and maintain high standards. Service providers have an obligation to implement national standards that are set by government. Progress is monitored by the Commission for Health Improvement.

Clinical guideline A series of systematically developed statements designed to assist practitioners and patients make decisions about appropriate health-care for specific clinical circumstances.

Clinical iceberg A way of illustrating the idea that most illness and disease is submerged and does not come to the attention of medical professionals.

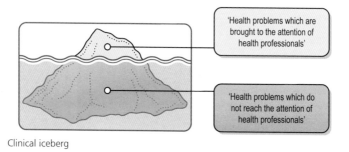

'Health problems which are brought to the attention of health professionals'

'Health problems which do not reach the attention of health professionals'

Clinical iceberg

Clinician A healthcare professional providing healthcare, for example doctor, nurse or physiotherapist.

Clone A group of genetically identical cells or organisms descended from a common ancestor.

Clonus Rhythmic contractions that occur when a muscle group is stretched rapidly, most commonly seen at the ankle when the foot is dorsiflexed. If pronounced it can interfere with function.

Closed fracture There is no communication between the fracture and the outside environment.
See *Open fracture* and *Fracture classification*

Closed kinematic chains See *Kinematic chain*

Cloward's spots Areas of referred pain in the thoracic spine, close to the scapula, often found in association with degenerative cervical spine disorders.

Clubbing Enlargement of the terminal phalanges of the fingers/toes. Clubbing occurs with heart, lung, liver and bowel disorders, in addition to being a congenital abnormality. If recent, clubbing may be related to sepsis, cryptogenic fibrosing alveolitis (CFA) or various carcinomata (including the lung). It may be evident in both suppurative, e.g. bronchiectasis and cystic fibrosis and infiltrative lung diseases, e.g. CFA. It is not a feature of COPD.

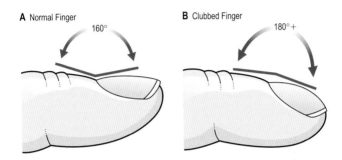

A Normal Finger   160°

B Clubbed Finger   180°+

Clunk test Tests for a glenoid tear at the shoulder.

Cluster A closely grouped series of events or cases of a disease or other related health phenomena with well-defined distribution patterns, in relation to time or place or both. Alternatively, a grouped unit for randomization (NICE 2004).

Coccydynia Pain around the coccyx. Often caused by trauma such as a fall onto the buttocks and often very painful.

Cochrane collaboration An international, non-profit, independent organization aiming to produce up-to-date, accurate information about the effects of healthcare readily available worldwide. It produces and disseminates systematic reviews of healthcare interventions and promotes the search for evidence in the form of clinical trials and other studies of interventions. The Cochrane Collaboration was founded in 1993 and named for the British epidemiologist, Archie Cochrane. The major product of the Collaboration is the Cochrane Database of Systematic Reviews, published quarterly as part of The Cochrane Library. Those who prepare the reviews are mostly healthcare professionals who volunteer to work in one of the many Collaborative Review Groups, with editorial teams overseeing the preparation and maintenance of the reviews, as well as application of the rigorous quality standards for which Cochrane Reviews have become known. Go to http://www.cochrane.org/index0.htm

Cochrane review A systematic review of the evidence relating to a particular health problem or healthcare intervention, produced by the Cochrane Collaboration. Available, via the internet, as part of the Cochrane Library.

Codes of ethics Guidelines that are produced by professional organizations that assist practitioners with ethical decision making and give guidance on duties, responsibilities and appropriate standards of behaviour. The guidance given is broad and general and does not absolve professionals from the responsibility of making ethical decisions. There is a tendency for ethical codes to mix genuine ethical issues with issues concerned with professional image and etiquette such as upholding the good name of the profession.

Coding Research term – a qualitative research term, it refers to the task of ascribing codes to concepts and themes that occur in an interview transcript.

Cognition The thinking processes that allow the individual to be aware of the self, objects and others and to rationally comprehend and interact within their surroundings.

Cognitive Pertaining to thought, awareness or the ability to rationally comprehend the world.

Cognitive behavioural therapy (CBT) This is a therapy based upon using thought processes to change behavioural responses.

Cogwheel rigidity When the limb is moved there is resistance that is released in an intermittent way giving the feeling of a cog wheel hence the name. This is common in Parkinson's disease and other disorders of the basal ganglia.

Cohort study Research term – A longitudinal study that begins with the gathering of two groups of patients (the cohorts), one which received the exposure of interest and one which did not. Then following this group over time (prospective) to measure the development of different outcomes.

Colectomy A term given to excision of all or part of the colon.

Colitis Inflammation of the large intestine characterized by bouts of colicky pain, diarrhoea or constipation often made worse by emotional stress.

Collagen The protein substance of the white fibres of skin, tendon, bone, cartilage and other connective tissue

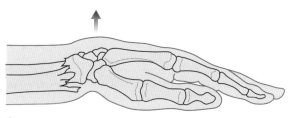

Colle's fracture

Colle's fracture A common fracture to the distal radius, usually brought about by a fall onto the outstretched hand, typically exhibits a dinner fork deformity.

Colloid A substance consisting of large molecules, which attract and hold water. Colloids are given to help correct hypovolaemia (a state of low circulating blood volume).

Colonoscopy The name given to the examination of the colon by an elongated endoscope (colonoscope).

Colostomy The creation of an artificial anus on the abdominal wall. A colostomy can either be permanent or temporary. A temporary colostomy may be created after surgery to allow the bowel to rest.

Colposcopy Examination of a living tissue, under magnification, to identify location and extent of a lesion or disease.

Coma A state of unconsciousness in which, despite sensory stimulus, the patient remains unresponsive, although cerebral cortical activity remains.

Combination therapy The simultaneous application of ultrasound with electrical stimulation is the most commonly applied form of combination therapy, though the term is not exclusive to this combination. The most frequently combined modalities are ultrasound with interferential therapy, or sometimes ultrasound with diadynamic current. There is very limited research evidence to support the modality, though there is reasoned evidence to explain how the ultrasound might be able to 'sensitize' a nerve such that when the electrical stimulation is delivered, a lower current intensity is required to reach the threshold and hence cause the nerve to fire. Whether combination therapy has the capacity to bring about and physiological or therapeutic effects over and above those that would have been achieved by the individual modalities remain uncertain. Anecdotal evidence would support its use in particularly recalcitrant lesions.

Comminuted fracture A fracture in which there are many small fragments of bone.

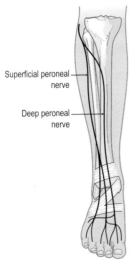

Superficial peroneal nerve

Deep peroneal nerve

Peroneal nerves

Common peroneal nerve The nerve that accompanies the tibial nerve, these two together form the sciatic nerve, the common peroneal nerve splits into deep and superficial peroneal nerves.

Communication The process of sharing and giving meaning in all social situations. It is most usually applied to one-to-one contexts, including face-to-face interaction. With technological advances (for example mobile telephones and email) interpersonal communication has become global for many people. Broader definitions include intrapersonal communication, or internal conversation, for instance in addressing the relationship between language and thought. Definitions also embrace group and mass communication. There are numerous modes of communication, including verbal, sign, written and non-verbal communication (facial expression, eye contact and paralanguage such as accent and tone of voice).

Community care   Care provided in diverse ways, mainly by family members, in the community. More formally, community care encompasses a diverse set of policies associated with de-institutionalization and the NHS and Community Care Act (1990) being central. It applies to groups including people with learning difficulties, people with mental illness and old people.

Community health council (CHC)   Statutory bodies independent from Health Authorities and NHS Trusts representing the health interests of local people and provide advice on health services.

Community mental health (CMH)   A treatment philosophy based upon the social model of psychiatric care that advocates a range of comprehensive mental health services made readily available to the community.

Community mental health centre (CMHC)   A community-based centre that provides a wide range of comprehensive mental health services.

Co-morbidity   Co-existence of more than one disease or an additional disease (other than that being studied or treated) in an individual.

Compartment syndrome   A pathological condition seen after trauma to muscle and soft tissue caused by progressive arterial compression and reduced blood supply. If left untreated it can result in permanent deformities such as Volkmans Ischaemic Contracture.

Signs and symptoms are the 5 Ps:

1. PALE
2. PAINFUL
3. PULSELESS
4. PARESTHESIAE
5. PARALYZED.

Complement   A group of proteins found in blood serum and plasma that, in combination with antibodies, causes the destruction of antigens.

Complex regional pain syndrome (CRPS)   A chronic pain syndrome with two forms. CRPS 1 currently replaces the term 'reflex sympathetic dystrophy syndrome'. It is a chronic nerve disorder that occurs most often in the arms or legs after a minor or major injury.

CRPS 1 is associated with severe pain; changes in the nails, bone and skin and an increased sensitivity to touch in the affected limb. CRPS 2 replaces the term causalgia and results from an identified injury to the nerve.

Complete blood count (CBC)   The calculation of the cellular elements of blood.

Compliance   This has two meanings. The first being the action of obeying or yielding to others. Healthcare professionals have frequently expected patients and clients to comply to their wishes with little consultation or negotiation. A greater partnership approach between healthcare professionals and patients and clients is now advocated and the term 'patient compliance' has largely been replaced by the less authoritarian term 'patient adherence'.

The second meaning refers to the ability to distend. Lung compliance is the ease with which the lungs inflate and is defined as the volume change per unit of pressure change (measured in l/cm of water). Conditions resulting in poor compliance include fibrotic lung diseases, e.g. fibrosing alveolitis, tuberculosis (TB) and acute respiratory distress syndrome (ARDS) and chest wall abnormalities such as severe kyphoscoliosis and pectus excavatum (stove-in chest). The lungs with low compliance are said to be 'stiff' and will yield a lower tidal volume for the same effort applied to respiration than 'normal' lungs. The lung compliance equation can be used to calculate how compliant the lungs are of a ventilated patient:

$$C = Vt/P$$

where

C = compliance; Vt = tidal volume and P is the driving pressure

For example:

Set Vt = 450 mls and P = 30 cmH$_2$O; then C = 450/30 = 15

This would indicate stiff lungs that are difficult to inflate (the normal value for compliance is 75).

Compound fracture – also known as open fracture A fracture in which the skin is broken.

Compression The term for pushing on the thorax during resuscitation or a technique of approximation the surfaces of a joint, it may be used as a diagnostic test or a treatment technique.

Compression garment These may be used following burns or other problems such as lymphoedema, they work by fitting the body very closely and exerting pressure on the tissues to limit build up of fluid.

Concordance This is the mutual agreement between patient and clinician to adhere to an agreed management regime/intervention.

Condyle A rounded usually articular projection.

Conference proceedings Compilation of papers presented at a conference.

Confidence interval (CI) A range of values for an unknown population parameter with a stated 'confidence' that it contains the true value. The interval is calculated from sample data and generally straddles the sample estimate. The 'confidence' value means that if the method used to calculate the interval is repeated many times, then that proportion of intervals will actually contain the true value (NICE 2004).

Confidentiality An ethical principle whereby promises are made to hold in strict confidence information about another person.

Confounding variable Any variable that may affect the results of a research study.
See *Extraneous variable* and *Bias*

Congenital Present from birth.

Congenital dislocation of the hip (CDH) A congenital orthopaedic defect in which the head of the femur does not articulate with acetabulum because it is abnormally shallow.

○ Clinical point Many people who have CDH eventually require hip replacement when they are young adults.

Congestive cardiac failure (CCF) A usually chronic condition characterized by circulatory congestion caused by cardiac disorders especially myocardial infarction of the ventricles. It can occur acutely after myocardial infarction of the left ventricle.

Coning This is where raising intercranial pressure leads to the brain herniating down through the foramen magnum. This is a neurosurgical emergency.

Connective tissue Tissue that supports and binds other body tissue and parts.

Consent Consent equals permission from a person to be treated, examined or other healthcare procedure undertaken upon them or a child under their care. Valid consent must be obtained before starting any such intervention. Patients have the right to determine what happens to their own bodies and consent is a fundamental part of good practice. A health professional who does not respect this principle may be liable both to legal action by the patient and action by their professional body. Employing bodies may also be liable for the actions of their staff.

Case law has established that touching a person without valid consent may constitute the offence of battery. Further, if health professionals fail to obtain proper consent and the patient subsequently suffers harm as a result of treatment, this may be a factor in a claim of negligence against the professional involved.

Consequentialism An approach to ethical decision making whereby the consequences of an action are viewed as more important than fundamental ethical principles such as respect for autonomy.

Consolidation The process of becoming solidified, seen especially in the lung when fluid solidifies.

CONSORT statement (Consolidated reporting of clinical trials) Recommendations for improving the reporting of randomized controlled trials in journals. A flow diagram and checklist allow readers to understand the conduct of the study and assess the validity of the results.

Constant current Electrotherapy term – current remains as set by the equipment operator. If set at 10 mA, the current output stays at 10 mA irrespective of changes in impedance or voltage. Ohm's law indicates that any changes to the resistance will, therefore, produce a change in the voltage. For example, if electrode contact is reduced, impedance will increase and so must the voltage. Disadvantage: current density will increase as contact area decreases (mA/cm^2), increasing any existing risk of skin damage.

See *Constant voltage*

Constant voltage Electrotherapy term – voltage remains as set. If set at 20 V it stays set at 20 V irrespective of any changes in impedance or current. Ohm's law indicates that any changes to the resistance will, therefore, produce a change in the current. For example, if electrode contact is suddenly increased and impedance decreases, current will increase. Disadvantage: changes in current level can increase the effectiveness of the stimulating technique too much and cause pain or an excessively strong contraction.

See *Constant current*

Constipation   Refers to infrequent or hard stools, or difficulty passing stools.

Constraint-induced therapy   See *Forced use*

Consumerism   The practice of buying and selling goods in a free market and at a market price. Government reforms, for example the NHS and Community Care Act (1990), have sought to give patients and clients (often referred to as customers and consumers) more choice within health and social services. Their choice is, however, limited because of restricted resources and lack of control. The health and social care market can thus be considered a 'quasi-market'.

See *Internal market*

Continuing professional development (CPD)   A process whereby professional workers, such as physiotherapists, continue to develop their knowledge and skills (by formal and informal means) once they are qualified. Evidence of continuing professional development will become mandatory for physiotherapists in 2006 in order to remain state registered and to practice within the NHS.

Continuous passive motion (CPM)   A form of passive mobilization.

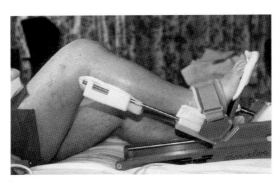

Continuous passive motion

Benefits of CPM

- Maintenance of synovial sweep and thus hyaline articular cartilage nutrition – useful after certain intra-articular fractures, e.g. tibial plateau.
- Regular rhythmical motion can act as an analgesic, can stimulate circulation and may assist in reduction of swelling.
- CPM has been used following anterior cruciate reconstruction particularly following patellar tendon graft – it is possible that this encourages more rapid revascularization and, therefore, strength of the donor graft.
- It is possible to increase the flexion/extension in a controlled manner that is immediately obvious to the patient and can assist in giving the patient a goal to strive for.

- Some units have counters so that the healthcare team can tell exactly for how long the patient has been using the unit.
- CPM units are now available for shoulder, wrist and other joints.
- CPMs may now be used in the patient's home.

Disadvantages of CPM

- It is passive and, therefore, by definition will not build muscle strength. Some patients mistakenly neglect active exercises in the belief that they no longer need to undertake them. It is the responsibility of the physiotherapist to ensure that this situation does not occur.
- Some patients are distressed by the appearance of and feel threatened by the unit (most units have a panic button so the patient can stop the unit for rest, meals or toiletting).
- The units can be bulky and expensive.
- If incorrectly positioned they can cause pressure problems and be uncomfortable.

They pose an infection risk if not properly cleaned and policies for their use followed.

Continuous positive airway pressure (CPAP) See *NIV*

This is the application of a positive airway pressure to the respiratory tract of a spontaneously breathing patient. It may be applied either invasively (via an endotracheal or tracheostomy tube) or non-invasively (via a face or nasal mask). The effects of CPAP are of a splinting nature in the respiratory tract causing the intrathoracic pressure to be held in a constant positive state even at the end of expiration, i.e. pressure does not return to atmospheric pressure at the end of the breathing cycle. Hence the airways are held open and thus allow more time for oxygen to diffuse across the alveolar capillary membrane, so improving the oxygenation status of the patient.

CPAP was first used non-invasively in the treatment of obstructive sleep apnoea (OSA), a condition in which the upper respiratory tract collapses during sleep, causing oropharyngeal obstruction and resulting in oxygen desaturation despite the presence of respiratory efforts. From its inception in this clinical area, it was noted that changes in daytime arterial blood gases resulted. Research into its application with COPD in combination with interface and machine development led to the extension of non-invasive positive pressure breathing support in the form of bi-level therapy (i.e. non-invasive ventilation or NIV).

Contracture Abnormal shortening of tissue.

Contraindication Any treatment known to cause serious adverse and possibly irreversible outcomes if used in the prevailing conditions. Some examples include: the use of SWD within 3–5 m of a patient with an indwelling stimulator such as a pacemaker; applying heat or cold to an area unable to adequately absorb and dissipate it (e.g. reduced local circulation); applying alternating current through the thorax; applying UVR or laser light (Class 3B) without therapist and patient wearing wavelength specific protective goggles.
See *Interactive effects*

Contralateral The limb on the opposite side of the body. Compare with ipsilateral, which refers to the same side.

Contrecoup injury This is where the brain tissue keeps moving when the skull has stopped resulting in an injury to the opposite side of the head to where the force was applied, i.e. a blow to the right side of the head will cause a contrecoup injury to the left side of the brain.

Control group Research term – The study patients that have not received the experimental manoeuvre or test.

Contusion A bruise.

COP Common medical abbreviation – Completion or change of plaster.

COPD Common medical abbreviation – Chronic obstructive pulmonary disease.

Coping strategies Commonly associated with cognitively and emotionally coming to terms with changed circumstances such as an acquired impairment. Therapeutic work may focus on helping people to acquire beneficial coping strategies.

Coronal plane The plane that divides the body into anterior and posterior portions.
  See *Anatomical position*

Coronary artery bypass grafting (CABG) A surgical procedure used to reperfuse an ischaemic myocardium. Internal mammary arteries and/or the long saphenous veins are grafted onto the myocardium to bypass the blocked and diseased coronary arteries post (or in patients who are at risk of) myocardial infarction. To enable this procedure the patient was traditionally placed on cardiopulmonary bypass, but developments in both technology and surgical techniques enable endoscopic procedures to be performed in some units.

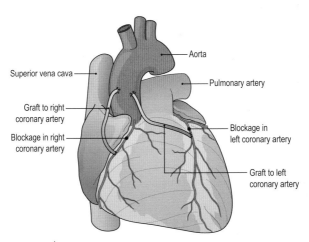

Coronary artery bypass

Coronary artery disease The term used to describe any abnormal condition that affects the arteries of the heart and produces a variety of pathological effects.

Coronary ligament The ligament that attaches the anterior horn of the medial meniscus to the tibial plateau.

Cor pulmonale This is right-sided heart failure secondary to a primary pulmonary disease. It is often associated with severe COPD and results from prolonged hypoxaemia due to the reflex response (to hypoxaemia) of pulmonary vasoconstriction. Other contributory and interactive factors to cor pulmonale include increased blood viscosity (with polycythaemia), myocardial hypoxia (causing poor ventricular contraction and function), destruction of the pulmonary vascular bed (in association with emphysematous lung disease changes) and acidosis (causing secondary retention of water and sodium).

Correlation (r) Research term – A statistical technique used to assess the relationship between two variables. Values of the r can range between −1 and +1.

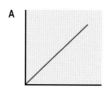

Positive correlation
e.g. between size of foot and shoe size.
Correlation of +1

Cortico-spinal tract This tract originates in the cortex of the brain and terminates in the spinal cord and is involved in the control of voluntary movement.

Corticosteroids Hormones (natural or synthetic) associated with the adrenal cortex that plays an influential role in the regulation of water and electrolytes and other key bodily functions, e.g. heart and renal function and metabolic processes.

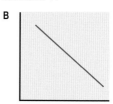

A negative correlation
As one gets larger, the other gets smaller
e.g. as age in adults increases, height decreases.
Correlation of −1

Cortisone See *Corticosteroids*

Costochondral Pertaining to the ribs and associated cartilage.

Costochondral junction The junction between the ribs and costal cartilages.

Costophrenic Pertaining to the ribs and diaphragm, e.g. the costophrenic angle on chest X-ray is the angle formed where the costal pleura meets the diaphragm.

Costovertebral Pertaining to the rib and vertebral column.

Cough One of the four cardinal symptoms of respiratory disease. It has been defined as follows: 'A spontaneous effective cough is a reflex mechanism utilizing maximum forced exhalation to clear irritants or secretions from the

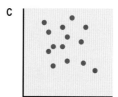

No correlation
e.g. the correlation between the colour of your socks and what you had to eat for breakfast.
Correlation of 0

airway' (AARC 1993). Closure of the glottis is a requirement for this action, so damage to the laryngeal nerve or vocal cords may result in loss of the explosive nature of the cough (normally a cough is performed when the raised intrathoracic pressure is suddenly released on relaxation of the glottis). Exploration of this symptom is vital and may yield significant clinical information to aid the path to diagnosis, e.g. when does the cough occur (asthmatics often report nocturnal cough), what triggers it (is there an allergic component), is it longstanding or productive of sputum (perhaps a smoker), etc.

Counselling In the informal sense, counselling is a relationship and communication that helps people explore and understand themselves and their personal circumstances and empowers them in determining their goals and resolving personal problems. In a formal sense, counselling is the application of psychological theories and communication skills by professional counsellors to help resolve clients' personal problems, distress or unwanted desires.

Counter irritant An irritant that is administered to a part of the body, in order to relieve an existing irritation in another part. We see the counter irritant effect in everyday life, if we bang our shin on a table, we rub the shin, this has a counter irritant (pain relieving) effect, when we stop rubbing the pain returns. In physiotherapy this is an important concept, heat sprays work on this principle by causing minor skin irritation, ice therapy may do the same and it is possible that so too do deep transverse frictions and TENS.

Course leader The person granted authority by the university (and sometimes professional body) to manage a specific course, e.g. physiotherapy.

CPK Common medical abbreviation – Creatine phosphokinase.

CPM Common medical abbreviation – Continuous passive motion.

Crank test A test for stability of the shoulder joint.

Cranial nerves These are twelve pairs of nerves that emanate from the nervous tissue of the brain and they exit/enter the cranium through small openings in the skull:

1. Olfactory
2. Optic
3. Oculomotor
4. Trochlear
5. Trigeminal
6. Abducens
7. Facial
8. Vestibulocochlear
9. Glossopharyngeal
10. Vagus
11. Spinal Accessory
12. Hypoglossal

Crash team Common medical abbreviation – Cardiac arrest team.

Crepitus A grinding noise or sensation within a joint or other tissue.

Creutzfeldt–Jacob disease (CJD) A disorder involving rapid decrease of mental function and movement. These are abnormalities believed to be caused by damage done to the brain by a protein called a prion.

Criterion (in audit) An explicit statement that defines a specific attribute of a standard that can be measured.

Critical appraisal The process of analyzing an article, or piece of work, and discussing the validity of its content.

Physiotherapists need to be able to read and more importantly assess and evaluate research literature if they are to make informed judgements about best practice, the following points are a guide for how to critically appraise literature.

Start

- Read the article carefully. Does the title give a clear guide for what is to follow?
- The title should be concise and precise
- What is the theme or the broad aims of the piece of work in front of you?
- Has the writer(s) explained or justified why they have done this study?
- Have they explained and summarized the previous literature in the subject area?
- Why did the author(s) decide to do this study?
- What is the research question? Is there a research question?
- What is the study design? Is it qualitative, quantitative, case study, systematic review or other format?
- More importantly, does the design fit the question?
- Have the researchers used 'the right tool for the right job'?
- How did the researchers collect their data?
- Did they perform a pilot study?
- Have they acknowledged any limitations of the study?
- Have they discussed validity and reliability?
- What was their sample size, do they note inclusion and exclusion criteria if relevant?
- How was sampling achieved?
- Ethics – Were there any ethical issues? Did they obtain consent?
- Presentation of the paper – How is the information presented?
- Are the statistical tests appropriate?
- Are any graphs clearly presented?
- Has any level of statistical significance been used?
- What are the findings of the paper?

- Did they answer their own research question?
- Does it add to the body of existing knowledge?

Conclusion
- How has the author(s) interpreted their results?
- Have they made unsupported claims or missed important points?

The 'so what' question
- Was it worthwhile? Will it change anything about your work as a physiotherapist?
- Could it be used in your own future clinical practice?
- How can you integrate the paper into your work as a physiotherapist?

The end

Critique   The academic process whereby a review is made of a piece of written or practical work.

Crohn's disease   A chronic inflammatory bowel disease usually affecting the ileum and/or colon. The disease is characterized by frequent attacks of diarrhoea, severe abdominal pain, nausea, fever, chills, weakness and weight loss.

Cross marking   The practice of markers marking the same piece of student work, usually blinded and comparing marks in an attempt at standardization of marks.

Crossover study design   Research term – The administration of two or more experimental therapies one after the other.

GROUP A TEST TREATMENT TEST NO TREATMENT

GROUP B TEST NO TREATMENT TEST TREATMENT

Cross-sectional study   Research term – Survey of an entire population for the presence or absence of a disease and/or other variable in every member (or a representative sample) and the potential risk factors at a particular point in time or time interval.

CRP   Common medical abbreviation – C-reactive protein.

Cryotherapy   Use of a local or general form of cooling. Most commonly used to reduce extent of acute pain or responses of the body to acute trauma (i.e. most effective in first few minutes or hours). Local methods include applications of a crushed ice pack or pre-made cooled gel pack in damp covering or an inflatable cuff through which cooled water can circulate. Ice packs are usually used in conjunction with rest, compression and depending on the region affected, elevation (RICE or CRIE depending whether the focus is on the cooling [ice] or compression). General or systemic methods include a reduced ambient air temperature, bathing in water containing ice or the surgical diversion of the blood supply through an external cooling system. Cooling reduces metabolic requirements during and after it.

Cryptogenic fibrosing alveolitis (CFA)   Unknown cause of fibrosing alveolitis.

C-section Common medical abbreviation – Caesarean section.
See *Caesarean section*

CSP Chartered Society of Physiotherapy, the professional body for physiotherapists in the UK.

CT Common medical abbreviation – Computerized tomography.

CT scan See *CAT scan*

Culture The values, beliefs, customs, norms, practices and ways of living in a society. Culture refers to everything within a society that is socially transmitted.

Current Electrotherapy term – flow of charged particles (ions or electrons) per unit time. Clinically current is usually at the mA level. If using microcurrent, μA. If treating over broken skin use very low current (e.g. for wound healing) as skin impedance is markedly reduced as broken skin effectively removes most of capacitive impedance component. As current passes through skin it spreads, more if electrodes are further apart and/or a higher intensity is used and very much less if close or a low intensity is used. Current spreading occurs because of the low resistance of subcutaneous tissues.
See *Current density*

Current density Electrotherapy term – current per unit area of electrode. Measured clinically in mA/cm². Current density increases if electrode size is reduced either intentionally or because the contact gel has dried out or the electrode is not firmly and consistently in contact with the skin. If current density is too high, the risk is of skin burns (e.g. specialized interferential suction cup containing four 1 cm² diameter electrodes reported to cause skin burns. The high current density with such small diameter electrodes combined with the high average IFT current markedly increases the risk of skin damage).
See *Constant current*

Cushingoid Caused by chronic overdose of glucocorticoids. Symptoms vary, but most people have upper body obesity and a rounded face, with increased fat around the neck.

Cushings syndrome A disorder in which ACTH levels are raised, it presents as myopathy, glucose intolerance and hypertension and psychological changes on occasion (Davies et al. 2001).

CVA(IN) Common medical abbreviation – Cerebrovascular accident (incident).

CVS Common medical abbreviation – Cardiovascular system.

C/W Common medical abbreviation – Consistent with.

CXR Common medical abbreviation – Chest X-ray.

Cyanosis This is a bluish discolouration of the skin/mucus membranes that is often classified into central cyanosis (the tip of the tongue loses its pink colour) indicating desaturation of arterial blood, or peripheral cyanosis (blueness of the fingers and toes) indicating possibly poor perfusion locally, or stasis of blood (not necessarily desaturation), e.g. as with peripheral vascular disease. Cyanosis is difficult to detect unless severe (SaO_2 <85%) with observer error being high. Influential factors include skin pigmentation, vessel patency, lighting (e.g. the presence of nail varnish), Hb and the eye itself. Its absence should not be misconstrued as falsely reassuring.

Cystic fibrosis (CF) CF is a genetically inherited disease involving primarily the respiratory and gastrointestinal tracts. CF is characterized by airflow obstruction and stasis of viscid respiratory mucus, malabsorption due to exocrine pancreatic insufficiency and high levels of sweat electrolytes. The respiratory problems frequently encountered include recurrent productive cough with thick tenacious secretions, repeated resistant bacterial bronchial infections, e.g. staphylococcus and pseudomonas, airway obstruction, haemoptysis, pneumothorax and respiratory failure. The management strategies include chest physiotherapy, postural drainage, bronchodilators, mucolytics, antibiotics, oxygen and transplantation for end-stage disease. The average life expectancy is around 30 years.

Cytotoxic Any agent or process that is toxic to cells that results in suppression of cell function or cell death.

Cytotoxic drugs The name used to describe any pharmacological compound that inhibits the growth of cells within the body.

DAS score Disease activity score, a useful tool for measuring disease activity on a scale of 1–10 based on the number of swollen and tender joints and the erythrocyte sedimentation rate (ESR).

Data (singular = datum) Research term – the pieces of information, facts and figures that have resulted from the study.

Data can be one of four types:

1. **Nominal** – naming data, e.g. male or female, yes or no
2. **Ordinal** – slightly more detailed, puts data into an order, e.g.:
   - Strongly agree
   - Agree
   - Neither agree nor disagree
   - Disagree
   - Strongly disagree.
3. **Interval** – as above, but assumes equal intervals between the categories
4. **Ratio** – as above, but also possesses a zero point.

This is important in research since the type of data dictates what statistical test can be undertaken.

DDD Common medical abbreviation – Degenerative disc disease.

Dead space The air present within the respiratory tract that is not involved directly in gas exchange, it is usually about 150 ml in humans.

Debridement Removal of foreign material from a wound to expose the underlying healthy tissue.

DECA Prefix meaning ten times.

Decerebrate rigidity Abnormal posturing that can follow head injury, resulting in a midbrain lesion. The patient usually forms a rigid posture with a clenched jaw, retracted neck, the body and both upper and lower limbs in a markedly extended position. Patients with decerebrate rigidity are at high risk of developing contractures.

DECI Prefix meaning one-tenth.

Decorticate rigidity Abnormal posturing that can follow head injury, resulting from a lesion above the superior colliculus, i.e. at the level of the thalamus or internal capsule. The patient usually forms a rigid posture with the body and lower limbs in a markedly extended position and flexor responses in the upper limbs. Patients with decorticate rigidity are at high risk of developing contractures.

Decortication Surgical removal of the pleura from the lung.

Deep tendon reflex See *Reflex*

Deep transverse friction (DTF) A technique pioneered by James Cyriax, it involves small amplitude massage to soft tissues. It has been suggested that they may have a local anaesthetic effect. Selective stimulation of mechanoreceptors by rhythmical movement over the affected area may close the pain gate. Another mechanism through which reduction in pain may be achieved is release of endogenous opiates. Friction massage may have a beneficial effect on all three phases of repair.

Gentle transverse friction, applied in the early inflammatory phase might enhance the mobilization of tissue fluid and, therefore, increases the rate of phagocytosis.

During maturation, scar tissue is reshaped and strengthened by removing, reorganizing and replacing cells and matrix. Internal and external mechanical stress applied to the repair tissue is the main stimulus for remodelling immature and weak scar tissue with fibres oriented in all directions and through several planes into linearly rearranged bundles of connective tissue. As transverse friction aims basically to achieve transverse movement of the collagen structure of the connective tissue adhesion formation may be prevented. Friction induces a traumatic hyperaemia or increased bloodflow to the area that may facilitate the removal of chemical irritants and increases the transportation of endogenous opiates.

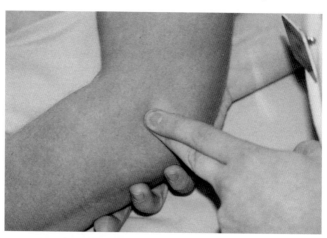

Deep transverse frictions for lateral epicondylitis (tennis elbow)

Deep vein thrombosis (DVT) The formation of a blood clot (thrombus), usually affects mainly the veins in the lower leg or the thigh. This thrombus may block blood circulation to the area, or it may break off and travel through the blood stream (embolize). The embolus thus created can lodge in the brain, lungs, heart, or other area, causing damage. Risks include prolonged sitting, bed rest or immobilization, recent surgery or trauma (especially hip, knee or gynaecological surgery), fractures, childbirth within the last 6 months and the use of medications such as oestrogen and birth control pills.

Most deep vein thromboses (DVTs) start in the calf and most resolve spontaneously. Proximal DVTs resolve slowly during treatment with anticoagulants and thrombi remain detectable in half of the patients after 1 year. Resolution of DVT is less likely in patients with a large initial thrombus or cancer. About 10% of patients with symptomatic DVTs develop severe post thrombotic syndrome within 5 years and recurrent ipsilateral DVT increases this risk (Kearon 2003).

Defecation The process of expulsion of faeces from the rectum.

Defibrillation The term given to the method of delivering an intentional electrical shock to the heart to bring it back into a regular pattern of beating when the cardiac muscle is in an uncoordinated haphazard pattern of contraction (fibrillation).

Degenerative joint disease (DJD) See *Osteoarthritis*

Degree classification The classification of an awarded degree is according to the total of marks gained over Levels 2 and 3 of a degree programme. They are usually expressed as follows:

- 1st class honours, 2.1, 2.2
- 3rd
- Pass.

Delayed-onset muscle soreness (DOMS) A dull, aching sensation that follows unaccustomed muscular exertion. Soreness usually peaks 24–48 h after exercise (Vickers 2001). Eccentric exercise seems to be the type of exercise that produces the greatest degree of soreness, although isometric exercise may also cause it (Byrnes & Clarkson 1986).

Delirium tremens (DTs) An acute reaction to alcohol or drug withdrawal characterized by sweating, tremor, restlessness, raised heart rate, fever, anxiety, chest pains, mental confusion and hallucinations.

Delphi technique A research technique that uses a group of people identified as experts in the field of interest. A group of experts are invited to give their opinions on a specific issue using a questionnaire. After data analysis they are then grouped into a series of statements that are then sent back to the participants who are asked to indicate their level of agreement with each statement. These are then returned to the researcher who provides an overall ranking of the statements that is then re-circulated.

Deltoid ligament Another name for the medial collateral ligament of the ankle joint, triangular in shape, hence its name. Much stronger than the lateral collateral ligaments; in fact, so strong that is it common for eversion injuries to cause fracture of the tip of the malleolus rather than rupture of the ligament itself.

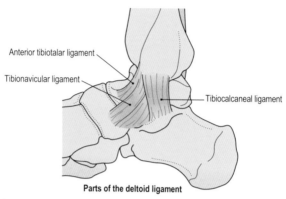

Parts of the deltoid ligament

The deltoid ligament

Dementia Progressive deterioration of memory, intellect and personality. The most common cause is Alzheimer's disease. Although not primarily affecting motor function it can lead to patients being unable to walk or undertake ADL as they lose the ability to plan and organize their activities.

Demyelination This is a pathological process in multiple sclerosis that results in damage to the myelin sheaths around nerves, such that nerve conduction is impaired.

Denervated muscle Peripheral nerve supply to a muscle disrupted. Responses to electrical stimulation markedly reduced, chronaxie increased, rheobase also generally increased.
See *Neuropraxia, Axonotmesis* and *Neurotmesis*

Dens – also known as otontoid The process projecting upward from the body of the axis, (C2) the atlas (C1) rotates about the odontoid.

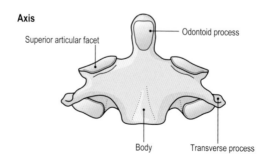

Deontology An approach to ethics whereby fundamental principles, such as respect for autonomy, are used to guide decision making.

Dependant variable Research term – the variable which alters as a result of manipulation of the independent variable.
See *Extraneous variable* and *Independent variable*

Depolarization This is where the membrane potential becomes less negative, resulting in an electric current passing down the nerve.
See *Action potential*

Depressed skull fracture This is where the skull fractures and forms a dent in the skull, which can be open (compound) or closed (simple). Although the patient may feel fine, it can require neurosurgery to correct and internal trauma may be present. Usually, the result of someone being hit on the head by an object.

Depression A mental state of sadness, despair and hopelessness with loss of interest that can be accompanied by insomnia, feelings of worthlessness, guilt and recurrent thoughts of death or suicide. Depression may be deemed clinical if it is persistent and severe.

De Quervain's tenosynovitis Inflammation of the tendons and sheath of abductor pollicis longus and extensor pollicis brevis.

Dermatitis Inflammation of the skin.

Dermatome Area of skin supplied by a particular spinal nerve level.

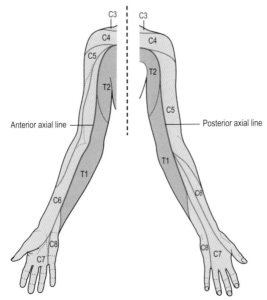

Dermatomes of the upper limb

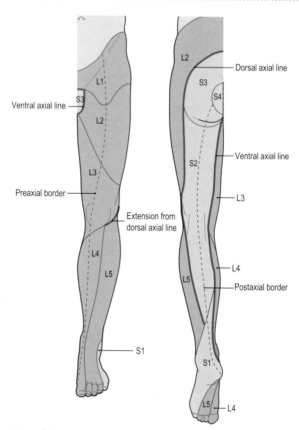

Dermatomes of the lower limb

Dermatomyositis A connective tissue disease that is characterized by swelling and inflammation of muscle tissue. An inflammatory myopathy of unknown cause, exhibits raised serum creatine kinase levels, electrophysiological abnormalities, and inflammation on muscle biopsy (Briemberg & Amato 2003).

Descending motor pathway Previously divided into pyramidal and extrapyramidal tracts, they may also be divided by anatomical location.

Descending (motor) spinal pathways

	Anatomical location in cord	Major function
Pathways of cortical origin		
Corticospinal		
Crossed pyramidal	Lateral ⎫	Voluntary movements of
Direct pyramidal	Anterior ⎭	the body
Pathways of brainstem origin		
Vestibulospinal	Ventromedial	Posture and balance
Tectospinal	Ventromedial	Motor component of visual and audio reflexes
Reticulospinal	Ventromedial	Muscle tone, autonomic system, regulation of sensory end-organs, e.g. muscle spindles
Rubrobulbar	Dorsolateral	Project to medulla
Rubrospinal	Dorsolateral	Extrapyramidal control of flexor muscles

Descriptive statistics A research term referring to statistics that convey information about and interpret large sets of numbers in an efficient way. Compare with inferential statistics, which can be used to make inferences from the data and express the confidence with which a generalization to a whole population can be undertaken.

Detrusor muscle The muscle of the bladder.

Deviance Refers to the breach of a norm of behaviour or the possession of an attribute or characteristic that violates a norm. A person with an impairment may be considered deviant, as may someone who refuses to engage in paid employment. However, precisely who or what is deemed deviant depends on the reasons for labelling and the social context. Deviance, from this perspective, is a label given to certain behaviours, characteristics or categories of people at certain times and in particular situations who, as a consequence, are devalued and often excluded. Divorced people and unmarried mothers were, for example, considered more deviant in the past than they are today in British society and the degree of deviance varies from country to country.

Diadynamic therapy Diadynamic currents (after Bernard) have been in use for over 50 years, though their popularity varies markedly. In the UK and USA they are used relatively infrequently, whilst in mainland Europe many more practitioners utilize them. There are two basic waveforms based on a half or full wave rectification of a sinusoidal waveform (usually at 50 Hz, though it can be of 60 Hz).

If the treatment application is based on a 50 Hz sinusoidal current with half wave rectification (MF or monophase fixe application), there will be a series of 10 ms pulses interspersed with 10 ms intervals. Each pulse will be a half sine wave shape. The second basic application is to use full wave rectification, thus generating 100 pulses per second, each at 10 ms and, therefore, presenting no interpulse interval. This application is referred to as DF (or diphase fixe). The other two forms of diadynamic therapy involve the combination of the basic waveforms. In the CP application (module en courtes periodes), the MF and DF currents are applied alternately (for 1 s each). The final form is to apply two MF currents with one current at a constant intensity and the other is surged. The surged current occupies the pulse intervals of the first waveform, thus each pulse is of 10-ms duration, there are effectively no interpulse intervals, but the surges are delivered at 5 s duration.

Diagnosis Determination of the nature or a cause of a disease, often shown in medical notes as the symbol Δ. The evaluation of a patient's medical history, clinical symptoms and laboratory tests that confirms or establishes an illness.

Dialysis The procedure that uses a machine to filter waste products from the bloodstream.

Diaphragm This is the major inspiratory muscle (dome shaped) constructed of approximately 50% type I fibres and 50% type II muscle fibres enabling fast, strong, prolonged low-tension contractions. It is attached at the crural portion to the upper lumbar vertebrae and at the costal portion to the inner aspect of the lower six ribs. On contraction (i.e. on inspiration), the diaphragm descends against the abdominal contents (pushing the abdominal wall outwards) so using the abdomen as a fulcrum on which to elevate the thoracic cage, causing a rise in intra-abdominal pressure. Inward movement of the diaphragm on inspiration (paradoxical movement) is indicative of diaphragmatic fatigue/weakness/paralysis. Higher lung volumes will reduce the resting length of the diaphragm and, therefore, provide a mechanical disadvantage to tension generation (as with hyperinflated states such as chronic airflow obstruction. These may result in an increased work of breathing and predispose diaphragmatic fatigue and respiratory muscle pump failure).

Diastasis rectus abdominis (DRA) Is an excessive gap between the muscle bellies of rectus abdominis at the level of the umbilicus, this can occur during pregnancy (Boissonnault & Blaschak 1988).

Diastole The period of dilatation of the heart.

Diathermy Electrotherapy term – deep heating produced clinically with short-wave diathermy (SWD), microwaves (MW) or ultrasound. Risks depend on the method used. For example, use of SWD or MW within 3–5 m of a patient with an indwelling stimulator or pump is contraindicated because the diathermy can alter functioning of the equipment. Ultrasound applied directly over the indwelling stimulator or pump is also contraindicated because of the risk of altering the equipment's functions.
  See *pswd*

Dichotomous question Research term – a question which enables a respondent to give one of two answers, e.g. yes/no, true/false.

Didronel A bisphosphonate drug specifically for the prevention and treatment of osteoporosis.

Differentiation test Differentiation tests help to determine the source of the patient's symptoms by objectively assessing different structures that may be the cause of the patient's complaint.

Differentiation of structures

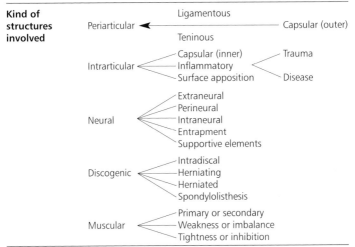

Kind of structures involved	Periarticular	Ligamentous ← → Capsular (outer) Teninous	
	Intrarticular	Capsular (inner) Inflammatory Surface apposition	Trauma Disease
	Neural	Extraneural Perineural Intraneural Entrapment Supportive elements	
	Discogenic	Intradiscal Herniating Herniated Spondylolisthesis	
	Muscular	Primary or secondary Weakness or imbalance Tightness or inhibition	

Diffuse idiopathic skeletal hyperostosis (DISH) A disease of elderly men characterized by ligamentous ossification and large osteophytes that bridge across the vertebrae.

Diffusion The movement of atoms or molecules from an area of high to low concentration/pressure.

Digitalis A family of drugs that increase the force of myocardial contraction. Digoxin is one such drug that is still very useful in patients with arrhythmias that can lead to heart failure.

Dilation – also known as dilatation The process of enlargement or expansion, e.g. vasodilation meaning increase in the diameter of a blood vessel.

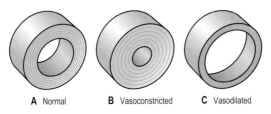

A Normal   **B** Vasoconstricted   **C** Vasodilated

Dilation

Dilation and curettage (D&C) A gynaecological procedure in which the lining of the uterus is sampled with a metal device called a curette. It is done to determine if there is an abnormality with the cells that line the uterus (endometrium).

Dinner fork deformity The typical deformity following a colles fracture where the hand is displaced posteriorly in relation to the forearm bones.
   See *Colles fracture*

Diplopia Double vision.

Direct current Electrotherapy term – one of three recognized categories of therapeutic currents (pulsed, direct and alternating currents). Current with a continuous (defined variously as in excess of 100 ms or 1 s duration) uni-directional flow of charge (electrons). The direction is traditionally described as being from the negative (cathode) to the positive electrode (anode). Used in iontophoresis and, if interrupted, to stimulate denervated muscle.

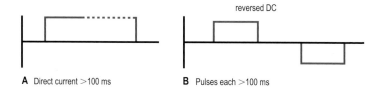

A Direct current >100 ms   **B** Pulses each >100 ms

Direct payments A process whereby people who require assistance in daily living can be assessed for a cash sum to purchase their own assistance. It was introduced in the Direct Payment Act (1996) and provides an alternative to relying on statutory workers to supply and deliver assistance. A forerunner was the Independent Living Fund which was introduced in 1988. It was closed in 1993 because of excessive demand.

Disability Can be defined from an individual model (including medical and tragedy models) or a social model. The individual model is dominant and assumes that the difficulties faced by disabled people are a direct result of their individual impairments and loss or lack of functioning. The social model of disability recognizes the social origins of disability in a society geared by and for non-disabled people. The disadvantages or restrictions, often referred to as barriers, permeate every aspect of the physical and social environment. Disability can, therefore, be defined as a form of social oppression.

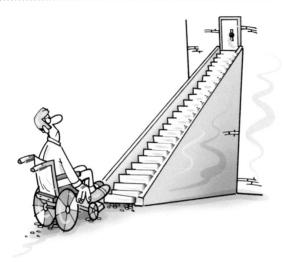

Whose problem?

Disabled role A role that disabled people are frequently expected to play that denies their own interests. It involves striving for 'normality' and 'independence' and 'adjusting' to and 'accepting' their situation within a disabling society. In this way the status quo is maintained and disabled people are kept in their disadvantaged position within society.

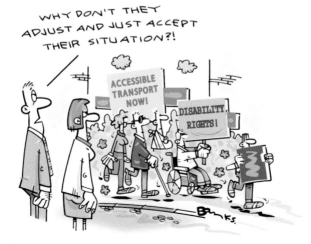

Disablism Stereotyped, negative beliefs about disabled people that may lead to discrimination. Disablism frequently leads to the denial of appropriate services and a lack of equal opportunities in comparison with other citizens.

Discectomy Surgical removal of the prolapsed portion of nucleus pulposus.

Disc herniation/protrusion Disruption to the normal integrity of an intervertebral disc, causing the nucleus pulposus to breach the annulus. There are varying degrees, from minor bulging, which may be asymptomatic, to bursting through the outer annular fibres into the spinal canal causing severe leg pain and nerve compression.

Protrusions can be classified as shown below (American Academy of Orthopaedic Surgeons 1987).

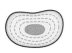 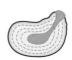

Normal disc	Bulge/protrusion	Extrusion	Sequestration
Nucleus is contained within the annulus	Posterior longitudinal ligament remains intact, the nucleus impinges upon the annulus	The nucleus escapes from the annulus but is still contained by the posterior longitudinal ligament	A portion of disc escapes and may become loose within the epidural space

Discrimination The identification of differences among individuals and groups of people. Discrimination can be positive or negative, though the term usually denotes negativity. Discrimination involves not only the recognition of differences, such as class, age, disability and sexual orientation, but also a negative response to an individual or group, whether this is attitudinal, behavioural or structural.

DISH Common medical abbreviation – Diffuse idiopathic skeletal hyperostosis.

Disinhibition This is where a patient loses the usual social inhibitions and as a result is inappropriate in the way they behave and what they say. It is associated with injury to the frontal lobes. For example, a patient may be sexually inappropriate.

Disorientation Inability to be orientated to time, place and person, sometimes seen following neurological injury, can be transient or long term.

Distal Anatomical term, remote, farther from any point of reference, opposite of proximal.

○ **Clinical point** The anatomical position is always the starting point for treatments and assessments, so, for example, no matter what position a person's arm is in, the hand is always distal to the elbow, even if it is raised above the head.

Distraction osteogenesis A surgical procedure designed to increase bone dimensions. Its origins are traced to a Russian orthopaedist named Ilizarov.
See *Ilizarov method*

Diuretic Any substance that encourages the formation of urine. They are often used in the management of heart failure.

DLCO This is an investigation of lung function, which details the diffusion capacity for carbon monoxide, i.e. a measure of the effectiveness of gas diffusion across the alveolar capillary membrane. It is measured in ml/min/mmHg.

DM Common medical abbreviation – Diabetes mellitus.

DMARD Common medical abbreviation – Disease modifying anti-rheumatic drug.

DNA (X2) Common medical abbreviation – Deoxyribonucleic acid or did not attend.

DOA (X2) Common medical abbreviation – Dead on arrival or date of admission.

Dopamine This is a neurotransmitter synthesized from dopa.

Doppler ultrasonography Doppler-corrected ultrasound enables real-time viewing of tissues, blood flow and organs.

Doman delecato technique A paediatric therapy technique. Repeated passive patterning accompanied by reverse hanging and developmental sequence of movement facilitates use of dormant pathways in CNS and brain.

Domiciliary care Medical and non-medical care that is provided for ill and disabled people in their own homes. It includes 'meals on wheels', community nursing and community physiotherapy.

Dorsal column The routes by which sensory afferent travel to the brain. Includes receptors for vibration, touch and proprioceptors.

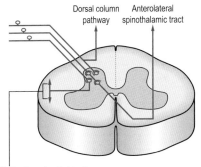

The major ascending sensory pathways in the spinal cord. The dorsal (or posterior) column conveys afferent information from mechanoreceptors (skin) and proprioceptors (muscle and joints) destined for the somatosensory cortex. The spinothalamic tracts in the anterior (ventral) and lateral white matter convey information mainly from nociceptors and thermoreceptors to the thalamus and on to the cortex. Spinocerebellar tracts in the lateral white matter route proprioceptive inputs to the cerebellum. Propriospinal tracts link the different segments of the spinal cord

Dorsal horn   The dorsal region of the spinal cord that contains cell bodies.

Dorsal root   A group of sensory axons from the spinal nerve and attaching to the dorsal side of the spinal column.

Dosage   Electrotherapy context. General dosage parameters include: intensity, wavelength, duration and frequency of treatments, location of application. Record all relevant parameters after every treatment – this enables appropriate modifications to repeat treatments and also helps in audits investigating the contribution of an electrophysical agent to an outcome.

Double blind   A research term that refers to the procedure in a clinical trial for issuing and administering treatment assignments by code number in order to keep study patients and all members of the clinical staff, especially those responsible for patient treatment and data collection, from knowing the assigned treatments.

Double-crush hypothesis   Proposes that a proximal lesion along an axon predisposes it to injury at a more distal site along its course through impaired axoplasmic flow (Morgan & Wilbourn 1998).

Dowagers hump   This is a curve on the upper spine. Often a symptom of osteoporosis.

Doxapram   This is a central respiratory stimulant useful in reversing opiate narcosis. (Its efficacy is not proven in the management of acute tachypnoeic respiratory failure patients.)

Draw tests   See *AP* and *PA draw tests*

Drop foot   See *Foot drop splint*

Drop-out cast   This is where part of a cast is cut away to allow the patient to undertake a movement while preventing movement in the opposite direction. Commonly used for the correction of contractures as it enables the patient to strengthen the opposing muscle group to the contracture.

In the arm, if the arm is contracted into flexion, then the posterior part of the splint is cut away above the elbow so that the arm can extend, but cannot flex any further due to the cast.

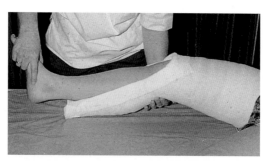

Drop-out cast

In the leg contracted into flexion, the anterior part of the splint is cut away below the knee so that the knee can extend, but cannot flex any further due to the cast.

DU Common medical abbreviation – Duodenal ulcer.

Dual X-ray absorptiometry (DXA) scan A diagnostic test for osteoporosis.

Duchenne muscular dystrophy An inherited muscular dystrophy affecting boys; it is rapidly progressive and severe. It is inherited recessively through the X chromosome. Usually apparent before the age of 5 years, it rapidly progresses with death usually in their teens due to cardiac or respiratory failure.

Dupuytren's contracture A fibrous contraction that occurs in the palmar fascia of the hand that may produce a flexion deformity of the metacarpophalangeal and proximal interphalangeal joints common in those of Anglo Saxon descent. The cause is unknown, but minor trauma and genetic predisposition may play a role, other risk factors include alcoholism, diabetes and liver disease. One or both hands may be affected. The ring finger is affected most often, followed by the little, middle and index fingers. A nodule develops within the connective tissue and eventually develops into a cord-like band. Finger extension becomes limited. The condition becomes more common after the age of 40 years and it is commoner in men than women.

Symptoms

- A painless nodule in the palm
- Thickening of the lines in the palms of the hands
- Difficulty in extending the fingers especially the 4th and 5th fingers.

Dura mater The thickest, outermost covering of the spinal cord and spinal nerves. Bleeding underneath this membrane is called a sub-dural haematoma.

Duty cycle Electrotherapy term – indicates the percentage of time for which there is an output. Formula:

$$\% \text{ duty cycle} = [\text{on time}/(\text{on time} + \text{off time})] \times 100$$

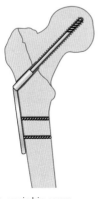

On and off times are usually measured in seconds. Used most commonly for electrical stimulation and pulsed ultrasound and pulsed SWD (PSWD).

Dynamic hip screw (DHS) An orthopaedic procedure undertaken on femoral neck fractures. It involves placing a plate on the femoral shaft and a screw that pierces the femoral head, the arrangement is such that when the person gets up to mobilize, there is some movement between the metal components and hence compression (and stimulation of bone healing) at the fracture site.

A dynamic hip screw

Dynamic stretching See *Stretching*

Dynamometer A mechanical instrument that allows for measurement of concentric and eccentric muscle action, muscle endurance and muscle balance ratios.

Dysarthria Problems with articulation, resulting in inability to speak caused by weakness, lack of co-ordination or spasticity. The patient has full understanding and knows what they want to say. This is commonly encountered in neurological disorders such as motor neurone disease.

Dysdiadochokinesia Inability to perform smooth rapidly alternating movements that requires actions of opposing muscle groups. This is often tested by asking the person to pat their hands on their legs, first palm down and then palm up rapidly.

Dyskinesia Impairment of voluntary movement, commonly results in fragmentary or incomplete movements.

Main causes of some dyskinetic movement disorders

Tremor	
Rest tremor	Parkinson's disease
	Drug-induced Parkinsonism
	Other extrapyramidal disease
Action tremor	Enhanced physiological tremor (e.g. anxiety, alcohol, hyperthyroidism)
	Essential tremor
	Cerebellar disease
	Wilson's disease
Intention tremor	Brainstem or cerebellar disease (e.g. multiple sclerosis), spinocerebellar degeneration
Myoclonus	
Without encephalopathy	Juvenile myoclonic epilepsy
	Myoclonic epilepsy
With encephalopathy	
Non-progressive	Post-anoxic myoclonus
Progressive	Storage disorders (e.g. Lafora body disease)
	Unverricht–Lindborg disease
	Metabolic encephalopathies (e.g. respiratory, renal and liver failure)
	Creutzfeldt–Jacob disease
Chorea	
Syndenham's chorea	
Pregnancy-associated chorea	
Contraceptive-pill-associated chorea	
Huntington's disease	
Thyrotoxicosis	
Systemic lupus erythematosus	
Drug-induced chorea (e.g. neuroleptics, phenytoin)	

Dystonia

Generalized	Idiopathic torsion dystonia
	Drug-induced
	Athetoid cerebral palsy
	Wilson's disease
	Metabolic storage disorders
	Dopa-responsive dystonia
Hemidystonia	Basal ganglia lesions (e.g. tumours, vascular, post-thalamotomy)

Dysmenorrhea Difficult and painful menstruation.

Dysmetria An inability to place the limbs accurately in relation to other objects.

Dyspepsia A term used to describe digestive upset.

Dysphagia Difficulties with swallowing commonly seen after stroke. Patients may aspirate their food and drink, i.e. it will go into their main bronchus and then into their lungs. This can lead to serious complications and so needs effective assessment and management by the MDT. Where present, alternative means of feeding must be established, such as via a naso-gastric tube or a percutaneous endoscopic gastrostomy (PEG), otherwise the patient will rapidly become malnourished.

Dysphasia A disorder of language and speech, this can be receptive (difficulty to understand speech) or expressive (difficultly expressing language). Strategies can be used to enable more effective communication. Speech and language therapists can advise on the best methods to use with each individual patient.

Dyspnoea Shortness of breath, often abbreviated to SOB, or SOBOE (short of breath on exertion).

Breathlessness or dyspnoea is a sensation perceived by an individual and should not be confused with tachypnoea (increased respiratory rate), hyperventilation (breathing which exceeds metabolic requirements) or hyperpnoea (increased breathing). Breathlessness has been described as the perceived intensity of stimuli produced with breathing (Altose 1989).

This conscious awareness of breathing becomes an overwhelming sensation severely affecting the existence of some chronic lung patients. Since the sensation is subjective and related to life experience, the clinician cannot fully appreciate nor judge the level of dyspnoea, as with other sensations e.g. pain, fear, hunger and grief (Borg 1982).

Dyspraxia Difficulty in carrying out purposeful voluntary movement in patients with good comprehension, normal sensation and some motor activity.

Dystaxia Difficulty in controlling voluntary movements.

Dystonia This describes an abnormal movement where the agonist and antagonistic muscles contract isometrically and involuntarily, leading to contorted posturing. This often occurs when the patient tries to initiate movement. Present in some neurological conditions and can affect the whole body or any part.

E

Early morning stiffness (EMS) This is a common feature of inflammatory conditions, particularly rheumatoid arthritis and refers to slowness or difficulty moving the joints when getting out of bed or after being still in one position for too long, it usually gets better with movement.

Eburnation The term for the polished appearance of articular cartilage affected by osteoarthritis. It refers to the dense, sclerotic appearance that the cartilage takes on in an attempt to remodel and deal with the extra stresses, it resembles ivory in that it is white and dense.

Eccentric Controlled, active lengthening of a muscle. For example, when placing a cup back on a table, the biceps muscle works eccentrically to lower the cup.

Ecchymosis A small haemorrhagic spot, on the skin or mucous membrane forming a blue or purplish patch.

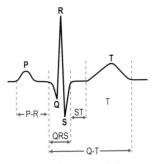

Configuration of a typical electrocardiogram or ECG. The P-wave signifies atrial depolarization, the QRS complex signifies onset of ventricular depolarization and the T-wave signifies ventricular repolarization. Reproduced from Berne RM, Levy MN 2000 Principles of physiology, 3rd edn. Mosby, London

ECG Common medical abbreviation – electro cardiogram.

A non-invasive test that is used to reflect underlying heart conditions by measuring the electrical activity of the heart by positioning leads on the body in standardized locations.

Echocardiography A diagnostic test which uses ultrasound waves to make images of the heart chambers, valves and surrounding structures. It can also measure cardiac output and detect pericarditis or abnormal heart valves.

Ectopic pregnancy A pregnancy elsewhere than in the uterus. Often occurs in the fallopian tube.

Eczema A type of dermatitis that occurs as a reaction to many agents.

It is characterized by erythema, a serous discharge between the cells of the epidermis and an inflammatory infiltrate in the dermis.

EDSS Expanded disability status scale is a classification scheme (rating scale) that insures all participants in clinical trials are in the same class, type, or phase of multiple sclerosis. It is also used to follow the progression of disability and evaluate treatment results.

EEG Common medical abbreviation – electroencephalogram.
A test that records the electrical activity of the brain using scalp electrodes.

Efferent Leaving the central nervous system, i.e. efferent axons are those taking information away from the central nervous system (CNS).

Effusion Joint Swelling, confined to a synovial cavity, it may also occur in the lungs = pleural effusion.

Ehlers–Danlos syndrome A connective-tissue disorder characterized by, amongst other signs and symptoms, hyperelasticity of skin, joints and other soft tissues.

Elastin A class of connective tissue fibres that can be readily stretched, found in walls of distensible vessels, e.g. veins, bladder, etc. Elastin is structural protein that gives our tissues and organs elasticity. It lines arteries, in our lungs, intestines and skin. In function it complements collagen, whereas collagen provides rigidity, elastin allows connective tissues to stretch and then recoil.

Elbow, tennis The terms for inflammation at the common extensor origin at the lateral epicondyle of the humerus (golfers elbow affects the medial epicondyle).

Electrically initiated torque (EIT) Electrotherapy term – the torque produced by stimulating a muscle electrically. EIT is usually less than the maximal voluntary torque (MVT), but can be greater. Developed as a way of comparing the comfort and effectiveness of different types of currents, e.g. pulsed versus alternating currents with a range of parameters. Used as a ratio with maximal voluntary torque to indicate change in fatigue and effectiveness of electrode positioning, but not a reliable measure (EIT/MVT).

Electrode Electrotherapy term – means of applying the output current from a machine to the part of the body to be treated by electrical stimulation or for when amplifying bioelectrical signals (e.g. EMG, EEC, ECG). **Types** of electrode for electrical stimulation include: reusable carbon rubber with purpose designed electrical stimulation gel or gel pads; metal (including aluminium and lead) used with moistened sponge or lint; self-adhesive; task-specific bare metal electrodes (e.g. anal or vaginal). **Size** varies according to the aims and area being treated, whether both are the same or different sizes also depends upon the type of current and the aims; size affects current density, so if it is too small with a high average current, there is a high risk of skin burns. **Location** will vary with the aims of treatment. **Number**: at least two per electrical circuit, four may be used (interferential or 2-channels concurrently) or, if using HVPS, may have one anode and two or more cathodes (bifurcated).

Electrodes for amplification

Type, number and locations are usually quite different for EMG, EEC and ECG than for electrical stimulation. For example, for EMG biofeedback three small electrodes are typically used (one ground, two active along the line of the fibres). They may be separate or comprise a single tri-electrode pre-amplifier.

Electrodiagnostic tests Tests that are used to record electrical activity of the brain or nerves, they include electroencephalography (EEG), nerve conduction tests and evoked potentials (EP).

Electrolytes Substances that become ionized in solution and acquire the capacity to conduct electricity. Normal electrolyte balance is essential for normal function.

Electromyography biofeedback Electrotherapy term – the use of amplified bioelectrical signals from motor unit activity as a form of feedback. Used to increase or decrease level of motor unit activity. For example, used to retrain movement after stroke and to decrease muscle activity associated with headaches.

See *Electrodes*

Electronic bibliography software Many undergraduate and postgraduate students now choose electronic reference management systems such as EndNote, Reference Manager or ProCite to help them search Internet libraries to capture relevant references to create their own personal databases and automatically generate and format in-text citations and bibliographies within their word processed papers. Rather than spending hours finding and managing references using traditional methods or creating and editing bibliographies manually, students may now turn to reference-management tools to save time, improve their accuracy and streamline the whole writing process.

For those already using bibliographic software, reference management has now been taken one step further with RefViz: a brand-new text analysis and visualization software package that lets the user visually evaluate the relevance of references. If documents feature technical or scientific content, it is worth considering investing in sciPROOF: the scientific author's proof-reading tool.

Electrophysical agents (EPAs) Electrotherapy term – methods of treatment using electrical stimulation or physical agents such as heat, cold, ultrasound, laser and ultraviolet radiations. Two also used diagnostically with appropriate equipment: ultrasound (for visualization of subcutaneous tissues) and ultraviolet radiations (for diagnosis of some skin conditions).

Electrotherapy The use of electrophysical agents (EPAs) for treatment. In the USA refers to the use of electrical stimulation only. Elsewhere more broadly understood as meaning all EPAs. Modalities used in the treatment of musculoskeletal disorders include, short wave diathermy, interferential therapy, transcutaneous electrical nerve stimulation or laser.

Ely's test A musculoskeletal test. Performed in cases of suspected rectus femoris tightness, the patients lets prone while the physiotherapist passively flexes the knee. If passive full knee flexion is attained the physiotherapist then passively moves the hip into extension, if during this the patient simultaneously flexes their hip then the rectus femoris is tight.

Emancipation The politics of eliminating or reducing oppression, inequality, injustice and exploitation. It is the liberation of individuals and groups from the constraints and unequal power relations that limit their life chances and quality of life.

Embolism The blocking of a blood vessel by a clot or other foreign material that has been brought to its site of lodgement by the blood flow, commonly seen are pulmonary emboli that have broken off from a previous deep vein thrombosis (DVT).

Embolization This is a technique that can be used to surgically block an arterio venous malformation to prevent it subsequently bursting. With the greater use of technology embolization is becoming more effective.

EMG Common medical abbreviation – electromyogram.

A test that records the electrical activity of a muscle. Normally carried out using needles inserted into the muscle, but can be undertaken using surface electrodes, in which case it is often described as a surface EMG. The latter is less accurate. Used in the diagnosis of many conditions and in the application of botulinum toxin injections.

Emotional lability An affective disturbance as a result of brain injury that results in the patient exhibiting very emotional behaviour, e.g. crying, in situations that such behaviour would not normally be expected. For example, a patient may cry every time she sees a family member. This can make normal social functioning very difficult.

Emphysema An obstructive lung disease characterized by enlargement of the terminal bronchioles and destruction of the alveolar walls without fibrosis. The total lung volume increases with added dead space due to air trapping, resulting in an increased work of breathing. The most common cause of emphysema is smoking, but some patients may have an inherited condition called alpha1 antitrypsin deficiency.

See *AAT* and *Bullae*

'Pink puffer' is an old term often used to describe the appearance of the emphysematous patient. Individuals classically have a wasted general musculature, a hyperinflated chest (elevated ribs with large lung fields, a flattened diaphragm and large antero-posterior thoracic diameter and tracheal tug), adopt a fixed posture breathing stance (i.e. fix the shoulder girdle in order to recruit the accessory respiratory muscles by leaning forward onto the arms) and automatically use pursed-lip breathing when physiologically stressed (to generate intrinsic positive end expiratory pressure, thus splinting the otherwise collapsible diseased airways open and facilitating oxygen uptake). This enables the emphysematous patient to maintain normal partial pressure levels of oxygen. Hence the term 'pink puffer'.

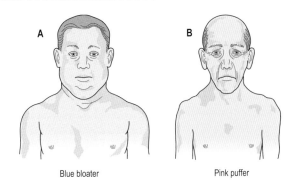

A

B

Blue bloater

Pink puffer

Empowerment A process of facilitating people in gaining greater control over their lives, life choices and the social and personal challenges they face. Though empowerment can be facilitated, it is changes experienced by those who gain a sense of control that are crucial to empowerment. In this sense empowerment cannot be 'given', but must be 'taken'.

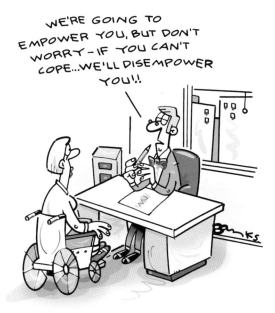

Empty can test – also known as supraspinatus test Performed in sitting or standing 90° of shoulder abduction bilaterally, full available medial rotation and 30° horizontal flexion. Supraspinatus is the main support for the suspended arm in this position. The physiotherapist resists abduction of the shoulder.

Abnormal finding Pain on resistance is a positive test for a lesion of the supraspinatus muscle or tendon.

Empyema The collection of pus within the pleural space, often as a result of bacterial infection or post pneumonia.

Encephalitis Inflammation of the brain.

End feel During passive movements, the end feel is noted. Different joints and different pathologies have different end feels. The quality of the resistance felt at the end of range was categorized by Cyriax (1982):

- Bony block to movement or hard feel is characteristic of arthritic joints.
- An empty feel or no resistance offered at the end of range may be due to severe pain associated with infection, active inflammation and tumours.
- A springy block is characterized by a rebound feel at the end of range and is associated with torn meniscus blocking knee extension.
- Spasm is experienced as sudden, relatively hard feel associated with muscle guarding.
- Capsular feel: a hardish arrest of movement.

Endocrine glands A series of glands each with specific functions listed in the table below.

Hypothalamus
Growth hormone releasing hormone, controlling growth hormone, corticotrophin releasing hormone, controlling adreno corticotrophic hormone (ACTH), thyrotrophin releasing hormone, controlling thyroid stimulating hormone (TSH), prolactin inhibiting hormone, controlling prolactin, gonadotrophin releasing hormone, controlling the gonadotrophins, luteinizing hormone and follicle stimulating hormone

Anterior pituitary
Growth hormone influences growth of all cells, ACTh controls the adrenal cortex, thyroid-stimulating hormone stimulates the thyroid to produce hormones, follicle stimulating hormone stimulates follicle growth in females and sperm production in males, and luteinizing hormone controls ovulation and production of oestrogen and progesterone and testosterone

Posterior pituitary
Anti diuretic hormone causes water reabsorption and, therefore, water balance oxytocin is involved in lactation

Thyroid gland
Controls metabolism in cells, calcitonin is involved in monitoring blood calcium levels

Parathyroid
Controls plasma calcium levels

Adrenal cortex
Aldosterone is involved in sodium and potassium regulation and cortisol is a key element in the body's defence system

Pancreas
Glucose metabolism and balance

Ovaries and testes

Endoplasmic reticulum The membrane system that courses through the cytoplasm.

Endorphins Substances implicated in the alleviation of pain, produced as a result of body stress or upon exercise.

Endoscopy Surgical procedure to view the inside of a body cavity with a device using flexible fibre optics.

Endotracheal intubation A procedure by which a tube is inserted through the mouth down into the trachea.

End plate – also known as vertebral end plate The end plates are found above and below each intervertebral disc, they are approximately 1 mm thick and have several functions: the end plate is thought to permit osmosis of nutrients between the vertebral body and the disc, it restrains the disc and may also protect the vertebra from pressure. Herniation or bulging of the nucleus into the vertebral body through the end plate may occur, but these are often asymptomatic (Giles et al. 1997).

End systolic volume The volume of blood at the end of systole, usually about 60 ml.

Energy The amount of work done, measured in joules (J). For example, for low level laser that also uses energy density:

$$= \text{Power density (W/cm}^2) \times \text{Time (s)} = \text{J/cm}^2$$

Enteric-coated tablet Tablets that are coated in order to delay release of the medication until after they leave the stomach.

Entonox An equal mixture of nitrous oxide and oxygen. It has pain-relieving properties and can be self-administered.

Enuresis Involuntary urination (bed wetting). It usually occurs at night and is quite common in children.

Enzyme A protein that triggers or accelerates chemical reactions, without itself being consumed.

Eosinophil White blood cells that can digest microorganisms.

Epicanthal fold A fold of skin that comes down across the inner angle of the eye. The epicanthal fold is more common in children with Down's syndrome.

Epicondyle An eminence on a bone above the condyle.

Epidemic A significant increase in the prevalence of a disease in a specific population or area.

Epidemiology The science of determination of the specific causes of a disease or the interrelation between various factors determining a disease, as well as disease trends in the population.

Epidermolysis bullosa A group of rare inherited disorders in which skin blistering occurs in response to skin trauma.

Epidural anaesthetic An anaesthetic injected into the epidural space which has the effect of numbing the abdomen and legs.

Epiglottis A cartilaginous lidlike structure that closes the glottis while food or fluid is passing through the pharynx.

Epiglottitis An acute and often life-threatening upper airways infection that causes major obstruction from supraglottic swelling, seen predominantly in children aged <5 years. The most common infective cause is haemophilus influenzae type B. Manifestations include fever, sore throat, stridor, increased work of breathing, swallowing problems. Emergency intubation/ tracheostomy may be indicated as a life-saving procedure.

Epilepsy This is a chronic disorder of the nervous system characterized by the patient experiencing episodic seizures – periods of loss of consciousness, impaired functioning or abnormal motor activity (fits). Between seizures that person will often function normally. Medication is the main treatment and enables many patients to live normal lives.

Epimysium The fibrous connective tissue envelope surrounding a skeletal muscle.

Epiphysis A bone growth plate, formed from a secondary centre of ossification, commonly found at the ends of long. Separated from the main portion of bone by cartilage (epiphyseal plate).

Episiotomy An incision performed between the vagina and the rectum that is used to increase the opening of the vagina to assist in the delivery of a baby.

Epistemology Research term – the theory of knowledge and how people achieve knowledge. It includes the possibility of attaining objective knowledge, and the psychological aspects of knowledge.

Epley manoeuvre This manoeuvre, which is also known as the particle repositioning manoeuvre (prm) or the canal repositioning procedure (crp), consists of a cycle of five positions for the treatment of BPPV (benign paroxysmal positional vertigo). The cycle of manoeuvres is to ensure that all the debris in the semicircular canals is transferred to the most dependent part of the canal.

Epstein–Barr virus The virus that causes glandular fever.

Equality The elimination of disadvantage, for example, in access to services, in opportunities to achieve socially desired ends and in rights to resources, property and power.

Equal opportunity policy Sets of practices and procedures within organizations and institutions designed to ensure that certain groups of people, such as women and disabled people, are not disadvantaged in terms of employment, housing, access to services and so on. Unless equal opportunity policies are robust they may serve as a 'smokescreen' to obscure discrimination.

Equal pressure point The point within the airways where the pleural and airway pressures are equal. This concept is used in the application of the forced expiration technique (FET) to facilitate clearance of pulmonary secretions (see FET) (West 1982).

Equilibrium reactions These are small involuntary changes in tone or movements that occur to enable balance. For example, when lifting the arm there is increased activity in the back extensors to stabilize the trunk. They are often impaired in neurological conditions.

Equinovarus Foot deformity in which the foot points down and inwards. Otherwise known as club foot or talipes equinovarus.

Equity A principle applied to the allocation of resources. The principle of equity demands that like cases are treated alike, but it also recognizes that equality is not achieved by treating everybody the same.

Erb's palsy – also known as obstetrical brachial palsy (OBP) and Klumpke's paralysis This is a paralysis or weakness of the arm in the newborn caused by damage to the brachial plexus.

ERCP Common medical abbreviation – Endoscopic retrograde cholangio-pancreatography.
  A diagnostic test to examine the duodenum, the bile ducts, the gallbladder and the pancreatic duct. The procedure is performed by using a long, flexible, viewing instrument.

Erector spinae The collection of muscles that are found in the posterior of the spine. Their actions are complex. The extensor muscles of the spine may be able to control individual vertebral movements and it seems likely that the erector spinae complex works in complex patterns to resist the tendency of the spine to flex in various postures.

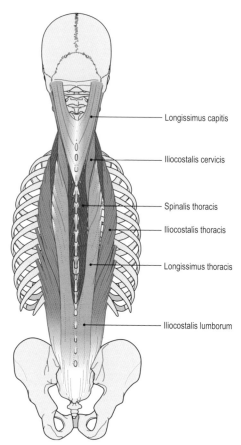

The erector spinae muscle showing its constituent parts

Ergonomics The study of how the workplace relates to the human and its function.

Erythema Reddening of the skin following an application of ultraviolet radiation (UVR) or heating or cooling. Used as the basis for dosage of UVR. Level of UVR required to produce minimal perceptible (MPE or E1) grade of erythema. Is established in a test prior to UVR treatment. Grades are E1 to E4 and based on depth of reddening, time until skin becomes red and for which it remains red, degree of subsequent pigmentation and any desquamation. Go to standard textbook for grades and method used to grade erythema.

Erythema nodosum A rheumatological disorder characterized by the formation of tender, red nodules on the front of the legs.

Erythrocyte sedimentation rate (ESR) A blood test that is used to detect and monitor inflammation. It is a measure of the red blood cells (erythrocytes) sedimenting in a tube over a given period of time. The normal sedimentation rate for males is 0–15 mm/h, females is 0–20 mm/h.

Escharotomy A term used in burn management where the surgeon releases the tension in the burned tissues via longitudinal incisions through the eschar along its full length.

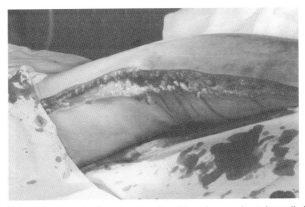

Full-thickness burns: inelastic leather-like skin with escharotomies to lower limb

Escherichia coli (E coli) A rod-shaped bacillus that is abundant in the large intestine.

ET Common medical abbreviation – Endotracheal tube.

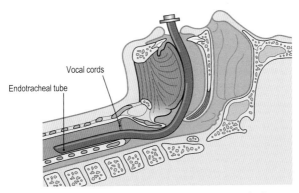

Positioning of endotracheal tube (ET). Proper ET tube placement in airway

Ethics A branch of philosophy which is concerned with the study of human values and morality.

Ethnicity A way of categorizing people who share common characteristics as defined by themselves or by others. Ethnicity can be an important aspect of identity for individuals and groups as it indicates cultural origins and differences. It can be the basis of national and political identity. Ethnicity is distinct from the contested term 'race', which categorizes people according to physical differences, such as skin colour, while ignoring cultural differences.

Ethnocentricity An attitude which presupposes that the beliefs, values and lifestyle of one's own group are superior to those of others.

Ethnography Research term – the description, study or interpretation of a culture.

Evidence Information on which a decision is based. This can be obtained from a range of sources including research trials (quantitative and qualitative), consensus of current practice, the expert opinion of clinical professionals and/or patients.

Evidence-based medicine/evidence-based practice (EBM/EBP) The conscientious, explicit and judicious use of current best evidence in making decisions about the care of individual patients. The practice of evidence-based medicine means integrating individual clinical expertise with the best available external clinical evidence from systematic research. Individual clinical expertise is the proficiency and judgement that individual clinicians acquire through clinical experience and clinical practice (Sackett et al. 1996).

It has been criticized for disregarding other factors involved in practice development, including financial resources and judgements based on experience and for ignoring important facets of practice that are difficult to measure.

EUA Common medical abbreviation – Examination under anaesthesia.

Euthanasia A process of painlessly killing a person who has a terminal or very distressing illness usually with their consent. Active euthanasia is against the law in Britain, but passive euthanasia, such as withholding physiotherapy treatment or drugs, is sometimes practised.

Eversion Turning outwards of the subtalar joint of the foot. The opposite of inversion.

Excitatory post synaptic potential (EPSP) A physiological term that refers to the effect that is produced when excitatory input to a neurone causes brief depolarization that spreads to the axon hillock, the balance between this and the inhibitory post synaptic potential determine the final output from the neurone.

Exclusion criteria Research term – the criteria by which members of the population of the sample will be excluded, for example in a study of heart rate, people with a history of cardiac problems would be excluded.

Executive dysfunction A loss of the normal high-level cognitive (executive) functions, due to brain injury. Patients can present as lethargic, poorly motivated, disinterested and with poor planning and organizational skills, however, superficially this deficit may not be immediately apparent unless the patient is asked to undertake complex tasks. They often also have disinhibition and so in social situations have great difficulties of which they are often not aware.

Exercise tests These tests provide valuable information concerning the cardio respiratory systems abilities to meet increased demands for gas exchange and oxygen transport during raised activity levels, the ability of the musculoskeletal system to generate effort and muscular activity and the ability to endure additional requirements over time. The tests may take a number of formats including treadmill and cycle ergometry tests, field walk tests, such as the 6- and 12-min walk tests, shuttle walk test and shuttle runs, etc.

The tests are aimed at detecting limitations to activity, identify levels of activity producing signs and symptoms, provide baseline values to enable reassessment and progression or decline in response to an intervention and form the basis for an individualized exercise prescription.

Expiratory reserve volume See *Lung volumes*

Extension Straightening of a joint – the opposite to flexion.

Extensor lag If a joint will extend passively but not actively, the resulting droop of the joint is known as an extensor lag.

Extensor response This is initiated by contact of the back of the head with a supporting surface with the result that the body and limbs extend. Normally seen in severe head injury or multiple sclerosis, this posturing is seen more markedly in supine lying.

Extensor thrust A compensatory response where the patient thrusts backwards into extension in an attempt to gain activity against gravity.

External fixation Method of fracture fixation whereby pins or wires are driven into the fragments and held by a piece of apparatus on the outside of the body.

Advantages of external fixation	Disadvantages of external fixation
Minimal disruption to the fracture site	Infection risk at pin sites
Enables inspection of the wound and fracture	Needs meticulous wound care
	Cosmetically ugly
Can be adjusted with minimal trauma	Functional impairment, e.g. adjacent joints may be restricted or soft tissues pierced by fixator
Can be used for limb-lengthening procedures	
Can be used to pin multiple fragments, e.g. comminuted fractures	Anaesthetic risk and its associated complications
It allows preservation of tissues in open or compound fractures, degloving injuries or burns	Patient will need several days in hospital
	Stresses taken by implant-decreased stimulus for callus formation
	Heavy

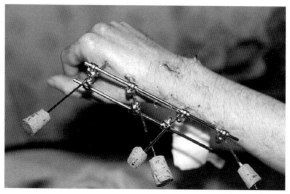

External fixator for comminuted fracture of the distal radius

Exteroceptive Receptors stimulated from the external environment.

Extra-articular Anatomical term referring to something that is external to a joint. For example, an extra articular feature of rheumatoid arthritis may be anaemia.

Extracorporeal membranous oxygenation (ECMO) This is a method of oxygenating the blood using an artificial lung (outside the body), thus enabling the actual lung to rest.

Extra-dural haematoma This is a bleed between the dura (the outer membrane of the meninges) and the skull following head injury. As there is nowhere for the blood to be absorbed it is very serious and rapidly leads to compression of the brain and death unless emergency neurosurgery is undertaken to stop the bleeding and remove the clot. Patients who receive neurosurgery in the early stages can make a full recovery and so it is essential that correct and frequent observations be undertaken on all head-injured patients to detect any deterioration.

Extrafusal fibres Skeletal muscle fibres innervated by a-motoneurones outside muscle spindle.

Extrafusal muscle Striated muscle fibre found outside the muscle spindle.

Extraneous variable – also known as confounding variable This is a factor other than the independent variable that may influence the outcome of a study. For example, if one is looking at knee joint goniometry, the temperature in the study room, previous level of patient exercise and degree of friction of the heel on the plinth may all be extraneous variables, an experimental design aims to minimize these by, for example, always using the same plinth, standardizing the pre-measurement exercise and the temperature in the room.

Extra-pyramidal This is a term used to describe the paired subcortical masses or nuclei of grey matter.

Extubation Removal of a tube from an organ, structure or orifice; specifically, removal of the tube after intubation.

F

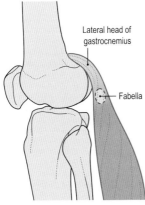

Lateral head of gastrocnemius

Fabella

Fabella on lateral knee X-ray

Fabella A sesamoid bone that sits within the lateral head of gastrocnemius, not always present.

➲ Student tip It may resemble a loose body on a lateral knee X-ray.

Faber test – also known as figure 4 or four test FABER stands for **F**lexion, **AB**duction, and **E**xternal **R**otation of the hip:

1. The patient lies supine.
2. The foot of the affected side is placed across the opposite knee.
3. The physiotherapist presses down on the flexed knee and the opposite anterior superior iliac crest.

A positive result is pain in the sacro-iliac area, which indicates a problem with the sacroiliac joint/ligaments.

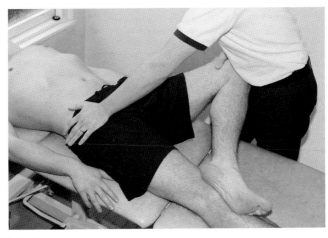

Faber test

Facet joint See *Zygapophyseal joint*

Facial Nerve The 7th cranial nerve, compression or lesion results in Bells palsy.

Facilitation Hastening or assistance of a natural process or the increased excitability of a neurone after stimulation. Facilitatory techniques can be used to either excite or inhibit activity. For example, a slow, smooth stretch to a muscle will tend to be inhibitory whereas a rapid sudden stretch would be excitatory. Techniques that can be considered as facilitatory are:

- brushing
- ice
- tapping
- passive stretching
- joint compression (approximation)
- vibration
- vestibular stimulation.

Facilitatory handling is where the therapist uses their hands in a graded manner to assist movement and changes in posture (Stokes 1998).

Faecal occult blood test (FOB) A laboratory test undertaken on stool samples to detect the presence of occult blood.

Fallopian tube The fallopian tubes normally transport the egg from the ovary, to the uterus.

Fallots tetralogy – also known as tetralogy of fallot This condition, which is a classic example of cyanotic form of congenital heart disease, gets its name from the French physician who first described it. It is a relatively uncommon malformation consisting of a ventricular septal defect, pulmonary valve stenosis, right ventricular hypertrophy and a shift of the aorta from the left to the right side so that it receives blood from both sides of the heart. A child born with this congenital disease can survive beyond infancy, but few survive to adulthood without surgery (Porter 2003).

False-positive reaction Research term – a mistakenly positive response. Positive test results found in subjects who do not possess the attribute for which the test is conducted.

FAM Functional Assessment Measure, an outcome measure mainly used by teams working in rehabilitation. This was a further development from the FIM (Functional Independence Measure), and includes cognitive and speech items, and so is particularly useful for neurological patients. Each item has seven levels. With training and using the decision-tree manuals it has good reliability and so is used widely both clinically and for research studies.

Familial hypercholesterolaemia Excess of cholesterol in plasma.

Faradic current Electrotherapy term – name used by some electromedical manufacturers to indicate a current designed for motor stimulation. Typically means a pulsed current with biphasic pulses, with a duration of less than 1 ms and a frequency between 30 Hz and 70 Hz. Variations include the use of monophasic pulses. 'Faradic' is not a helpful term as it was coined on equipment producing parameters no longer in use and, does not have a universally agreed definition.

F(A)ROM   Common medical abbreviation – Full (active) range of motion.

Fascia   The flat layers of fibrous tissue that separate different layers of tissue.

Fasciculation   A localized contraction of muscles, that can be observed through the skin as a flickering or twitching, they represent a spontaneous discharge of a number of fibres innervated by a single motor nerve filament. It is common in motor neurone disease.

Fasciotomy   Surgical division of fascia. Often performed to relieve pressure following compartment syndrome.
See *Compartment syndrome*

Fast motor unit   A motor unit containing an alpha motor neurone, which innervates quickly contracting and fatiguing muscle fibres.

Fast-twitch muscle fibre   Skeletal muscle fibre type that contracts rapidly and fatigues quickly. Has a high level of glycogen and relies on anaerobic metabolism for energy supply. Compare with slow-twitch muscle fibre.
See *Muscle fibre types*

Fat embolism   The release of fat from the bone marrow into the circulation. Can follow long bone fractures or crush injuries, diagnosed by increasing confusion, decreased oxygen saturation in the blood and occasionally petechial haemorrhages on the arms and chest, this can be fatal.

Fatigue   This is used to describe:
- the inability of a muscle to perform a strong contraction due to weakness bought on by repeated work
- a general affective disturbance resulting in tiredness and lethargy.
General fatigue is difficult to quantify and assess. It is common in many chronic diseases, multiple sclerosis for example, in which advice on energy conservation may be needed.

FEF   Common medical abbreviation – Forced expiratory flow
It is measured spirometrically. This is used as a diagnostic tool in airflow obstruction, at different stages of the expired breath, e.g. through 25–75% (written as FEF_{25-75}).

Felty's syndrome   Felty's syndrome is a complication of rheumatoid arthritis where there is enlargement of the spleen and leukopenia.

Feminism   A social movement concerned with exposing and challenging the disadvantage women experience because of their gender. It is a set of ideas based on the assertion that women are structurally subordinated to men within society. As a perspective feminism has a number of forms within the social sciences.

Femoral nerve

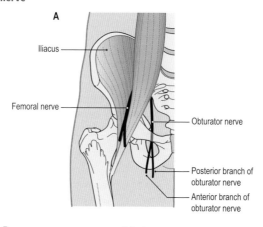

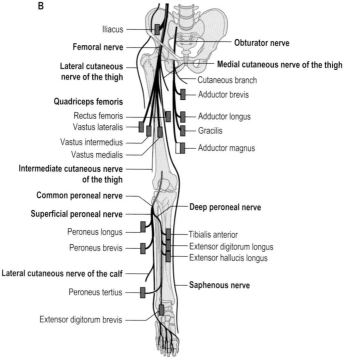

Femoral and obturator nerves

Femoral nerve stretch See *Neurodynamics*

The patient lies prone. The physiotherapist flexes the person's knee and then extends the hip.

Abnormal finding   Pain in the back or distribution of the femoral nerve indicates femoral nerve irritation. Comparison is made with the other side.

Femur   The thigh bone, the longest bone in the body:

- bent to aid shock absorption
- vascular (fractures may haemorrhage a great deal)
- consists of cancellous (each end) and tubular (central region) bone.

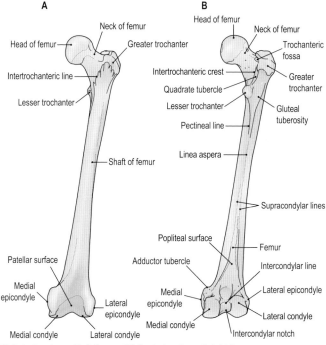

(**A**) Anterior view of left femur. (**B**) Posterior view of right femur

FER   Common medical abbreviation – Forced expiratory ratio.

This is a spirometric term used to detail the ratio of the FEV_1 to FVC. This ratio is diagnostic of restrictive, obstructive and combined lung diseases. Where the ratio is <70%, airflow obstruction is diagnosed.

See *Spirometry*

Festinating gait A gait characterized by small shuffling steps, the centre of gravity stays very central with prolonged double stance. Typically exhibited by a person with Parkinson's disease. Patients may lean too far forward and appear to be chasing their own centre of gravity.

FET Common medical abbreviation – Forced Expiration Technique or huff.

The forced expiration technique is used to facilitate the expectoration of pulmonary secretions and is an augmentation of normal bronchial tree movement during expiration (Pryor 1991). The intrathoracic pressures produced during the FET are less than those produced with a cough and, therefore, less exhausting.

The FET or huff is based on West's equal pressure point principle (1982). The EPP is the point at which the airway and pleural pressures are equal. Hence, during a forced expiration, collapse and compression of the airways occurs toward the mouth, thus moving secretions in a peripheral direction as lung volume decreases. Hence, FET from low lung volumes will shift secretions from the more peripheral airways; while a huff at a high lung volume will clear secretions from the upper airways.

This technique is integral to the active cycle of breathing techniques as first described by Webber (1988).

FEV Common medical abbreviation – Forced Expiratory Volume.

See *Spirometry*

FH Common medical abbreviation – Family history.

Fibrillation Two meanings in medicine:

1. Irregular uncoordinated contractions of heart muscle.
2. The term for minute cracks that are seen in the early stages of osteoarthritis.

Fibrillation, atrial An abnormal irregular heart rhythm whereby electrical signals are generated chaotically throughout the upper chambers (atria) of the heart. Many persons with atrial fibrillation have no symptoms, the most common symptom is palpitations, an uncomfortable awareness of the rapid and irregular heartbeat.

Fibroblast A cell that resides within connective tissue that secretes procollagen, fibronectin and collagenase.

Fibromyalgia A disorder characterized by muscle pain, stiffness and fatigue.

The aetiology and pathogenesis of fibromyalgia still remain uncertain. The myopathological patterns in fibromyalgia are non-specific: type-II-fibre-atrophy, a slight increase in lipid droplets and proliferation of mitochondria (Pongratz & Spath 2001).

Fibrosing alveolitis An inflammatory condition starting with diffuse alveolar damage and resulting in fibrosis commonly seen in collagen-vascular diseases.

Fibrositis A benign, intermittently recurring and protracted disease process, with a lack of underlying pathology. The condition is often associated with muscular pain and stiffness.

Field Electrotherapy term – the force surrounding a charged particle or object. The size, distribution and magnitude of a field are represented by field lines around an object or, between objects (e.g. capacitor plates used for SWD). The magnetic field is the force surrounding a wire carrying an electric current. It depends on the magnitude of the current and the distance between adjacent loops of wire carrying current.

See *Electric field*

Field notes/Fieldwork diary Research term – the records or reflections kept by the researcher that act to enrich the data obtained or put them into some sort of context, commonly used in qualitative research.

Finger-nose test A test of voluntary eye-motor coordination of the upper limbs. The patient is asked to slowly touch the tip of his nose with an extended index finger; it may be used to assess cerebellar function.

FIM Common medical abbreviation – Functional Independence Measure.

An outcome measure extensively used in the MDT treatment of neurological patients. There is a paediatric version called the WeeFIM. More items have been developed leading to the FAM assessment, which is often preferred by teams treating neurological patients, as it has cognitive and speech items.

Fine-needle aspiration Procedure to remove cells or fluid from tissues using a needle with a syringe.

Finkelstein's test The test for de Quervain's syndrome, whereby the patient clenches his or her fingers over the thumb and performs ulnar deviation. Pain in the region means a positive result.

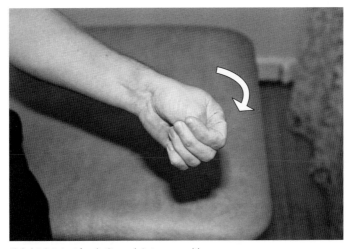

Finkelstein's test for de Quervain's tenosynovitis

Fistula An abnormal connection between tissues.

Flaccidity A term used to describe muscle tone below the normal tone, i.e. more floppy and the absence of movement. Hence there is a lack of resistance to passive movement.

Flags This refers to information obtained during patient assessment that highlights findings that need monitoring and/or referral to a consultant (red flags) and determines a method of specific physiotherapy management (yellow flags).

Red flags

These are findings from both subjective and objective examination that could indicate serious pathology such as fracture, tumour or infection and possible cauda equina syndromes.

Subjective findings
These would include:

- Mode of onset – major trauma, road-traffic accident (RTA), sudden onset of severe symptoms, such as acute unremitting pain or bilateral weakness of the lower limbs.
- History suggestive of tumour or infection, anyone aged over 50 years or under 20 years, history of carcinoma, unexplained weight loss, recent fever, frequent urinary tract infections, history of drug abuse or HIV.
- Possible cauda equina syndrome – bladder disturbance, such as urinary retention, increased frequency or overflow incontinence and bowel dysfunction such as unexpected laxity of the anal sphincter, saddle anaesthesia (numbness in the saddle region), bilateral parasthesia and/or weakness of the lower limb.

Objective findings
- Limping or coordination problems.
- Neurological signs such as diminished or brisk reflexes, positive Babinski and clonus.

Yellow flags

These include:

- Psychological factors such as – maladapted attitudes and beliefs about pain, behaviours including reduced activities, poor compliance with physical exercise, extended rest periods, lack of satisfaction from previous interventions and avoidance of normal activity.
- Social factors – prolonged absence from work, withdrawal from hobbies/social activities and overly dependent on family.

Flail Unstable chest wall after fractures of the ribs or sternum.

Flail chest This occurs through thoracic trauma involving multiple rib fractures resulting in a destabilized segment of thoracic cage with paradoxical movement during breathing, i.e. the segment moves in during inspiration and outwards on expiration. Pulmonary contusion, haemothorax and pneumothorax frequently accompany this type of injury.

Flat-back posture Posture typified by cervical spine extension, upper thoracic spine flexion, an absent lumbar lordosis, posterior pelvic tilt, hip extension and slight ankle plantarflexion.

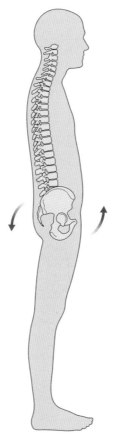

Flat back posture. Elongated and weak: hip flexors, paraspinal muscles. Short and strong hamstrings. Reproduced from Kendall FP et al. 1993 Muscles testing and function, 4th edn. Williams and Wilkins

Flexion reflex – also known as a withdrawal reflex When a noxious stimulus is applied to an arm or leg, there is an automatic withdrawal of the limb as a protective mechanism, flexors contract whilst extensors simultaneously relax, there may be simultaneous extension in the opposite limb – known as a crossed extensor reflex (Davies et al. 2001).

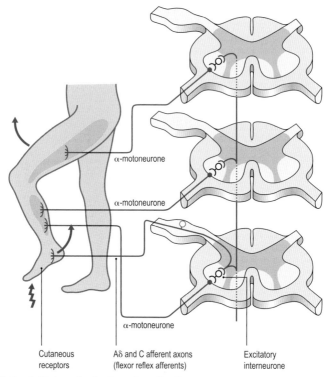

α-motoneurone

α-motoneurone

α-motoneurone

Cutaneous
receptors

Aδ and C afferent axons
(flexor reflex afferents)

Excitatory
interneurone

Flexion (withdrawal) reflex to noxious stimuli

Flexor spasm A spasm (involuntarily contraction of the muscles) in the flexor muscle group, commonly seen in the lower limb with the result that the leg jumps up flexing at the hip and knee and dorsiflexing at the foot. Following the spasm the leg drops back down. Spasms can be painful and can lead to poor positioning and abnormal postures.

Floxacillin/flucloxacillin A common antibiotic.

Fluid displacement test Is performed by squeezing excess fluid out of the suprapatellar pouch, then stroking the medial side of the knee joint to displace any excess fluid to the lateral side of the joint. Repeat this procedure by stroking the lateral side of the joint. A positive finding is any excess fluid will be seen to move across the joint and distend the medial side.

FMRI (Functional magnetic resonance imaging) A scanning technique, which can illustrate brain activity during functioning.

Focus group Research term – the term for a group of people who have been gathered together in order to gain some insight into their ideas and attitudes towards a particular subject. A useful technique used in conjunction with other research methods to achieve triangulation. The topic can then be pursued using research that is more quantitative in nature, they can help to clarify quantitative results or generate hypotheses for future research.

Foot angle – also known as angle of gait Biomechanical term – the angle of foot orientation away from the line of progression during walking.

Foot-drop Paralysis or weakness of the ankle dorsiflexors, it may indicate several pathologies including: common peroneal nerve damage from a fracture or a plaster cast that is too tight around the neck of the fibula, a disc prolapse in the lumbar spine or other neurological conditions. The tibialis anterior primarily has the role of decelerating the foot following heel strike, so a person with a foot drop may slap the foot on the floor during walking or may adopt a high stepping gait in an attempt to ensure that the foot still clears the ground on swing through phase of gait.

Foot drop splint A splint that is usually made to fit into a standard shoe. Can be trimmed or moulded with heat. They are used in cases of drop foot or gross instability at the ankle.

See *Drop foot*

Foramen Anatomical term meaning an opening or passage especially through a bone.

Foramen magnum The large hole at the base of the skull where the spinal cord meets the brain.

Force couple Where two or more muscles combine to work together to produce a single movement, a good example is scapular rotation:

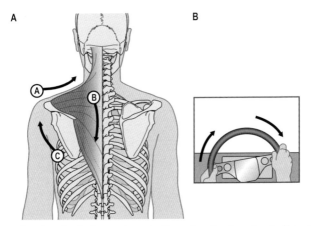

(**A**) A = direction of pull of upper trapezius fibres; B = direction of pull of lower trapezius fibres; C = direction of pull of serratus anterior. (**B**) Combined force couple result is scapular rotation, rather like steering a car by using two opposite movements on either side of the wheel

Forced-use – also known as constraint induced　This is a term used to describe treatment techniques where the patient is forced to use one limb due to restraint of the other limb, also called constraint-induced therapy. Used in neurological patients, for example, one arm may be tied up forcing the patient to use the affected hand. Is thought to be useful in breaking habitual disuse of a limb where the patient has regained motor control, but continues not to use the affected limb.

Fossa　Anatomical term meaning a trench or channel, a hollow or depressed area.

Fracture　A break in the continuity of a bone, same as a break in medicine. See *Open fracture* and *Close fracture*

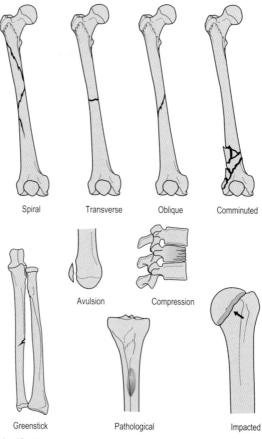

Spiral	Transverse	Oblique	Comminuted

Avulsion	Compression

Greenstick	Pathological	Impacted

Fracture classification

Fractures – complications
- Pulmonary embolism
- Deep vein thrombosis

  Shock – caused by hypovolaemia or loss of blood. Femoral shaft fractures may bleed as much as 3 pints and pelvic fractures may lose 6 pints. Clinical signs of this are tachycardia (rapid heart rate), pallor reduced peripheral perfusion, hypoxia (decreased oxygen saturation) confusion and a state of semi consciousness.

- Infection/tetanus – especially following open or compound fractures. Osteomyelitis (bone infection) can be stubborn to respond to treatment.

- Fat embolism (ARDS – acute respiratory distress syndrome) – If a person sustains multiple fractures of large bones, crushing injuries, or if large amounts of marrow become exposed, there may be leakage of microscopic fat globules into the circulatory system. These may become trapped in the lungs. Symptoms include respiratory distress, shortness of breath, drowsiness, decrease in saturation of oxygen levels and petechiae (tiny haemorrhages that appear on the chest). ARDS can be potentially fatal.

- Plaster sores – Reassure the patient that large amounts of dry flaky skin following removal of plaster is normal. Reddened areas or sores caused by plaster of splints must be reported to the relevant team member.

- Muscle damage and atrophy – Muscle fibres may be torn, crushed or ruptured as a result of the injury and this will cause additional bleeding and swelling. Tendons may be severed, particularly in the case of open fractures or sometimes there may be a rupture following a fracture. Surgical intervention is usually necessary to repair a rupture.

- Compartment syndrome – If muscles become damaged or inflamed at the time of injury and intra muscular pressure builds up with no means of release, death (necrosis) of the tissues from ischaemia (lack of blood supply) may result. It is defined as the condition in which high pressure within a closed fascial sheath reduces capillary blood perfusion below the level necessary for tissue viability. Grill a sausage without pricking it first and the pressure inside rises to the point where problems occur. This analogy is useful when explaining compartment syndrome to patients. Compartment syndrome is seen most commonly in the anterior tibial muscles or forearm muscles. Treatment revolves primarily around accurate diagnosis, check colour, sensation and movement after any injury or surgery, elevate and cool the limb. Surgical decompression (fasciotomy) may be necessary as an emergency procedure. Clinical signs of a limb with compartment syndrome are the five **P**s:

  Pale

  Painful

  Pulseless

Paresthesiae

Paralyzed.

- Avascular necrosis – Bone receives its blood supply by the soft-tissue structures attached to it or by intra-osseous vessels. In certain instances one part of the bone is very dependent on the intra-osseous (within the bone) vessels for its blood supply and if this is interrupted because of a fracture, avascular necrosis may occur (part of the fractured bone may die). It can occur in fractures of the neck of the femur leading to avascular necrosis of the head and in fractures of the scaphoid bone where the proximal pole may be affected. This may be a cause of non-union of the fracture and, as the fragment usually includes an articular surface, it can lead to osteoarthritis.

- Delayed union – May occur if the gap between the bone ends is too big, blood supply is poor (lower one-third tibia), the area is infected, or if internal fixation is used (this sometimes removes the stimulus for callus formation).

- Non-union – In this case there are distinct pathological changes and radiological evidence of non-union. There appears to be no callus formation and the fractured ends of bone become dense and the outline clearcut. The gap between the bone fragments may be filled with fibrous tissue and form a pseudo arthrosis. The lower one-third of the tibia has notoriously poor healing capabilities, even occasionally in the young and healthy.

- Malunion – A fracture may heal in a less than perfect position. Overlapping of the fragments could lead to shortening and this would affect function. Angulation or rotation of the fragments may impair function because of the resulting altered biomechanics.

- Growth disturbance – If the fracture includes the epiphysis (growth plate).

- Sudecks atrophy/reflex sympathetic dystrophy (RSD)/algodystrophy/causalgia – The term complex regional pain syndrome is now being used to describe these pathological states. This is a complication where the patient complains of severe pain on movement or at rest out of proportion to the initial injury and the limb is swollen. The skin appears shiny, discoloured and the skin feels cold, in extreme cases this may lead to the limb becoming exquisitely tender and discoloured. Osteoporosis and permanent contractures may follow. Management is difficult. Vasodilator drugs such as guanethedine are occasionally successful. It may also respond to nerve blocks, local analgesia, TENS and other local therapies, but recovery is slow and may take several months. Fortunately this complication is comparatively rare.

- Intra-articular fractures – Fractures involving the articular cartilage predispose the joint to osteoarthrosis in the future, e.g. fractures of the tibial plateau. This is due to the area of roughness that inevitably results after a fracture and also because the immobilization of the fracture results in cartilage death (see below). For the latter reason one will now find that some fractures are treated aggressively by physiotherapists from an early stage.

Another problem with intra-articular fractures is that if callus is attempting to form within a joint cavity, it is constantly being washed away by synovial fluid, for example after a fractured neck of femur.

- Visceral injuries – For example, a fractured pelvis may also damage the bladder or urethra. A fractured rib may cause a pneumothorax. A skull fracture may cause brain injury.
- Adhesions – These may be within the joint (intra-articular) or around the joint (periarticular).
- Injury to large vessels – If a large artery is occluded in such a position as to cut off the blood supply to the limb, this may lead to gangrene or if there is a partial occlusion an ischaemic contracture may develop. These injuries must be dealt with as an emergency by the surgical team. Thrombosis of veins may occur in the neighbourhood of the fracture. This presents as a sudden development of a cramp-like pain in the part, by an increase of swelling and by marked tenderness along the line of the vein. Anything that appears to be abnormal in the circulatory system must be reported to the surgeon immediately. Blood vessels may sustain damage, e.g. following supracondylar humeral fractures the brachial artery may be damaged.
- Nerve injury – Certain fractures, e.g. mid shaft humerus, may lead to radial nerve palsy. If a plaster is too tight it may cause nerve damage, the common peroneal nerve is vulnerable to this if a plaster cast is moulded too tightly around the fibular head, resulting in foot drop as the tibialis anterior muscle is affected and unable to perform its function of decellerating the foot upon heel strike and permitting toe clearance during the swing through phase of gait.

Frank–Starling relationship This states that the greater degree of tension in myocardial fibres at the end of diastole, the more forceful the subsequent myocardial contraction.

FRC Common medical abbreviation – Functional Residual Capacity
See *Spirometry*

Fredrich's ataxia An inherited form of ataxia.

Freiberg's disease Osteochondritis dissecans, with avascular necrosis of the bone, usually involving the head of the second metatarsal.

Freshers week The period of time allocated to new students in a university to register, orientate and socialize.

Fresnel zone/Franhofer zone Therapeutic ultrasound has a near field (Fresnel zone) and a far field (Franhofer zone).

In the near field the intensity of the beam is irregular, but towards the far field, these irregularities are less pronounced. Most of the therapeutic benefits of ultrasound are thought to occur in the near field (Lowe et al. 1990).

Frequency Electrotherapy term – the rate per second, recorded as hertz (Hz). A parameter relevant to a number of electrophysical agents. For example, the frequency of ultrasound used therapeutically is usually between 0.8 and 3 MHz and 1.5 MHz for fracture healing. For a twitch response to electrical stimulation (e.g. for strength duration testing), a frequency of 1 Hz is ideal. For a tetanic contraction (a fused response of individual motor units) a frequency of 30–50 Hz is required, depending on the muscle. Torque increases as the frequency of pulsed current is increased, peaks soon after 50 Hz and does not increase much after about 70 Hz. A carrier frequency is a frequency of alternating current pulses.

See *Russian current*

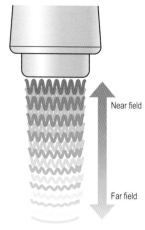

Fresnel zone/Franhofer zone

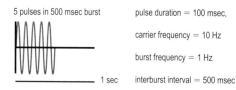

Frequency

Frequency, urinary Urinating too often, at too frequent intervals.

Froments sign A test for ulnar nerve paralysis.

The person grips a piece of paper between the thumb and index finger, the paper is pulled out and if the test is positive the IP joint of the thumb flexes.

Frontal lobe The lobe most anterior in the cerebrum.

Frozen shoulder Alternate name for capsulitis of the shoulder.

Fugel–Meyer Known as the FM. An assessment of the Sensorimotor recovery after stroke. Frequently used measure of motor recovery, balance, sensation, joint motion and pain. Does not test fine or complex movement.

Functio laesa Loss of function; a fifth sign of inflammation added by Galen to those proposed by Celsus, i.e. (rubor, tumour, calor and dolor).

Functional bracing (cast bracing) Functional braces have hinges to allow movement. The soft tissues of the limb squeeze against the inside of the brace and in conjunction with the use of a heel cup, permit weight to be taken through the substance of the brace. This has reduced many of the problems that were seen as a direct result of prolonged immobilization. Another benefit of allowing movement of joints, provided that it does not unduly stress the fracture site, is that it may promote union by improving the area's blood supply.

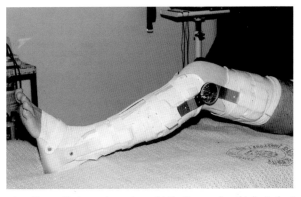

A functional brace. Photograph courtesy of Mike Somervell and Julie Butler Senior Occupational Therapists

Functional electrical stimulation (FES) FES is a specific type of NMES in which to aim is to enhance function rather than just muscle contraction. It has been argued that FES should be considered as a subgroup within NMES. Simple forms of FES include electrical stimulation of the ankle dorsiflexors following stroke or other central-nervous-system (CNS) lesions. The stimulation is activated by some form of foot-switch device located in the shoe. This enables the timely stimulation of the dorsiflexors, raising the toes and preventing a trailing foot during the swing phase and promoting a better heel strike (drop-foot stimulators). More complex forms of FES include the standing and walking systems used for patients with more severe neurological deficits, e.g. paraplegic patients. These systems are usually multi-channel stimulators, computer controlled and, in the more advanced systems, using implanted electrodes. By stimulating numerous muscle groups in a carefully timed sequence, a pattern of stimulation can be achieved that mimics a functional activity, e.g. sit-to-stand or basic-gait patterns. Recent advances in the computer control systems required to manage complex stimulation patterns together with significant advances in implanted electrode technology has moved these complex applications forward and they are becoming more widely used in specialist centres.

Functional reach (FR) test A measure used to assess dynamic postural control used clinically as a performance test to assess the postural responses to the patient reaching forwards. It is essential that the procedure be properly standardized for the data to be reliable. Mainly used in assessing neurological patients and patients with balance problems.

Forced vital capacity (FVC) Lung capacity measured with the subject exhaling as rapidly as possible.

G

Gag reflex Also known as the pharyngeal reflex, an involuntary contraction of the pharynx and elevation of the soft palate to protect the airway. This may be impaired in neurological conditions and is associated with dysphagia.

Gait The pattern of locomotion.

Typically divided into the following stages:

- Loading response: the initial double support stance.
- Mid stance: from the time the opposite limb leaves the floor until body weight is aligned over the forefoot.
- Terminal stance: the time from heel rise until the other limb makes contact with the floor. During this phase body weight moves ahead of the forefoot.
- Pre-swing: from the time of initial contact with the contralateral limb to ipsilateral toe-off.
- Initial swing: from toe-off to when the swing limb foot is opposite the stance limb.
- Mid swing: from the time the swing foot is opposite the stance limb to when the tibia is vertical.
- Terminal swing: from the time when the tibia is vertical to initial contact.
- Push off: when there is an ankle plantar flexor moment.

Galeazzi fracture Fracture of the radius and subluxation of the lower end of ulna.

Galvanic current Electrotherapy term – this is an old name for direct current, still often used by some electromedical manufacturers. Also have interrupted galvanic – unidirectional pulses that may be rectangular, trapezoidal, triangular, etc., in shape, with durations ranging from approximately 10 µs to 600 ms, a frequency of 1–1.5 Hz and used for strength-duration testing.

Ganglion

1. A group of nerve cell bodies located outside the nervous system.
2. Benign tumour of synovium arising from the joint or tendon sheath, commonly found around the wrist.

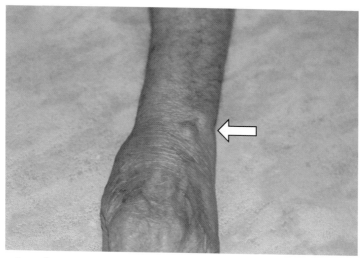

A ganglion

Gantt chart A project-planning tool. The anticipated timing of specific tasks within a project are identified. Project stages comprise the vertical column, dates run from left to right and each task is represented by a horizontal bar, the left end of which signifies the expected beginning of the task and the right end the planned completion date.

Gap junction These provide means of electrical and chemical communication between cells of the body.

Garden classification A method used to classify severity and subsequent management of fracture of the femoral neck.
Garden classification of femoral neck fractures:

- Type 1 Inferior cortex is not completely broken

- Type 2 Cortex is broken but there is no angulation

- Type 3 Some displacement and rotation of femoral head

- Type 4 Complete displacement.

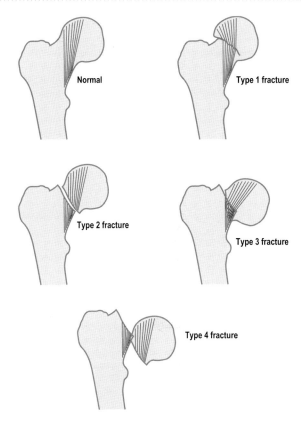

Garden classification. Any displacement should be assessed along the lines laid down by Garden which, amongst other things, take into account the disturbance of the weight carrying trabeculae radiating from the calcar femorale.

Type 1 fracture: The inferior cortex is not completely broken, but the trabeculae are angulated (abduction fracture).

Type 2 fracture: The fracture line is complete and the inferior cortex is clearly broken. The trabecular lines are interrupted, but are not angulated. In both type 1 and 2 fractures, there is no obvious displacement of the major fragments relative to one another.

Type 3 fracture: Here the fracture line is obviously complete. There is rotation of the femoral head in the acetabulum, the proximal fragment being abducted and internally rotated. This may be apparent from the disturbance in the trabecular pattern. The fracture is slightly displaced.

Type 4 fracture: In this, the severest grade, the fracture is fully displaced and the femoral head tends to lie in the neutral position in the acetabulum. Garden type 3 and 4 fractures of the femoral neck carry the worst prognosis.

Gas exchange This is the exchange of the metabolic gases oxygen and carbon dioxide during respiration.

Gastrectomy Surgical excision of the stomach.

Gastric Relating to the stomach.

Gastroenteritis Inflammation of the stomach and/or intestines.

Gastrointestinal (GI) Relating to the stomach and intestines.

Gate-keeping A process whereby resources are rationed by restricting access to equipment or services. For example, general practitioners are the gate-keepers of specialist medical services and physiotherapists may be the gate-keepers of wheelchairs and other equipment.

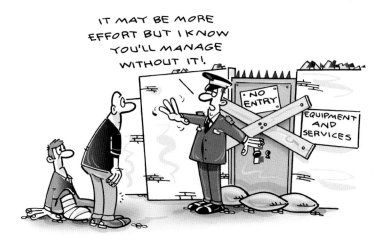

Gate theory See *Pain gate*

Gel Electrotherapy term – water-soluble substance used to complete a circuit or to couple an output to the skin.
  Electrical stimulation gel: is used between the electrodes, if flexible reusable carbon rubber type and the skin to complete the circuit.
  Ultrasound gel: enables ultrasound to pass from the applicator to the skin, not otherwise possible given the high acoustic impedance of air to MHz frequency ultrasound. Ultrasound gel is typically cheaper and with a higher resistance than electrical gel (usually labelled ECG gel or electrical stimulation gel) and should not be used as a replacement.

Gender A social identity. The perceived differences between the two sexes that generates social differentiation, inequality, discrimination and prejudice.

The term 'gender' is distinct from the term 'sex', which denotes biological differences between males and females.

Generalizability The extent to which the results of a study based on measurement in a particular patient population and/or a specific context hold true for another population and/or in a different context.

Genome The DNA map that comprises the complete genetic composition of the human.

Genu recurvatum See Genu figure.

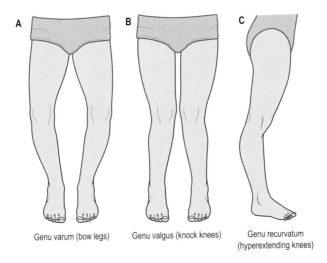

Genu varum (bow legs)   Genu valgus (knock knees)   Genu recurvatum
(hyperextending knees)

Genu valgum Seen at the knee. Commonly known as 'knock knees'. See Genu figure.

Genu varum Seen at the knee. Commonly known as 'bow legs'. See Genu figure.

Gerdy's tubercle Lateral tubercle at upper end of tibia, the site of partial insertion of iliotibial band. Common site of pathology due to friction of iliotibial band on bone.

GH Common medical abbreviation – Gleno-humeral (the shoulder).

Giant-cell arteritis An inflammatory condition of the temporal artery. It is a serious chronic vascular disease, characterized by inflammation (vasculitis) of the blood vessel walls.

Glasgow coma scale (GCS) The Glasgow Coma Scale is the most widely used scoring system used in quantifying the level of consciousness following traumatic brain injury.

Glasgow coma score

Eye opening (E)	Verbal response (V)	Motor response (M)
4 = Spontaneous 3 = To voice 2 = To pain 1 = None	5 = Normal conversation 4 = Disoriented conversation 3 = Words, but not coherent 2 = No words...only sounds 1 = None	6 = Normal 5 = Localizes to pain 4 = Withdraws to pain 3 = Decorticate posture 2 = Decerebrate 1 = None

Total = E + V + M

Glaucoma A condition where there is increased fluid pressure inside the eye that damages the optic nerve and causes partial vision loss and can progress to blindness.

Gliomas A fast-growing malignant tumour of the glial cells of the CNS. These are graded 1–4 according to malignancy with 4 being the most aggressive.

Globin The protein portion of haemoglobin.

Glossopharyngeal Pertaining to the tongue and pharynx.

Glottis This is the opening between the vocal cords, which is variable in size. In order for a cough to have its explosive nature and be effective in clearing debris from the respiratory tract, the glottis must be closed.

Glyceryl trinitrate (GTN) A drug that can help to dilate the coronary vessels temporarily, as well as reducing the resistive load on the heart. Often taken as a spray or under the tongue (sub lingual).

Goal setting See *SMART goals*

Goblet cell A mucus secreting cell within the airways. The cell has a protective mechanism since the mucus secreted acts to trap particles that have entered the respiratory tract, which are then transported via the mucociliary escalator to the mouth for clearance.

Goitre An enlargement of the thyroid gland.

Golgi tendon organ (GTO) A proprioceptive receptor located within tendons. It responds to excessive muscle tension by inhibiting further muscle contraction. In so doing it protects against muscle damage. They are made up from extrafusal muscle fibres that enter a funnel-like capsule that is filled with collagen fibre bundles. Nerve endings are triggered when tension in the muscle is transferred to the collagen fibres of the Golgi tendon organ. Golgi tendon organs are arranged in series with the extrafusal muscle fibres. The Golgi tendon organ is designed to monitor the load or tension on a muscle, independent of its length.

Goniometer Apparatus for measuring range of motion at a joint.

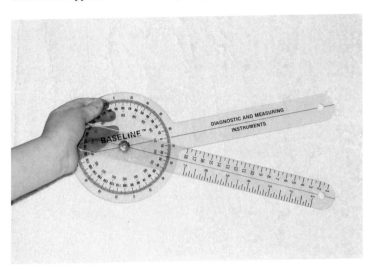

Goniometer. Thanks to J, Al, and CB

Gout A metabolic rheumatological disease associated with hyperuricaemia (increased uric acid in the blood) with symptoms occurring as a result of uric acid crystals being deposited within the tissues.

Grand mal This is a major seizure involving the whole body with generalized shaking and tachycardia, normally preceded by an aura. Trauma frequently occurs due to the violent movements; sufferers may bite their own tongue.

Grasp reflex When the palm of the hand is touched it induces a flexor response, it can be seen in infancy, patients with neurological damage and older patients with dementia.

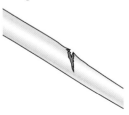

A greenstick fracture

Greenstick fracture A fracture sustained by children, the bone does not break across its diameter, rather it behaves as a green twig and partially snaps.
See *Fracture classification*

Grey literature Reports that are unpublished or have limited distribution and are not included in the common bibliographic retrieval systems.

Grief An intense and prolonged feeling of sadness when somebody who is highly valued is lost. The loss of objects, status, identity and lifestyle can also give rise to grief, for example, the loss of a job, a country or a home.

Grounded theory Research term – a research approach that generates theory from the data.

Ground reaction force The force that acts on a body as a result of the body resting on or hitting the ground.

Group therapy Group exercise is a widely used method of exercise delivery. Especially with more recent moves towards physiotherapists working in primary care as part of their educational or advisory role, as with any technique there are benefits and drawbacks.

Advantages of group exercise

- Competitive element can be useful in increasing a person's performance.
- A variety of exercises is possible.
- Group exercise can be fun if properly organized.
- Helps the individual to feel less isolated if they meet people with similar problems.
- Provide a good opportunity for the physiotherapist to educate and inform the group about their condition.
- Specialist groups, such as ankylosing spondylitis or cardiac rehabilitation groups, provide social support.

Disadvantages of group exercise

- No two human beings are identical, this means that it is difficult to pitch the exercises at a level that is suitable for all group members.
- There may be a temptation to put inappropriate individuals in the group to save time and relieve overburdened staff.
- It is difficult to monitor all of the people all of the time.
- It may be difficult to progress all the members of the group appropriately.
- The competitive element may be counterproductive or dangerous.
- Some people do not respond well in a group situation, they may be embarrassed, afraid to ask advice.

Group work Academic work that is produced by a group of students working together and sharing resources – it is often assessed.

Grunting An abnormal respiratory sound heard in expiration (more commonly in children). It is a sign of respiratory distress, which is thought to occur in order to generate a backpressure (positive expiratory pressure) by closure of the glottis, thus preventing alveolar collapse.

Guillain–Barre syndrome (GBS) This is also known as acute inflammatory demyelinating polyneuropathy.

An acute type of nerve inflammation that damages portions of the nerve cell, resulting in muscle weakness or paralysis and sensory loss. Initial weakness can progress rapidly to complete paralysis requiring ventilation. GBS is often preceded by a respiratory or gastric upset before the onset of symptoms. Today with the advances in medication it is possible to prevent deterioration in many patients. Complete recovery occurs in many patients, although some are left with residual weakness.

Gymnastic balls These are large air-filled balls that can be used in treatment to provide a mobile support, enabling smooth movements and stimulation of postural mechanisms. The balls need to be well inflated to withstand the weight of the person with minimum deformation.

Habituation To become used to a stimulus or to reduce awareness of it for duration of stimulation (e.g. to TENS output after first 10 min).

Haemangioblastoma This is a tumour of vascular origin.

Haemarthrosis Bleeding within a joint. Found commonly following anterior cruciate rupture or in cases of haemophilia – a disorder of the normal clotting mechanism of the blood.

Haematocrit A laboratory measurement that determines the percentage of packed red blood cells in a given volume of blood.

Haematoma Bleeding into tissues. A localized collection of blood, usually clotted, in an organ, space or tissue, due to a break in the wall of a blood vessel.

Haemodialysis The process of withdrawing blood, passing it through semipermeable tubing that is permeable to smaller molecules but not to larger proteins and cells.

Haemoglobin (Hb) This is a protein within the erythrocyte, consisting of: the 'globin' part (four linked polypeptide chains) in combination with the 'heme' complex (containing a ferrous iron ion). The polypeptide chains are coiled together and alterations in their shape, determine Hb's affinity for oxygen. Hence, when the first oxygen molecule binds to Hb, it becomes easier for the second to bind and so on. In its deoxygenated state, Hb becomes an important blood buffer of H+ and is, therefore, important in the transport of CO_2. When oxygen binding is complete, Hb is referred to as oxyhaemoglobin. In blood (which has an average Hb content of 15 g/dl), each gram of Hb carries ~1.34 ml of oxygen. Thus, the oxygen-carrying capacity of the blood is increased by almost 70-fold in the presence of Hb (in comparison to the amount of oxygen carried in its dissolved state directly in the blood itself). The saturation of Hb determines how much of its oxygen-carrying capacity is used. The saturation of Hb varies with changes in the PaO_2 and this is demonstrated by the oxyhaemoglobin dissociation curve.

Haemopoiesis The process whereby blood cells are produced.

Haemophilia A disorder of the blood's clotting mechanism.

Haemophilus influenzae A common cause of respiratory infection, particularly seen in patients with underlying lung pathologies such as chronic obstructive pulmonary disease (COPD) and bronchiectasis.

Haemoptysis The presence of blood in sputum. It may signify several states including carcinoma, trauma from intubation following surgery, infections, cystic fibrosis and other conditions.

Haemorrhage The escape of blood from the vessels that normally contains it.

Haemorrhoids A dilatation of a vein of the superior or inferior haemorrhoidal plexus. Presents as a painful swelling formed by the dilation of the blood vessels around the margin of, or within, the anus. Haemorrhoids may occasionally bleed.

Haemothorax Blood within the pleura of the lungs.

Half penetration depth (half depth) See *Penetration depth*

Electrotherapy term – the depth at which 50% of energy applied to an object or body remains. The preferred term now is penetration depth. The half value penetration depth of a 1 MHz beam is 4 cm whereas for a 3 MHz beam it is 2.5 cm. Physiotherapists use this knowledge by selecting the appropriate frequency to penetrate to the desired depth. Let us say that we treat the skin with 1 watt/cm.

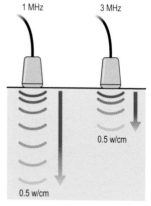

Half penetration depths of a 1 MHz and 3 MHz ultrasound beam.

Look how the 1 MHz beam penetrates almost twice as far as the 3 MHz beam before it has lost half of its intensity.

Hallpike manoeuvre This is a diagnostic test for **BPPV**, if positive nystagmus in the eyes is seen and vertigo is provoked. The head and neck is rotated to 45° and then extended to 30°.

○ Clinical note Great care must be taken to exclude neck pathology before undertaking this specialist procedure.

Hallux rigidus Loss of movement of the metatarsophalangeal joint of the first toe, particularly extension.

Hallux valgus Deformity of the MTP joint of the first toe, whereby the toe deviates into the lateral position.

Haloperidol An antipsychotic drug used to calm patients.

Halotraction Application of skeletal traction to the head by means of a halo device.

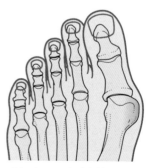

A bunion on the left big toe.

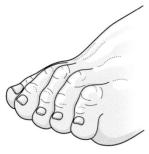

Hammer toe

Hammer toe Deformity of the toe whereby the PIP flexes and DIP extends. The MTP is usually extended or remains in the neutral position.

Handicap This is a term used to describe the individual's inability to be involved in normal life situations within society and used to be a category within the World Health Organizations model for describing Health: Impairment, Disability, Handicap. The WHO redefined these definitions in 1997, with a result that the term 'participation' is now used replacing the term handicap.

Previous terminology	Current terminology
Impairment	Function
Disability	Activity
Handicap	Participation

Handling This is a common therapeutic term used to describe assisted movement and physical contact with the patient.

Hangman's fracture A type of cervical spine fracture. Bilateral fracture of pedicles of the axis (C2).

Harms Adverse effects of an intervention.

Harvard referencing A style of referencing used in an academic piece of work where strict protocols operate. The authors name takes precedence in the text, followed by the year of publication, and references are listed alphabetically in the reference list at the end of the work. It is the system used in the professional journal Physiotherapy and is commonly the one used on physiotherapy courses.

Haversian canals The small canal's that run longitudinally through the centres of haversian systems of compact bone.

Hawthorne effect Research term – refers to the phenomenon whereby subjects alter their behaviour when they know that they are being observed.

HDL Common medical abbreviation – High-density lipoprotein.
See *Low-density lipoprotein*

Healing by second intention Delayed closure of two granulating surfaces.

Healing by first intention Healing by fibrous adhesion, without suppuration or granulation tissue formation.

Health Definitions differ between individuals, cultural groups and social classes. One view is that health is the absence of disease or illness. Within the medical model health can be defined by reference to certain physical and biochemical parameters. From broader perspectives, health includes the physical, psychological, behavioural, social and spiritual aspects of a state of well-being and recognizes the importance to individuals of realizing aspirations and needs.

Health assessment questionnaire (HAQ) A useful measure of outcome in chronic arthritis (Fries et al. 1980).

Health belief model The central feature of this model is that people tend not to adopt health behaviours unless they believe they are susceptible to the disease or disorder in question, that it is serious, that the recommendations will be effective and that the advantages of following the advice will not outweigh the disadvantages. The individual may also require a trigger (for example the diagnosis of a friend with the disease) before any change of behaviour occurs.

Healthcare commission (commission for healthcare audit and inspection) Established to promote improvement in the quality of NHS, private and voluntary healthcare across England and Wales. Formed by the Health and Social Care (Community Health and Standards) Act 2003 and launched on April 1st 2004.

Healthcare outcome The results of healthcare processes.

Health education Measures that are designed to improve health through education, such as giving advice on diet and exercise. Health education is a facet of health promotion.

Health Professions Council The Health Professions Council (HPC) is an independent, UK-wide regulatory body responsible for setting and maintaining standards of professional training, performance and conduct of the 12 healthcare professions that it regulates. Registration with the HPC means that agreed professional standards of training and proficiency have been met and that if any registrants do not uphold these standards they may be subject to having their fitness to practise investigated and dealt with by HPC. The Council of the HPC is responsible for developing strategies and policies and consists of 24 members (made up of one representative from each of the professions regulated and 12 lay members) plus a president. In addition, the HPC runs committees, which help the Council with its work. For more information on the committees of the HPC, please see the committees section of the website. http://www.hpc-uk.org

The HPC regulates the following professions: Arts Therapists, Orthoptists, Biomedical Scientists, Prosthetists & Orthotists, Chiropodists/Podiatrists, Paramedics, Clinical Scientists, Physiotherapists, Dietitians, Radiographers, Occupational Therapists, Speech & Language Therapists.

With thanks to Niamh O'Sullivan. The Health Professions Council

Health promotion A broad range of activities that aim to improve health. These include health education such as teaching correct lifting techniques, environmental measures such as the control of pollution, preventative medicine such as cervical screening, fiscal measures such as financial benefits and legal measures such as seat belt legislation.

Health-related quality of life A combination of an individual's physical, mental and social well-being; not merely the absence of disease (NICE 2004).

Health technology Any method used by those working in health services to promote health, prevent and treat disease and improve rehabilitation and long-term care.

Heart attack See *Myocardial infarction (MI)*

Heart murmur The sound caused by turbulence as blood passes through a faulty heart valve.

Heart rate This is the number of heart beats per minute. The normal resting adult heart rate is 60–100 beats per minute (bpm) and should be monitored for rate, strength and rhythm.

Heart sounds Normal heart sounds correspond to the closure of the four valves of the heart.
- First heart sound = 'LUB' sound, closure of the mitral and tricuspid valves.
- Second heart sound = 'DUP' sound, closure of the aortic and pulmonary valves.
- Third heart sound = cardiac failure in adults (may be normal in children and corresponds to vibration of ventricular walls).
- Fourth heart sound = vibration of ventricular walls in late diastole, heard in heart failure, hypertension and aortic valve disease (Pryor & Prasad 2002).

Heat therapy See *Ice/cold therapy*
  The physical effects of adding heat to an object:
  1. Rise in temperature (the average kinetic energy of the molecules increases).
  2. Expansion of the material (molecules vibrate more and move further apart. Gases expand more than solids and liquids more than solids).
  3. Change in physical state.
  4. Acceleration of chemical reactions (van't hoffs law = any chemical reaction capable of being accelerated, is accelerated by a rise in temperature) this is of major importance to physiotherapists.
  5. Decrease in viscosity of fluids, e.g. synovial fluid.
  The distribution of heat depends on:
- the size of heated area
- the depth of absorption of specific radiation
- the duration of heating
- the intensity of heating and method by which it is applied.

Heat and cell metabolism
A lot of what we do as physiotherapists is aimed at speeding up or slowing down the metabolism within a cell or group of cells. Metabolic rate increases by 13% for every 1°C rise in temperature. This means that the cells require

more oxygen and nutrients and accordingly there is an increased production of metabolites or waste products. This is one of the reasons that one develops a fever when fighting an infection such as the common cold, the body is trying to kill the bugs more effectively. The same logic accounts for the fact that a boil or spot is red.

See *Inflammation*

Physiotherapists often use this principle. For example, a ligament that has been injured may become chronically inflamed, this means that the inflammatory response almost grinds to a halt and healing ceases. By applying a treatment such as ultrasound, the metabolism to the area can be selectively increased, the inflammation changed to an acute response and the healing process recommenced.

There is a limit to how far the temperature of tissues can be effectively raised. Proteins actually coagulate above a certain temperature (that is what happens to the white of an egg when it is fried). Generally speaking, irreversible tissue damage occurs at approximately 45°C.

Heat and cold therapy simplified

Consider a typical cell in your body. At normal body temperature it is content to receive a trickle of nutrients, oxygen and other essential items such as hormones. The surrounding lymphatic and blood supply is responsible for clearing away any metabolites.

If a hot pack were to be placed on it, as it heated up its chemical and biological processes would speed up and the trickle of nutrients would no longer be enough to meet its demands. It would need much more and at a faster rate; it would also make more waste products which would need to be removed, since they would be toxic if they were allowed to build up too much. As a result, the surrounding blood supply would increase.

If an ice pack were to be placed on it, as it cooled down gradually, its chemical and biological reactions would slow down and only a very small amount of oxygen and nutrients would be needed; it would also produce almost no waste products. The surrounding blood vessels would constrict and some local capillaries would close off.

Heberdens nodes Bony swellings that affect the fingers.

See *Bouchards nodes*

Heel lock A technique of strapping, thought to ensure of the stability of the sub-talar joint.

Heel to shin test This is a test where the patient is asked to run their heel of one foot down the shin of the other leg. This is a test of co-ordination. Poor responses may suggest a lesion of the cerebellum and results in reduced co-ordination.

Hemianopia Defective or loss of vision in half of the visual field of one or both

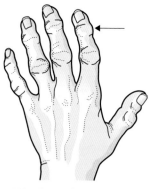

Heberdens nodes

eyes due to brain injury. The patient may bump into things on the affected side or ignore objects or people on that side of them.

Hemiparesis Paresis affecting one side of the body. Common presentation of stroke.

Hemiplegia Paralysis of one side of the body.

Henderson–Hasselbach Equation A formula used to calculate the bicarbonate concentration in the arterial blood when pH and $PaCO_2$ are known.

Heparin A drug that prevents blood from clotting, used after diagnosis of deep vein thrombosis, relevant to physiotherapy since it affects clotting, bruising and healing.

Hepatic Pertaining to the liver.

Hepatitis Inflammation of the liver, often accompanied by jaundice, enlargement, fever, fatigue and nausea and abnormal liver function blood tests (LFTs).

Hepatitis B A viral liver disease that can be acute or chronic and even life-threatening, particularly in people with poor immune resistance. Hepatitis B virus can be transmitted by sexual contact, contaminated needles or contaminated blood products.

Hepatitis C A viral disease that causes liver inflammation, and may cause severe, life-threatening liver damage.

Hepatomegaly Enlarged liver.

Hepatosplenomegaly Enlarged liver and spleen.

Hereditary Transferred via genes from parent to child.

Hering–Breuer reflex An inhibitory inspiratory reflex initiated by overstretching of the stretch receptors in the smooth muscle of the large and small airways. This reflex is only activated by large tidal volumes (around 900 mls) so is unimportant in quiet tidal breathing, but vital for regulation of breathing in moderate/strenuous exercise.

Hernia The protrusion of a loop or part of organ or tissue through an abnormal opening, hiatus hernia for example is herniation of the stomach through the diaphragm.
See *Hiatus hernia*

Heterotophic ossification (HO) This is where bone is laid down in soft tissues. There are a number of types, neurogenic HO is found following neurological insult. Maintaining active movement and the use of medication can prevent it. Where it does occur surgery may be required (Knight et al. 2003).

Hiatus Anatomical term for a gap.

Hiatus hernia Protrusion of the stomach upwards into the opening normally occupied by the oesophagus in the diaphragm.

High-frequency ventilation This is mechanical ventilation provided at more than four times the usual frequency, in order to reduce peak airway pressures by reducing the delivered tidal volume. Ventilation occurs through the movement of gases from a high to a low concentration gradient rather than through the exchange of gases via tidal volume changes. This type of ventilation can be delivered in three ways, classified by the method of gas delivery to the lungs: high-frequency positive pressure ventilation (HFPPV), high-frequency oscillation (HFO) and high-frequency jet ventilation (HFJV).

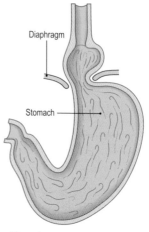

Hiatus hernia

High-voltage pulsed stimulation (HVPS) Electrotherapy term – a type of pulsed current with very short monophasic pulses, shape is usually either a pulse with twin peaks or a double pulse with no interpulse interval. Duration is typically less than 50 µs, so the current is comfortable and little risk of skin irritation. HVPS (also known as HVPC) has a

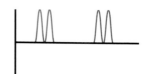

HVPS twin peak pulse

low average current, ideal for use in a battery-powered portable stimulator, charge per pulse may be too low for effective large-muscle stimulation even using multiple cathodes (option: use an alternating current or longer duration pulsed current).

Hill–Sachs lesion/deformity Following anterior dislocation of the shoulder, the head of the humerus can sustain a compression fracture from contact with the glenoid and its labrum. This consequent depression of the humeral head is known as a Hill–Sachs lesion.

HIV Common medical abbreviation – Human immunodeficiency virus.

Hinged ankle foot orthosis (AFO) This is an AFO with a hinge at the ankle joint so that the patient can dorsiflex their foot, but not plantarflex it further than plantargrade. It allows for a more normal gait pattern than a fixed AFO, but can be heavy and bulky for patients to wear.

Hip pointer A contusion of the iliac crest. Usually due to some form of trauma.

Hip replacement (total hip replacement = THR) The hip joint is the largest and deepest joint in the body that takes the form of multi-axial spheroidal joint with three degrees of freedom of movement with high levels of congruency (stability and surface area for stress transmission) and extensive range of movement:

- Metal alloy femoral head and stem (e.g. stainless steel, chromium cobalt) with high-molecular-weight (high-density) polyethylene cup. Where the small head of the Charnley prosthesis is used the procedure is known as the low-friction arthroplasty (LFA).

- Operating time = 90 minutes.

- The surgical approach to the hip-joint depends on surgeon's preference and impacts upon post operative rehabilitation. Commonly used approaches include the lateral transtrochanteric division necessitating trochanteric rewiring at closure and posterolateral intermuscular division. The femoral neck is divided, the joint dislocated (where possible) and the head removed.

- The femoral canal and acetabulum are reamed down to fresh bleeding bone and prepared for component implantation. Cavity size depends on fixation technique.

- If the components are to be cemented in situ, trial components are inserted and size/fit determined. These are then removed and the quick-setting cement, available impregnated with antibiotics, is pushed into the cavities. The implants (surfaces protected) are pushed into the cement – a complete cement mantle between the implant and the bone is essential for even distribution of forces and therefore implant life/procedure success. Significant pressure is applied to ensure this.

- The joint is then relocated and tested for stability. Once the surgeon is satisfied, the joint is adducted, flexed and medially rotated to dislocate the joint. The surface protection is removed, the joint relocated and closure commenced.

- If the greater trochanter was sawn off for access then it is rewired back onto the femur with specialized wiring techniques, developed to resist breaking.

- Soft tissues are repaired in their layers.

- Deep and superficial drains may or may not be used.

- The patient is usually catheterized for fluid balance measurement in the early days.

- The patient has intravenous fluids and possibly a PCA (patient controlled pain relief) through a venflon inserted into a hand or forearm vein.

- Many people now undergo epidural anaesthesia for hip replacements, this means that they are generally fitter in the post-operative period and many 'fast track' wards now exist where discharge at 5 days is common (Birch & Price 2003).

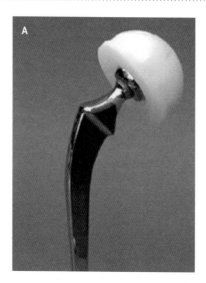

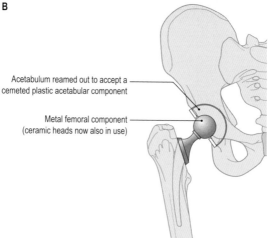

Acetabulum reamed out to accept a
cemented plastic acetabular component

Metal femoral component
(ceramic heads now also in use)

Hip replacement

Holistic The holistic approach to patient care is where consideration is given
to an individual's lifestyle, social functioning as well as any pathological
presentation in selection of treatment and management.

Homan's sign A test for a deep vein thrombosis (DVT). The person lies supine
or prone or sitting, the physiotherapist passively extends the knee, then
dorsiflexes the ankle. The calf also may be palpated, pain in the calf suggests

a DVT, this test may give false-positive results as the movement may be painful for other reasons.

Homophobia A prejudiced attitude or fear of people who are gay or lesbian.

Hoover's sign The patient lies supine, when asked to raise one leg, they involuntarily make counter pressure with the heel of the opposite leg. This sign is not present in cases of malingering.

Horner's syndrome Caused by interruption to the sympathetic nerves to the face and eye. A common feature is ptosis (drooping) of the eyelid.

Hospice A facility for people who are terminally ill. The hospice movement started in the 1970s and was pioneered by voluntary organizations. Many of its principles and values have now spread to the NHS, although hospices still remain independent of it. Hospices provide residential and domiciliary care.

Hotpacks A form of superficial heating. Types of hotpacks heated in a hydrocollator include canvas packs (moist heat) and plastic packs (dry heat). Other types of hotpacks: gelpacks and wheatpacks heated in a microwave oven and chemical packs in which the user bends or breaks apart to initiate an exothermic reaction. Duration of heating depends on method and initial temperature. Dangers are mainly of burns or tissue damage if applied to an area with an insufficient blood supply.

Housemaid's knee Inflammation of the infrapatellar bursa.

Humerus The bone of the upper arm.

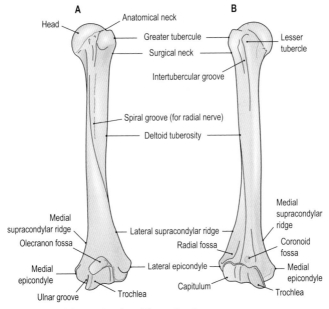

Right humerus: (**A**) posterior view, (**B**) anterior view

Humidifier A machine that puts moisture in the air.

Huntington disease An inherited degenerative disease that affects the basal ganglia and cerebral cortex leading to loss of cognitive function and choreiform (jerky, involuntary) movements.

Hyaline membrane disease A respiratory disease of the newborn.

Hydrocephalus An increase in the volume of cerebro-spinal fluid (CSF). Usually resulting from impaired absorption and occasionally from excessive secretion. It may be congenital or acquired.
  Hydrocephalus can be classified into:

- Obstructive – obstruction of CSF flow within the ventricular system
- Communicating – this occurs where there is obstruction within the subarachnoid space.

  Patients may present with enlarged head, prominent forehead, brain atrophy and convulsions; they may also be confused and have developed a flexed posture and shuffling gait. Ultimately, they will lose consciousness. Treatment usually requires the neurosurgical insertion of a shunt that takes the excess fluid into the peritoneal cavity. Hydrocephalus is a common complication following sub-arachnoid haemorrhage.

Hydrophilic Readily absorbing moisture, or having an affinity for water.

Hydrotherapy Rehabilitation exercises performed in water.

Hydroxychloroquine A drug used to treat and prevent malaria. It is also used to treat rheumatoid arthritis.

Hypaesthesia Abnormally decreased sensitivity to stimulation.

Hyperalgesia A lowered threshold for the interpretation of pain, or hypersensitivity

Hyperbaric chamber A pressurized chamber that allows for the delivery of oxygen in high concentrations for therapeutic benefit.

Hyperbaric oxygen This is the administration of oxygen therapy at pressures greater than 1 atmosphere, e.g. for air embolus and decompression sickness.

Hypercalcaemia Too much calcium in the blood.

Hypercapnia An excess of carbon dioxide in the blood.

Hyperextension Active or passive force that takes the joint into extension, but beyond its normal physiological range. Since human movement encompassess a wide spectrum of variations. A degree of hyperextension may be considered normal especially in the elbows of the knees.

Hyperinflation A state of overinflation of the lungs or chest wall, resulting in an increase in dead space, higher work of breathing and mechanical disadvantage of the respiratory muscles. Hyperinflation characteristics include an increased antero-posterior thoracic diameter, elevated horizontally positioned ribs and a flattened diaphragm.

Hyperkinesia Excessive involuntary movements seen in some neurological conditions, they include such phenomena as tremor, clonus and tics.

Hypermetria A disorder of movement where the patient tends to overshoot the intended target.

Hypermobility An increase beyond the 'normal' range of joint movement.
N.B. 'normal' actually comprises a broad spectrum and hypermobility is one end of this spectrum, as such it may not be a sign of any pathology or even produce any symptoms.

Hypernatraemia An excess of sodium in blood plasma.

Hyperpnoea Ventilation, which is appropriately increased to maintain a normal $PaCO_2$.

Hyperreactivity A state in which a reaction is greater than the normal response to a stimulus.

Hyper-reflexia Presents as exaggerated reflex activity, demonstrated on EMG. This is part of the upper motor neurone syndrome; it may be seen following stroke or brain injury. It is thought to be related to plastic changes in the nervous system.

Hypertension Persistently high arterial blood pressure. It may have no known cause (essential or idiopathic hypertension) or be associated with other primary diseases (secondary hypertension). Persistently high blood pressure is a risk factor in cardiovascular disease, heart attack and stroke.

Hyperthermia A raised body temperature.

Hypertonia Increased tone or tension within muscles. The opposite of hypotonic. There are two types of hypertonia: spasticity and rigidity.

Comparison of spasticity and rigidity

	Spasticity	Rigidity
Pattern of muscle involvement	Upper limb flexors; lower limb extensors	Flexors and extensors equally
Nature of tone	Velocity-dependent increase in ton; 'clasp-knife'	Constant throughout movement; 'lead pipe'
Tendon reflexes	Increased	Normal
Pathophysiology	Increased spinal stretch reflex gain	Increased long-latency component of stretch reflex
Clinical significance	Upper motor neurone (pyramidal) sign	Extrapyramidal sign

Hypertrophic scar An elevated scar often seen after severe burns.

Hypertrophy An increase in the size, the opposite of atrophy.

Hyperventilation This is a state of over breathing that results in an abnormally low level of $PaCO_2$ (hypocapnoea), i.e. <4.5 kPa (35 mmHg). The chronic hyperventilation syndrome, is a breathing pattern disorder that is often underdiagnosed, resulting in the movement of patients between departments for investigation of the many disabling physical symptoms experienced.

Hypnosis The induction of a dreamlike state of heightened suggestibility in a person by a hypnotist. Some people may, for example, have dental treatment under hypnosis.

Hypocalcaemia Too little calcium in the blood.

Hypocapnia Deficiency of carbon dioxide in the blood, if prolonged it can eventually lead to alkalosis.

Hypoglycaemia An abnormally diminished concentration of glucose in the blood.

This occurs when a person with diabetes has injected too much insulin, eaten too little food, or has exercised without extra food.

Hypokinesia Poverty of movement.

Hypometria A disorder of movement where the patient tends to fail to meet the intended target.

Hypomobility A decrease in the normal range of movement at a joint. This may include the loss of accessory movements.

Hyponatraemia A deficiency of sodium in the blood plasma.

Hypopharynx This is the area between the epiglottis and larynx.

Hypopnoea This is an appropriate reduction in ventilation, which maintains a normal $PaCO_2$. When occurring during sleep, hypopnoea is defined as a reduction in ventilation of 10 s or more (SIGN 2003).

Hypotension Low blood pressure, postural hypotension is a low blood pressure that only emerges upon the adoption of a particular posture by a person.

Hypothermia A lowered body temperature.

Hypothesis Research term – the proposed answer to a research question.

The wording of a hypothesis may be two-tailed hypothesis (no direction implied) or it may be more specific and indicate the direction of the effect, i.e. a one-tailed hypothesis.

An example of a two-tailed hypothesis would be if there were a difference in intelligence between students and their lecturers.

An example of a one-tailed hypothesis would be if the students were more intelligent than their lecturers.

⮑ Student tip Not all research requires a hypothesis; indeed, many qualitative studies only generate hypotheses upon their completion.

Hypotonia Lack of muscle tone. Reduced resistance to passive stretch, patients may have difficulty in maintaining a given posture or position against gravity. Muscles appear floppy.

Hypoventilation This is alveolar hypoventilation or under breathing, resulting in an elevated $PaCO_2$ level.

Hypovolaemic shock Shock caused by a decrease in the amount of blood that is in the circulation.

Hypoxaemia This is defined as insufficient oxygen content in the blood. There are four major causes of a reduced partial pressure of oxygen in the arterial blood. These are:

1. hypoventilation
2. impairment of diffusion
3. shunt
4. V/Q inequalities.

Hypoxia This is an inadequate amount of oxygen availability at tissue level for cellular respiration (Weilitz 1993).

If sustained, normal cellular function is disrupted and the result may be complications such as cardiac arrhythmias, hypotension and cardiac arrest. Hypoxia occurs as a result of an imbalance between the availability of oxygen in the blood and the demands of oxygen consumption.

Hysterectomy A surgical procedure whereby the uterus (womb) is removed.

Iatrogenic Induced inadvertently by medical treatment or procedures. For example, an infection caused during surgery is iatrogenic.

I band The portion of the muscle filament that extends from the z line to the a bands.

> See *Muscle structure*

IBS Common medical abbreviation – Irritable bowel syndrome.

ICD-10 The International Statistical Classification of Diseases and Related Health Problems, tenth revision. The latest in a series that was formalized in 1893 as the Bertillon Classification or International List of Causes of Death.

Ice therapy See *Heat therapy*

What happens to a blood vessel when it is cooled?

If a physiotherapist places an ice pack on a typical blood vessel, to minimize contact with the cold environment and the loss of any further heat, the vessel's smooth-muscle-wall lining contracts, thus causing the vessel's diameter to shrink (vasoconstriction). After about 5 min, the muscle in vessel wall begins to become paralyzed. If this vasoconstriction were to continue, the tissues that the vessel feeds would start to die. The vessel, therefore, reopens ([CIVD] cold-induced vaso dilatation). However, this does not help, because as it reopens it comes into contact with more cold. For as long as the ice pack is in situ, the vessel is constantly switching between vasoconstriction and vasodilatation in an attempt to 'hunt' for the most suitable diameter. This is known as Lewis's hunting reaction.

Ice is best thought of as a damage-limitation procedure immediately following an injury to soft tissues such as a haematoma, sprain or strain. Ice should probably be applied for little more than 2–3 min and then regularly reapplied to emphasize the vasoconstriction element of its effects. There is also little evidence about the anti-inflammatory effects of ice once the immediate acute period is over.

Other effects of ice

Application of ice stimulates pain and cold sensation, but if the cold is intense enough, both of these sensations are suppressed. Small-diameter non-myelinated group 4 fibres are least affected and myelinated a fibres are most affected.

Muscle strength is decreased, by cooling, but increases beyond its initial value 1 h later. Cold is useful in decreasing muscle spasm and spasticity.

As skin temperature decreases, the need to produce internal heat increases, this is partly achieved by muscle contractions (shivering). Also, adopting a foetal position assists in reducing heat loss. Finally, do not forget that ice can be quite unpleasant, e.g. to the hands, feet, abdomen – bear this in mind when applying cold therapy to your patients.

The effects of cold have been studied on canine and human blood vessels. The following conclusions were found concerning the phenomenon of the hunting reaction seen in human extremities on their exposure to severe cold:

- On exposure to cold there is a marked increase in the affinity of the postjunctional alpha-adrenoceptors for norepinephrine. This results in a powerful constriction of the blood vessels and a cessation of blood flow to the distal tissue.

- As the temperature of the tissues rapidly falls, sympathetic nerve conduction is interrupted and vasodilatation occurs, due to the cessation of norepinephrine release and the depressor action of cold on the contractile machinery. The resultant return of blood flow rewarms the tissue, nerve conduction is re-established, and this, combined with the increased affinity of the alpha-adrenoceptors for norepinephrine, leads to renewed vasoconstriction.

- Repetition of this cycle could result in the hunting reaction (Shepherd & Rusche 1983).

ICP Common medical abbreviation – Intracranial pressure.

ICU Common medical abbreviation – Intensive care unit ([ITU] intensive therapy unit).

Identity The knowledge of individuals and groups concerning who they are in relation to others in their group or society. It involves not only feelings and understandings about themselves in relation to others, but also feelings and understandings about others in relation to themselves. People may have multiple identities, for example British, parent, physiotherapist and musician.

Idiopathic Without any well defined physiological cause.

IF Common medical abbreviation – Interferential therapy.

IGG Common medical abbreviation – Immunoglobulin G.

Ileostomy Surgical creation of an opening into the ileum, with a stoma on the abdominal wall.

Ileus An obstruction of the intestines.

Illness The subjective feeling of being unwell. Illness may or may not be associated with disease or impairment.

Illness behaviour The ways in which people respond to illness and impairment and the type of help if any, that they seek. Illness behaviour depends upon a multitude of factors including how symptoms are perceived and evaluated, the severity of the symptoms, past experience of illness, social support and how convenient or inconvenient it is to be ill at any given time.

Iliotibial band A strong band of connective tissue situated laterally in the thigh. It has action over the knee (can act as a flexor at >30° of knee flexion and as an extensor at <30° of flexion) and can be affected by overuse (iliotibial band syndrome). Pain presents over the lateral compartment of the knee where the iliotibial band passes over the femoral condyle. Pain is usually brought on by running, and there may be associated crepitus or clicking.

Ilizarov method The Ilizarov method of fracture fixation had its origins in Russia in the 1940s. It incorporates an axial system of wires or pins fitted through the bone and connected to a circular ring. It is sometimes used in cases of non-union. This method also incorporates the principle of distraction osteogenesis and can be used in the restoration of large skeletal defects, limb lengthening and the correction of skeletal deformities (Schwartsmann et al. 1990).

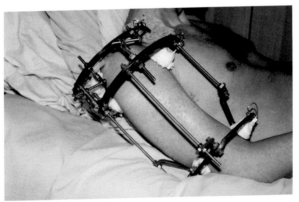

Ilizarov fixation for fractured humerus and scapula

IM (X2) Common medical abbreviation – Intramuscular or intra-medullary.

Immobility A general term clinically used to describe a lack of movement either locally (i.e. at a joint or muscle) or globally (e.g. unable to walk).

Immobilization Prevention of movement, either intentional, e.g. enforced in a plaster of Paris cast to allow for natural healing to take place. Or unintentional, e.g. following the flu.

Immune system Elements of the body that recognize foreign agents or substances, eliminate or neutralize them, and recall the response when faced with the same challenge in the future.

Immunoglobulin A protein that acts as an antibody to help the body fend off disease.
    There are five classes: IgG, IgA, IgD, IgM and IgE.

Impacted fracture A fracture where one fragment has been driven into another.

See *Fracture classification*

Impact factor The value ascribed by the academic community to the importance of a journal:

- high impact = important
- low impact = less important.

Impairment This is a term used to describe the loss or abnormality of psychological, physiological or anatomical structure or function. Impairment also has a social dimension as it means different things in different societies at different times. The term was used within the World Health Organization's model for describing health: impairment, disability and handicap. The WHO redefined the definitions in 1997, with a result that the term 'function' is now used replacing the term impairment.

See *Handicap* (table)

Impetigo A common skin infection. It is most common in children. In adults, it may follow other skin disorders.

Incentive spirometry An approach to enhancing lung expansion through the use of a simple flow or volumetric device, e.g. the Triflo and Voldyne incentive spirometers, which gives visual feedback as to whether the desired predetermined target has been met. The devices encourage a sustained and maximal inhalation, which decreases pleural pressure thereby encouraging alveolar inflation. There are few complications associated with their use, but these include hyperventilation, pain in poorly analgesed patients, hypoxaemia secondary to breaks in therapy and fatigue.

Inclusion criteria (in clinical study) Research term – criteria that define who is eligible to participate is a clinical study.

Incomplete lesion A lesion in which there is a partial preservation of sensory and/or motor function is found below the neurological level and includes the lowest sacral segment.

○ Clinical note With the advancement of acute intervention, more spinal injured patients are now presenting with incomplete lesions. This is important to recognize as rehabilitation for incomplete and complete spinal injured patients takes a different approach.

Independence Predominantly associated with the ability to do things for oneself, being self-supporting and self-reliant. In some cultures independence is also associated with life transitions, particularly the transition from childhood to adulthood. Independence is less valued in some cultures than others who may have a collectivist orientation. The meaning of independence in terms of 'doing things for oneself' has been increasingly challenged by disabled people on a number of grounds. The Disabled People's Movement views independence in terms of self-determination, control and managing and organizing the assistance that is required. In a very real sense we are all dependent on each other for our survival so nobody is independent.

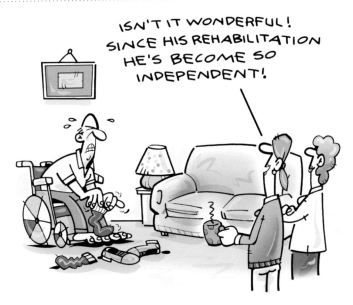

Independent living A set of ideas, sometimes referred to as a movement, developed by disabled people to establish their right to participate fully within society. The concept is broad and embraces the full range of human and civil rights. A key focus in the Independent Living Movement has been the availability of direct payments to buy services (Direct Payments Act 1996) and the employment of personal assistants rather than relying on statutory services. The philosophy of independent living is practised in centres of integrated (or independent) living (CILs), which are controlled by disabled people and which challenge the practice and philosophy of statutory services.

Independent variable Research term – the variable which is changed (manipulated) so that its effects on the dependant variable can be seen.

Inertia The reluctance of a body to start moving, or stop moving once it has started.

Infarction See *Myocardial infarction*

Inferential statistics Statistics that can be used to make inferences from the data and express the confidence with which generalization to a whole population can be undertaken.

Inferior Anatomical term towards the feet in the anatomical position.

Inferior draw test (Sulcus test) A sulcus sign is established by pulling the patient's arm distally while relaxed. If the humeral head slides out of the glenoid an indentation will occur underneath the acromion. The sulcus sign is positive in patients with shoulder laxity.

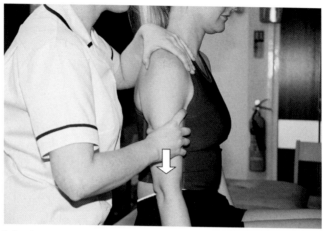

Inferior draw test

Inflammation A complex stereotypical reaction of vascularized living tissue to local trauma. The four cardinal signs of inflammation are:

1. rubor
2. dolor
3. calor
4. tumour.

Some authorities add loss of function.

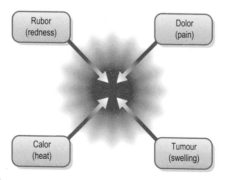

Inflammation

Inflammatory myopathies This is a disorder of muscle in which there is clinical and laboratory evidence of an inflammatory process. It is an acquired muscle disorder.

Informal care Care and assistance that is provided by unpaid carers (usually kin, but sometimes friends and neighbours) who have an emotional attachment to the person in need of assistance or a sense of obligation. Volunteers may also provide informal care.

Informed consent A process whereby patients, clients and research participants are fully informed of the procedures they will undertake in order that they can make an informed choice. Ensuring informed consent is a moral and legal duty of health professionals.

Infrapatellar fat pad This lies deep to the patellar tendon and fills the space between the tibial condyles and the femur.

Infrared radiation (IRR) Infrared radiation is a form of electromagnetic radiation, lying in the EM spectrum between visible light and microwaves. The wavelengths are between 760 nm and 1.0 mm and are subdivided into:

$$\text{Near IRR} = 760-1500\,\text{nm}$$
$$\text{Far IRR} = >1500\,\text{nm}$$

There are both natural and artificial sources, though for therapeutic purposes, the artificial source is usual. It was previously widely used in therapy, but is much less common now. Infrared generators can be 'luminous' or 'non-luminous'. The spectral output of the non-luminous source is from 760 to 15000 nm (usually peaking at 4000 nm). The luminous generator tends to produce a shorter wavelength spectrum of IRR and also produces some visible emission. The emission spectrum is typically from 350 to 4000 nm (with a peak at 1000 nm). The red bulb (which is common) filters out short visible and any UV lights, therefore, the patient is exposed to IRR and red visible light. Near IRR (e.g. 1200 nm – luminous source) penetrates to dermis (few mm).

Far IRR (>1200 nm – non-luminous source) can only penetrate superficial epidermis (1 mm or less). The EM waves penetrate the tissues and are absorbed and as a result of the absorption, heat is generated in the tissues. The therapeutic effects of Infrared include: pain relief, muscle relaxation and improved local blood flow.

INH Common medical abbreviation – Inhalation.

Inhalation therapy This is the use of drugs administered via the respiratory tract. Commonly, bronchodilators (drugs used to open up the airways by relaxing the bronchial smooth muscle) are given via this method. In order to be taken into the lung the particle size is of extreme importance and should, ideally, be 5 μm in diameter (i.e. the thickness of a human hair) to ensure adequate pulmonary deposition. Particles larger than this will hit the upper respiratory tract while smaller particles will be exhaled.

Inhibitory post-synaptic potential (IPSP) A term that refers to the effect that is produced when excitatory input to a neurone causes brief hyperpolarization that spreads to the axon hillock. The balance between this and the excitatory post-synaptic potential determine the final neurone output.

Innervation ratio The term used to describe the ratio between the number of α motor neurones and the total number of skeletal muscle fibres.

- Small innervation ratio = muscles such as the eye muscles that need very fine control
- Large innervation ratio = limb muscles.

The innervation ratio increases with age as neurones die, this is one of the reasons for a loss of hand control in elderly people.

Insight This term relates to the patients cognitive ability to understand their situation. Insight can be impaired following brain damage. Patients with poor insight may present as difficult and non-compliant, as they fail to recognize their own problems.

Inspiratory muscles These are the muscles used during inspiration and consist of the diaphragm and intercostals.

Instability The term used to describe an excessive range of abnormal movement for which there is no muscular control (Maitland 2001).

Institutionalization The adverse social and psychological effects on individuals of residence in institutions, including long-stay hospitals for people with learning difficulties or mental illness. The effects can include passivity, enforced dependency and depression. Small home settings, as well as large establishments, can create institutionalization if they are run rigidly with little regard for the needs of residents.

Insulin The substance that has key importance in glucose metabolism, the factors that affect its secretion and its actions are summarized in the figure below.

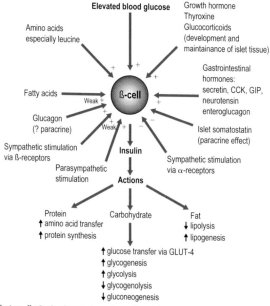

Factors affecting insulin secretion and an outline of the actions of insulin.
GLUT-4 = glucose transport protein-4

Integrated care pathways (ICPs) This is where a team gets together and writes down how a patient should be cared for and what should happen when and by whom. The best care pathways integrate all of the health professionals' input to maximize effectiveness and are based on best available evidence and national guidelines, but applying these within the local resources and context. ICPs were initially introduced for elective-surgery patients, but now their use is widespread. Standards in the care pathways should be monitored and audited as part of a commitment to ongoing evaluation of clinical care. This is often undertaken by using a core document in which all health staff record their care.

Intelligence Can be formally defined as that which is measured by standardized intelligence tests. Such testing, though still widely used, has been strongly criticized, in terms of objectivity, reliability and validity. There are different psychological models of intelligence, though they generally include verbal ability, problem solving and practical intelligence. More recently, the notion of emotional intelligence has emerged, which refers to the ability to interpret and use emotions in oneself and others. Intelligence, as an overall concept, has never been satisfactorily defined.

Intention-to-treat analysis – also known as analysis by intention to treat Research term – in a randomized control trial patients can be randomly assigned to different treatments. After randomization, patients who have been assigned conservative therapy may decide to have surgery instead; conversely, patients assigned to the surgical treatment may decide not to undergo surgery. In an intention-to-treat analysis, patients would be analyzed according to the groups for which they were originally assigned.

Intention tremor A tremor that occurs when the individual attempts voluntary movement, caused by a disorder of the nervous system.

    ⬆ Clinical note It can be seen in patients with multiple sclerosis and this tremor is more incapacitating than a resting tremor (as seen in some Parkinson's patients) as it interferes with function.

Interactive effects Electrotherapy term – applying two different electrophysical agents concurrently or sequentially may increase the risks to the patient. For example, applying ice or TENS or electrical stimulation over a region before or with ultrasound can reduce a patient's capacity to report if it becomes too hot and can lead to skin burns.

Interburst interval Electrotherapy term – time during which no current flows following a burst or between successive bursts (continuous train of alternating pulses).
    See *Alternating current* and *burst*

Intercostal chest drain (ICD) These drains are used to remove air or fluid from the pleural space enabling lung re-expansion to occur, e.g. post trauma, post operatively or after pneumothorax. Such drains require an underwater seal drain to allow restoration of the integrity of the pleural space. Suction may be added to the drain where the air leak is brisk, but this should not be so high that it prevents the lung from sealing itself. Regular monitoring of such drains is required, with the amount type and colour of drainage noted. Water in the tubing should fluctuate during breathing, while bubbles in the underwater seal during breathing or coughing would be indicative of an air leak (from the lung). The drains are removed when the fluid drainage and fluctuations have ceased and X-ray and breath sounds have returned to normal (indicating the lung is reinflated).

Intercostal muscles Muscles between ribs, employed in breathing.

Inter-disciplinary team A type of team where professionals and other workers meet regularly and work very closely together. There is considerable blurring of professional boundaries in order to deliver holistic and integrated care. Such teams tend to be relatively informal and are characterized by relationships of equality among members. Patients and clients should be considered central in such teams.

Interferential therapy (IFT) Electrotherapy term – for 'true' or 'quadripolar' IFT, two channels of alternating current are crossed, producing an amplitude modulated current in the subcutaneous area between the four electrodes. Alternatively, the current can be premodulated, so only one channel with two electrodes is required. Each burst of modulated current is called a 'beat'. While not as popular, research suggests premodulated IFT is as effective as true IFT used with large electrodes and has fewer risks and a considerably lower average current.

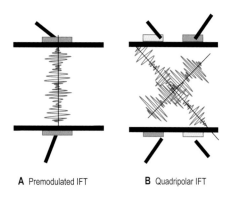

A Premodulated IFT   **B** Quadripolar IFT

Interleukin A chemical hormone (cytokine) secreted by and affecting many different cells in the immune system.

Intermediate care This refers to the type of care that patients can be given after coming out of an acute hospital and includes day hospitals, intermediate care wards and community-based care, although its definition is often locally interpreted. It is often given to patients who are unable to return home immediately and require some form of rehabilitation. It is usually time limited (6 weeks). Its aim is to bridge the perceived gap between acute medical care and independence in the community.

Intermittent claudication A condition characterized by leg pain and weakness brought on by exercise or walking, symptoms disappear following a brief rest. It is most often caused by atherosclerotic narrowing of the iliac and femoral arteries, often combined with lesions in distal arteries of the leg.

Internal capsule A band of fibres that runs between the basal nuclei and the thalamus, in the brain.

Internal market The simulation of market conditions within state services such as the NHS and social services. There is a separation between the purchaser and the provider of the services (the purchaser/provider split). Services are purchased on behalf of patients and clients by care managers (usually social workers) and come from a variety of providers within the private, voluntary and statutory services.

See *Purchaser/provider split* and *Mixed economy of welfare*

Internal oppression Oppression is internalized when those who experience it (for example, through injustice, discrimination, harassment) come to accept the views and beliefs of those who oppress them. Thus, the child with learning difficulties who is treated as worthless comes to believe that he or she is worthless. Internal oppression is rarely complete and can often be dispelled if the individual is presented with alternative ideas.

See *Oppression*

International classification of functioning, disability and health (ICF) Classification system of health and health-related domains that describe body functions and structures, activities and participation. Used for describing how people live with their health condition. The domains are classified from body, individual and societal perspectives and include a list of environmental factors. It can be used in clinical settings, health services or surveys at the individual or population level. Go to http://www3.who.int/icf/icftemplate.cfm?myurl=homepage.html&mytitle=Home%20Page

International normalized ratio (INR) The time taken for blood to clot compared to a control. The INR is should fall between 0.9 and 1.2.

Interprofessional (Multiprofessional) education Where a number of different professional groups learn together in a structured way.

Interpulse interval Electrotherapy term – time between separate pulses.

See *Pulsed current*

A frequency of 50 Hz means there are 50 pulses/s with equal interpulse intervals between (except if catchlike current). For a pulsed current with a 50 Hz frequency and pulse duration of 300 μs, the combined interpulse intervals:

$$= 1\,\text{s} - (50\,\text{Hz} \times 300\,\mu\text{s}) = 985\,\text{ms}$$

Interstitial lung disease (ILD) This categorization refers to a number of lung conditions grouped together due to similarities in their clinical presentations, radiological and physiological features. The abnormalities are more consistent with changes in the interstitium rather than the airspaces. Within this category are a number of diseases with diverse causes, treatments and prognoses. Such diseases include those associated with occupational, allergic, soft tissue and idiopathic causes, e.g. asbestosis, rheumatoid lung. Sarcoidosis, drug-induced fibrosis, fibrosing alveolitis, etc. However, the usual impairment is that of a physiological restrictive deficit with reduced lung volumes (but a preserved spirometric forced expiratory ratio [see *Spirometry*]) and diffusing capacity for carbon monoxide (see *DLCO*). Clinical symptoms include worsening dyspnoea, cough, weight loss, lethargy, fever and arthralgia. Examination findings may include dyspnoea, clubbing, fine inspiratory crackles, cyanosis and rheumatoid arthritis, with death occurring as a result of a gradual deterioration terminating in respiratory failure over a 4/5 year period. However, prognosis can be varied from months to years. Management regimes (dependant upon the diagnosis of the specific ILD) may include exposure avoidance, corticosteroids, cytotoxic agents, oxygen therapy, transplantation, vaccinations and pulmonary rehabilitation.

Intervertebral disc   See *Annulus fibrosus* and *Nucleus pulposus*

The disc forms a cartilaginous joint between the vertebral bodies, made up of the annulus fibrosis, nucleus pulposus and the cartilage end plates. It is the most common cause of lumbar spine disorders. Intervertebral discs (referred to as the disc) are often described as shock absorbers, allowing load to be transmitted from one vertebra to the next, this is only part of their function. An equally important role of the disc is to permit controlled small-amplitude movements between the vertebra above and below it. Between two adjoining vertebrae, only small movements are possible. When added together, the result is a column that is extremely mobile without sacrificing stability. The normal spine is self-stabilizing and for humans to stand erect takes very little muscle action, illustrated by the fact that persons who have spent prolonged periods in bed can sit upright with relative ease.

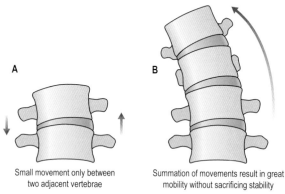

A   Small movement only between
two adjacent vertebrae

B   Summation of movements result in great
mobility without sacrificing stability

The role of intervertebral discs (**A**) Small movements only; (**B**) summation of movements results in greater mobility

Interview A research method, interviews may be open, structured or semi structured.

Structured interview
Here the interviewer will aim to use short specific questions, read the question exactly as on the schedule, ask the questions in the identical order specified by the schedule.

Semi-structured interviews
Here the investigator has a set of questions on an interview schedule, but the interview will be guided by the schedule rather than be dictated by it. So there is an attempt to establish rapport with the patient/person the interviewer is free to probe interesting areas that arise, the interview can follow the respondent's interests or concerns.

Intra-articular Being within the joint. For example, the anterior cruciate ligament is intra-articular.

Intracranial haemorrhage (ICH) A bleed into the cerebral tissue, commonly called a stroke, although the more common cause of a stroke is an infarct. An ICH can also be caused by an aneurysm, arteriovenous malformation, trauma or hypertension.

Intracranial pressure This is the pressure within the cranium. If you consider the cranium (skull) as a box there are basically three components: brain tissue, blood and cerebrospinal fluid. Any increase in any of these three components will result in a raised intracranial pressure. An increase in intracranial pressure is common after head injury when the brain tissue swells and causes a resulting raise in pressure. It is a serious condition monitored clinically using the Glasgow Coma Scale and by a ventricular shunt in critical cases in intensive care units (ICU) or high-dependency units. The brain can 'compensate' initially for a small increase in volume of one of the components but a continuing increase results in a rapid 'decompensation' (i.e. where the brain cannot accommodate any more swelling) and may result in death. Normal values are between 0 and 15 mmHg, treatment of a raised intracranial pressure is usually required above 20 mmHg.

⊕ Clinical note The main consideration for physiotherapy is not to undertake treatment that might raise intracranial pressure (ICP), in patients where a raised ICP is present. So minimizing the use of suction, avoiding positioning that might raise ICP (patients should be in 30° of head and trunk elevation) and avoiding other noxious stimuli is important. However, ICP is affected by changes in respiratory blood gases so maintaining good lung function is also very important. For this reason careful clinical decision-making needs to take place for each individual patient as if respiratory treatment is indicated.

Intractable pain Pain which proves difficult to control.

Intra-disciplinary team A team consisting of members of the same profession who may have different levels and types of experience and expertise. Patients and clients should be considered central in such teams.

Intrafusal fibre The bundle of fibres found within the muscle spindle; they are divided into nuclear bag and nuclear chain fibres.

Intramedullary (IM) nail Intramedullary nailing has revolutionized management of long bone fractures. Here a hollow metal rod is introduced at one end of a long bone, travels down the medullary canal and may be locked with screws distally and proximally. The proximal aspect of the nail is threaded and this permits a tool to be threaded onto the nail at a later date for its removal. IM nailing for fractures of long bones has revolutionized management of many fractures, which up until a few years ago would have been managed by prolonged bed rest. The trauma is less than open techniques and results in decreased hospital in-patient stay, more rapid patient mobilization and rehabilitation with minimal risk of complications associated with immobility. The implant rather than the bone may take stresses and strains and for this reason the surgeon may choose to remove the locking screws

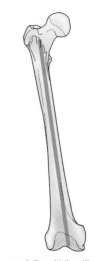

Intramedullary (IM) nailing for fractured shaft of femur

at a later stage. This permits the nail to move slightly and cause compaction of bone ends, this is known as dynamization. This allows the bone to once again take its normal stresses and strains and adapt in accordance with Wolff's law. Fractures of the shaft of tibia and humerus may also be nailed in this way.

Intramuscular Into the muscle: frequently in reference to the administration of injections, but can also refer to a haematoma that is situated between muscles, e.g. intramuscular haematoma.

Intraneural Within neural (nerve) tissue.

Intraobserver variability Research term – variability between the observations of the same observer on repeated occasions; for example, does the same physiotherapist give the same reading of knee flexion when goniometry is performed on more than one occasion?

Intrapulmonary receptors These are receptors within the lung that facilitate the regulation of breathing, e.g. J receptors, which detect stretch.

Intubation The process of introducing a tube to assist respiration, there are various means of so doing, these are listed below in the table along with their indications and advantages.

Intubation

Site of tube	Indications and advantages	Type of tube
Oral	Most commonly used in adults Used in emergency situations	Endotracheal tube – cuffed (adults) – uncuffed (paediatrics
Nasal	Used when oral intubation impossible or impractical, e.g. trauma Commonly used in paediatrics	
Tracheostomy – temporary – permanent	Used for long-term ventilation Improved comfort, reduces need for sedation, facilitated normal eating and drinking Maintains and protects airway where a neurological or anatomical abnormality is present	Portex® – cuffed or uncuffed – single lumen – speaking valve Shiley® – cuffed or uncuffed – fenestration for speech – long-term use – inner cannulae Silver – uncuffed – permanent use – single lumen – phonation tube

Inverse care law This law states that those who are most at risk of acquiring illness and disease are least likely to receive medical and social services. This is due to a wide variety of factors relating to social inequalities and the availability of services.

Inversion Turning the sole of the foot inwards.

Investigator bias Research term – occurs when the interviewer is aware (not blinded) of the outcome variable. An unblinded interviewer may be more vigorous in searching for the exposure of interest.

In vitro Latin for 'in glass': an artificial environment created outside a living organism.

In vivo Latin for 'in life': the term usually refers to studies conducted within a living organism.

Ions Charged particles. May be positive or negative.

Iontophoresis Electrotherapy term – the use of direct current to push therapeutically active ions through the skin. The ionized medication is placed under the electrode (cathode or anode) with the same charge. The repulsion between like charges forces the ions through the skin directly to the area being treated. It is used with some local anaesthetics, steroids, antiinflammatories, etc.

IPPB Common medical abbreviation – Intermittent positive pressure breathing.
This device became known more commonly as 'the Bird' (the name of the manufacturer). The device is a simple breathing device that responds to a spontaneous or timed trigger to deliver positive pressure to the airway throughout inspiration via a mask or mouthpiece. Its uses include delivery of bronchodilator-inhaled drugs, reduction of the work of breathing and reinflation of atelectatic pulmonary areas through increases in functional residual lung capacity. The device can be used in conjunction with other therapies, such as positioning and thoracic expansion exercises.

INTERMITTENT POSITIVE PRESSURE BREATHING (IPPB)

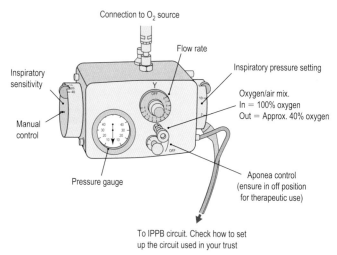

Diagram to show an example of intermittent positive pressure breathing (IPPB) dials

IPPV Common medical abbreviation – Intermittent positive pressure ventilation.
This is the application of positive pressure to the airways to facilitate breathing.
See *Ventilators*

Irritability (see SIN factors) The amount of activity necessary to worsen the condition, the extent of the exacerbation and the duration of the response. Forms part of a patient assessment along with irritability and nature. These three items form what is known as SIN factors, which are a valuable aid in planning frequency and duration of treatment. This has implications for the amount of assessment and treatment provided to the patient.

IRQ Common medical abbreviation – Inner range quadriceps.

Ischaemia Deficiency of blood in a part, e.g. ischaemic heart disease or transient ischaemic attack (TIA).

Isokinetic Applies to muscle contraction in which a constant joint angular velocity is maintained by accommodating resistance.

Isometric Contraction of muscle without movement at the joint, when there is no change in the length but tension increases.

Isotonic contraction Constant loading of a muscle, with variable velocity.

Isotonic solution A solution with the same concentration as plasma.

ITU Common medical abbreviation – Intensive therapy unit.

IV Common medical abbreviation – Intravenous.

°**Jaccol** Common medical abbreviation – No jaundice, anaemia, clubbing, cyanosis, oedema, lymphadenopathy.

Jaundice Yellow colouration of the skin and eyes due to accumulation of bile. It is usually associated with some form of liver damage or disease. The sclera (white outer portion) of the eye may also become yellowed.

Johnstone approach A treatment approach developed by Johnstone for the treatment of stroke patients. It is based on the use of developmental sequences of movement and on sensory stimulation through the use of pressure splints. Pressure splints are used to enable weight bearing in patterns that are thought to inhibit spasticity.

Johnstone splints These are air filled splints that envelop a limb or part of a limb they are used in the Johnstone approach to treat patients with neurological deficit.

 ❂ Clinical note They can also be used as a temporary measure to help with limbs that are showing signs of contractures. As with all splints they require careful monitoring.

Joint classification The main types of synovial joint.

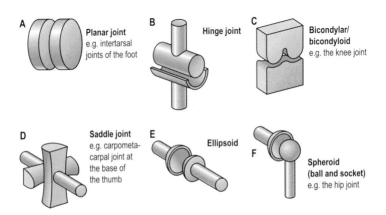

A **Planar joint** e.g. intertarsal joints of the foot

B **Hinge joint**

C **Bicondylar/bicondyloid** e.g. the knee joint

D **Saddle joint** e.g. carpometacarpal joint at the base of the thumb

E **Ellipsoid**

F **Spheroid (ball and socket)** e.g. the hip joint

Joint hypermobility syndrome A common childhood condition involving hypermobile joints (that can move beyond the normal range of motion).

Joint locking A condition, usually caused by trapping of a loose body within the joint, such as a fragment of torn meniscus at the knee. The person typically describes a history of having to push or jiggle the joint in order to unlock it.

Joint position sense The awareness of the joints in space. Often tested by getting a patient to close their eyes and then the therapist places the impaired limb in a position and the patient tries to copy with the other. This is often impaired in neurological patients.

Joint replacement – also known as arthroplasty There is no 'typical' patient who is appropriate for a joint replacement. As with all modern medicine a decision has to made that balances the risks of surgery against the potential improvements. Patient age per se is not an acceptable clinical decision making tool. Generally, the surgical team will wait until pain or disability is severe enough to cause a significant impact on the person's quality of life, where surgery would make things significantly better or prevent a major deterioration. It is quite feasible, for example, to replace the hips of a 16-year-old with severe rheumatoid arthritis. At the time of writing, an artificial joint are still not as efficient as their organic counterparts. If a synthetic joint becomes worn or damaged, it does not repair itself as a normal joint does. It will also not be as efficient at absorbing the stresses and strains of daily life as an organic joint. The field of joint prosthetics is making remarkable improvements, however.

Joint space The term for the space that appears on an X-ray of a joint, it is not, in fact, a space since it is occupied by articular hyaline cartilage, but this is invisible to a traditional X-ray.

Jugular venous pressure (JVP) This is a reflection of the pressure within the right side of the heart. It is estimated by assessing the blood column in the jugular veins with examination performed with the patient lying supine, with the bed head elevated to a 45° angle. When JVP is raised, the neck veins may be distended as high as to the angle of the jaw. In the position described above, venous distension greater than approx 4 cm above the sternal angle is considered to be abnormal. However, examination and

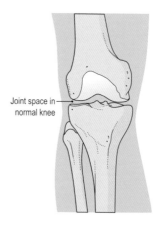

Joint space in normal knee

assessment in the obese patient can be difficult. Raised JVP may occur with hyperinflation, right-sided heart failure and hypervolaemia.

Jumper's knee A musculoskeletal condition. Associated with a small area of degeneration at the tendon attachment at the lower pole of the patella, symptoms are pain and local tenderness.

Justice principle An ethical principle that dictates that we should treat people in the same way unless there are relevant differences among them. It may be considered just, for example, to wait in a bus queue on a 'first come, first served' basis. If, however, somebody in the queue feels unwell and needs to get home, it may be considered just to allow that person to jump the queue.

Juxtacapillary (J) receptors These are stretch receptors located in the lung parenchyma close to the pulmonary capillaries, stimulated by inflammatory processes, congestion and oedema. Tachypnoea, dyspnoea and glottic narrowing result from stimulation of these receptors.

K

Kaposi's sarcoma (KS) A tumour of blood-vessel walls or the lymphatic system. Usually appears as purple spots on the skin, but may also occur internally in addition to or independent of lesions.

Keller's arthroplasty also known as Keller's excision arthroplasty Keller's excision arthroplasty is performed to correct severe hallux valgus deformity.

It involves the excision of the bunion on the first metatarsal and the excision of the proximal part of the first proximal phalanx. Following this operation the great toe is left shorter and more floppy than normal.

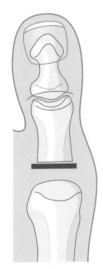

Keller's arthoplasty

Keloid An overgrowth of scar tissue at the site of a skin injury.

Keratin The protein that is a primary constituent of hair, nails and skin.

Keratoderma blennorrhagica Pustules and crusts associated with Reiter's syndrome (Reiter's syndrome is a type of reactive arthritis).

Kernig's sign A sign of meningeal irritation, having placed the hip in full flexion, an attempt to passively extend the knee results in pain and spasm of the hamstrings.

Ketosis Metabolic production of abnormal amounts of ketones. A consequence of diabetes mellitus.

Key points of control These were described by Bobath (1990) as areas of the body from which movement can most easily be controlled. A point in the upper thoracic region is described as the central key point, the pelvis and shoulder girdles as the proximal key points and the hands and the feet as distal key points.

Kilo Prefix meaning a thousand times.

Kinaesthetic sense The sense by which position, weight and movement are perceived. One should be able to tell the difference between perceiving static positions and joint motion.

Kinematic chain exercises See *Closed/open chain exercises*

A kinematic chain is an engineering term used to describe a system of links connected by joints. They may be open or closed.

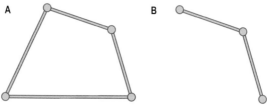

(**A**) Closed kinetic chain; (**B**) Open kinetic chain

The open-chain exercise is defined as an exercise where the distal end of the segment is not against a constraint or a resistance. In a closed-chain exercise, the terminal segment is restrained. For example, a squat is an example of a closed-chain exercise.

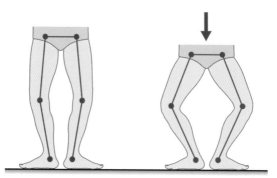

A squat

A leg curl from sitting in a chair is an example of an open-chain exercise.

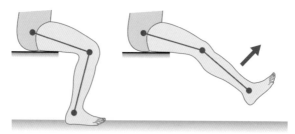

A leg curl

Kinematics Is the science concerned with reporting the exact description of the diverse positions and motions of the body in space.

Kinesi- Pertaining to motion.

Kinesiology The study of body movement.

Kinetics A branch of dynamics that looks at forces that lead to, stop or modify motions of the body.

Kinetic tremor An oscillation that occurs during movement.

Knock knees See *Genu valgum*

Knowledge of performance (KP) A term used to describe the patients awareness of how the movement was performed. Reference to this term is made in the 'motor relearning approach' (Carr & Shepherd 1998) to the management and treatment of neurological patients.

Knowledge of results (KR) Improved information provided about success or mistakes made in achieving functional movements. It is a term used to describe the patient's awareness of the achievement, or not, or of the task. Reference to this term is made in the 'motor relearning approach' (Carr & Shepherd 1998) to the management and treatment of neurological patients.

Kromayer Electrotherapy term – a type of mercury vapour ultra-violet ray (UVR) lamp. UV tube is water cooled to remove infrared radiations so applicator used in contact with skin or in cavities using special applicator.

Kussmaul's breathing This is the over breathing associated with diabetic ketoacidosis (a metabolic acidosis resulting from the build up of excessive ketones from deranged carbohydrate metabolism).

Kyphoscoliosis A postural deformity characterized by anteroposterior and lateral spinal curvature, which may result in a restrictive breathing pattern.

Kyphosis An exaggerated curvature of the spine, in the flexion/extension axis. In the elderly, the most common cause of kyphosis is osteoporosis. This may result in a restrictive lung defect as detected by spirometry.

○ Clinical note If fixed as opposed to adaptive/compensatory then seating and cushions need to be adjusted to ensure appropriate support.

Labelling theory A long-standing and much discussed and criticized socio-logical theory. The central assumption is that deviance is created by society in that social groups create rules and those who infringe these rules are labelled as outsiders. Precisely who is labelled and why depends on the social context. Behaviour may, for example, be considered criminal at one time or in one culture but not at another time or in another culture. Patients and clients may be labelled 'difficult' if they do not comply with the wishes of health professionals.

Labrum Anatomical term meaning edge, rim or lip.

Labyrinthine righting reflexes Stimulation of the labyrinth proprioceptors causes contraction of the neck muscles which bring the head back into its natural position in space.

Labyrinthitis Inflammation of the inner ear and semicircular canals. The structures that normally maintain balance and the perception of body position. Inflammation results in nausea, vomiting and vertigo especially on movement.

Lachman's test (Modified Anterior Draw Test) The patient is supine with the knee resting over the therapists' thigh at around 20–30° of flexion. The physiotherapist grasps around the medial proximal aspect of the tibia with the right hand. The lateral aspect of the patient's femur is stabilized by the therapists left hand. Anterior and posterior translation of the tibia is produced by the physiotherapist's right hand. The Lachman test has been shown to be a sensitive test for the diagnosis of anterior cruciate injury (Kim & Kim 1995).

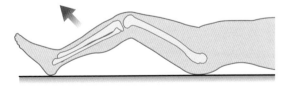

Lachman's test

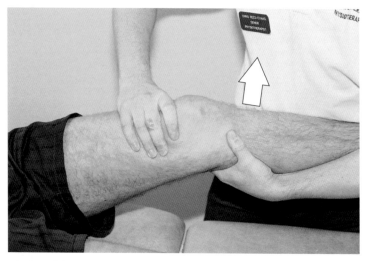

Lachman's test

LACI Lacunar infarction which is a type of stroke.

Lactic acid A byproduct of anaerobic metabolism. It is an intermediate product of carbohydrate metabolism derived mainly from muscle cells and red blood cells. Lactic acid levels may be measured in the bloodstream in conditions of metabolic acidosis.

Lactose intolerance A disorder characterized by abdominal cramps and diarrhoea after the consumption of food containing lactose (for example, milk, ice cream).

Lamina A thin flat plate or layer usually describing part of a vertebrae.

Laminectomy Surgical removal of a portion of the lamina, to provide more room in the vertebral canal. Usually for disc herniation or spinal canal stenosis.

Laparoscope A fibreoptic flexible tube that allows the internal refraction of light for viewing. This device is used in laparoscopic surgery.

Laparotomy General term for abdominal surgery.

Lasegues sign/test See *Neurodynamics*

Laser Electrotherapy term – an acronym for Light Amplification by Stimulated Emission of Radiation. A form of electromagnetic radiation. Wavelength is from 780–904 nm (GaAlAs diode laser) to 904 nm (GaAs diode laser) to 623.8 nm (HeNe gas laser). Three properties distinguish laser from visible light or infrared radiations: it is monochromatic (one wavelength), collimated (minimal divergence of beam) and coherent (in phase). Penetration depth varies from approximately 3 or 4 mm (GaAlAs) to 2 mm (HeNe). Clinical uses are for wound healing and pain control. Dosages measured as energy density, J/cm^2. Clinical utility still not known. Dangers are primarily to eyes and, depending on class of laser, if 3B, 4 or 5, wavelength specific protecting lenses must be warn by patient and therapist.

Lateral Anatomical term meaning further from the midline.

Lateral epicondylitis Also described as 'tennis elbow', but often with no history of sport, it is associated with the origin of the common extensor tendon at the lateral humeral epicondyle.

Lateral longitudinal arch of foot Formed by the calcaneus, cuboid and two lateral metatarsals, it is supported normally by ligaments, intrinsic muscles, and the tendons of extrinsic muscles of the foot.

Lateral release Surgical division of the lateral patellar retinaculum, from the patellar tendon to within the muscle fibres of vastus lateralis. Usually as a treatment of patellofemoral dysfunction, following failed conservative measures.

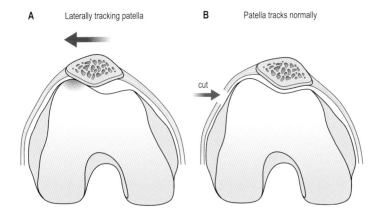

A   Laterally tracking patella   B   Patella tracks normally

cut

Lay referral system A process whereby people who experience signs and symptoms of illness and disease seek the advice of lay people (for example relatives and friends) before, or instead of, seeking medical advice. If medical advice is obtained, the lay referral system may be used to evaluate the advice that is given.

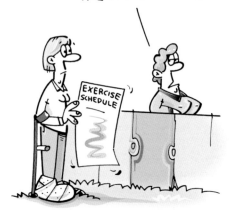

LBP Common medical abbreviation – Low back pain.

LCL Common medical abbreviation – Lateral collateral ligament.

LDL Common medical abbreviation – Low-density lipoprotein.

Lead pipe rigidity A phenomenon encountered in people with Parkinson's disease and other extra pyramidal disorders, it manifests as a uniform resistance to movement throughout the available range of movement.

Learned non-use This is a term used to describe a state where a patient has some recovery in an affected limb, but is not using it functionally as they have habitually learnt to not use it. It is often used to describe patients with recovery in the arm following stroke, where the patient is not using the motor activity they have in daily ADL. Some researchers, for treatment of this presentation advocate the use of constraint-induced therapy.

Learning The acquisition of knowledge and understanding, or the development of skills or behaviour.

Learning difficulties The definition of learning difficulties has been dominated by the medical model of disability. Criteria for the diagnosis of learning difficulties include low intelligence (as measured by standardized IQ tests) and 'social incompetence' in terms of norms in many areas of social life. More recently, this has been challenged in a number of ways by people with learning difficulties and their supporters who have questioned the labelling and associated marginalization of people who are labelled in this way.

Lecture The traditional form of university teaching where the teacher talks to the assembled students and presents all of the material they feel the students should have.

Legionella pneumophila An acute bacterial pneumonia characterized by a flu-like illness with fever, chills, muscular aches and headache.

Leg length See *True* and *apparent leg length*

A measure from the anterior superior iliac spine, to the tip of the medial malleolus, although this may be inaccurate in the presence of pelvic rotation or asymmetry. Leg-length discrepancies may not be significant if they are less than 6 mm, many asymptomatic patients have a leg length difference of up to 12 mm.

With the person stood or lying with their feet 18 inches apart:

- true leg length – measure from ASIS to medial malleolus
- apparent leg length – measure umbilicus to medial malleolus.

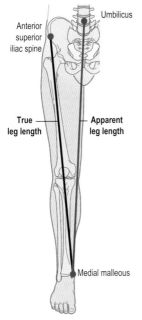

True and apparent leg lengths

Length–tension curve This relates to the relationship between a muscle's ability to contract and its length. Muscles that have been lengthened for example by being immobilized in a plaster, generate tension more slowly than muscles that have been shortened. Short muscles are able to generate tension quickest and so tend to be recruited first. This is a fundamental principal to serial casting. Imagine an elastic band held around your index fingers, it would generate tension as you pull your fingers apart; now if you take a smaller elastic band it will generate tension quicker.

Length–tension relationship This refers to the fact that isometric tension generation in skeletal muscle is a function of the magnitude of overlap between actin and myosin filaments. Maximum force is generated within the muscle when there is maximum overlap between actin and myosin filaments.

Leukaemia A disease characterized by an abnormal increase in the number of leucocytes in the tissues with or without a corresponding increase of those in the circulating blood. It is classified according to the type of leucocyte most prominently involved.

Levodopa A drug that crosses the blood–brain barrier and is used in the treatment of Parkinson's disease.

Lewis hunting reaction See *Ice therapy*

Lewis triple response The changes, which make up this vascular component were described in 1927 by Lewis and are known as the Lewis triple response. This flush, flare and wheal effect can be demonstrated by drawing a blunt instrument firmly across the skin (for convenience the forearm is often used) and watching the following sequence of events, which are similar irrespective of the type of injury:

1. Instantly, a white line forms following the 'injury'. This is due to vasoconstriction of the underlying arterioles as a direct response to the injury and is only transient. This vasoconstriction is not considered to be fully part of the inflammatory process.

2. A flush rapidly follows, seen as a dull red line which occurs as the capillaries dilate. To the naked eye, the vasodilation can give the impression that the effected tissue actually contains a greater number of blood vessels. This dilation may last for as long as the inflammatory process persists.

3. The flare where an irregular red zone develops. This has occurred due to the response of the surrounding arterioles, which have been affected by both nervous and chemical mediators.

4. The formation of a 'wheal' (a raised area of skin) occurs owing to the fluid passing out of the blood vessels and into the extravascular space, so leading to oedema.

Secondly (though it occurs at the same time as the above process), the endothelial cells that form the internal wall of the blood vessels retract such that they no longer form a completely continuous lining of the vessel. Consequently, the vessels become 'leaky' to the extent that fluid, namely water and some of the salts and smaller proteins (one of these is fibrinogen), contained in plasma may pass out directly into the extra cellular spaces of the damaged area.

Thirdly, the fluid exudate becomes transformed into a cellular exudate. This is achieved through circulating neutrophils leaving the blood vessels and entering the extra cellular spaces in the area of tissue damage. In the first 6–24 h of an inflammatory response it is the neutrophils that predominate; between 24 and 48 h, however, they are superseded by monocytes and lymphocytes acting in a similar way (Court & Lea 2003).

LFA Common medical abbreviation – Low-friction arthroplasty.

LFT (X2) Common medical abbreviation – Lung- or liver-function tests.

Lifelong learning (LLL) Lifelong learning is defined as learning that continues throughout an individual's lifetime. A theme that aims to ensure that the workforce is equipped to do the jobs that will contribute to high-quality public services and promote prosperity in the UK. Lifelong learning can range from the most highly formal and structured educational activities to the most informal modes of learning. Lifelong learning encompasses many different levels, purposes, contents, outcomes and motives for learning. Lifelong learning can be provided in a variety of learning styles and approaches.

With kind permission of Dariel Terry. Assistant Professor of Information System Technology. Northern Virginia Community College. USA

Lifestyle A term with different meanings. It can denote the contrasting ways of living of different groups in society, such as young affluent people, old people and unemployed people. It also conceptualizes alternative ways of living, evident in values, behaviour, dress, food and consumption generally.

Life-years gained Average years of life gained per person as a result of the intervention.

Likert scale A form of gathering data whereby a respondent circles or ticks a category, such as in the table below.

Likert Scale

Strongly Agree	Agree	Undecided	Disagree	Strongly Disagree

The answers may then be coded, e.g. 1-2-3-4-5, but this remains just a coding. The data collected are ordinal, i.e. they have an inherent order or sequence, but one cannot assume that the differences between each answer are equal in size, i.e. the scale is not linear.

Limbic system Collective term for a collection of brain structures at or near the edge (limbus) of the medial wall of the cerebral hemisphere, includes the hippocampus, amygdala and fornicate gyrus. The limbic system exerts an important influence upon the endocrine and autonomic motor systems; its functions also appear to affect motivational and mood states.

Limits of stability The range within which a person can move the furthest in any direction without losing their balance or making a postural adjustment, i.e. stepping.

Linea alba A band running vertically the entire length of the anterior abdominal wall, receiving the attachments of the oblique and transverse abdominal muscles.

Literature review See *Electronic bibliography software*

A literature review is an attempt to classify and evaluate what researchers have written about a particular topic, it must be organized according to a guiding theme such as your own research project, dissertation or problem. A good literature review does not merely list as many articles as possible; rather, it should recognize relevant information and synthesize and evaluate it according to the guiding concept you have determined for yourself, i.e. an informed evaluation of the literature. Physiotherapy students need to be able to scan the literature efficiently using manual or computerized methods to identify useful articles and books. You will need to have the ability to apply principles of analysis to identify those studies that are unbiased and valid. Your readers or examiners will want more just than a descriptive list of articles and books.

Organize your review into logical, informative sections that present themes or identify trends, do not begin every paragraph of your review with a list of names of researchers.

Tips for conducting a good literature review

- Organize the information and relate it to the research question that you are asking.
- Synthesize results into a summary of what is generally accepted and which areas are not so clearly understood.

- Identify controversy whenever it appears in the literature.
- Develop questions for further research.

Liver function test (LFT) A test that measures the blood serum level of several enzymes produced by the liver. Elevated liver-function test results can be a sign of liver damage.

°**LKKS** Common medical abbreviation – No liver, kidney, kidney, spleen.

Lobectomy Removal of a lobe usually refers to the lung or brain.

Lobes Divisions of the lungs. The lungs are divided into lobes; the right lung contains three (upper middle and lower) and the left contains two (the upper which has a subdivision called the lingular segment and the lower lobe).

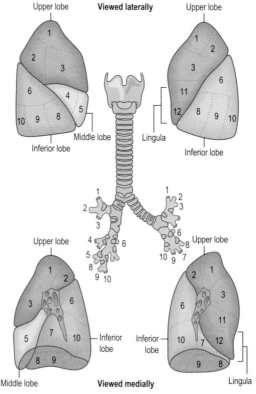

The trachea and the distribution of the main and segmental bronchi.
Bronchopulmonary segments: 1: apical; 2: posterior; 3: anterior; 4: lateral;
5: medial; 6: apical basal; 7: medial basal; 8: anterior basal; 9: lateral basal;
10: posterior basal; 11: superior; 12: inferior

Locked-in syndrome This is where a person has intellectual functioning, but is unable to express this either verbally or through movement due to neurological damage. Such patients are described as 'locked in' – they are locked in their body and unable to express thoughts or emotions. Often such patients can learn to communicate through eye movements, or other small movements. This may be a transient stage.

Locus of control A term from psychological theory referring to a person's generalized sense of responsibility and control over his or her life. People with an internal locus of control feel responsible for their lives and expect their behaviour to have an effect on events. People with an external locus of control are more inclined to believe that life events occur through fate or chance rather than their own actions. People may have an internal or an external locus of control in different spheres of their lives. Locus of control can be measured on a standardized questionnaire.

Long-term memory Information that is retained relatively permanently.

Longwave ultrasound (LWUS) Traditionally therapeutic, US employs a frequency of 1–3 MHz. Claims have been made that LWUS, with a frequency of 45 kHz, is superior to MHz US for treating soft tissue injuries. These claims have been refuted by others, who state that the beam divergence and the energy reflection of LWUS result in a more superficial effect. By employing a lower frequency, the wavelength will be greater (assuming the velocity in tissue is approximately constant) and, hence, the theoretical penetration depth will be greater. This is estimated at around 20 times more than traditional MHz ultrasound, though it is argued that because the majority of this energy will be absorbed in the near field, the modality will actually be more effective in the superficial tissues. This can account (in part at least) for the superficial heating effect experienced by many patients.

The divergent beam means that the US energy will be more diffuse at depth with LWUS. It has been estimated that the energy content of the beam has reduced to 50% at 0.5 cm and down to 10% at 2 cm from the surface. There is little clinical research evidence with regards LWUS and no substantive evidence to determine whether its physiological and cellular effects are the same as traditional MHz ultrasound. Anecdotal evidence from clinical practice is largely supportive.

Loose body An object, located within a joint that has become detached and is able to move around within the joint. A common cause of locking of a joint.

Lordosis Curve of the spine, whereby there is hollowing. Normal lordosis is seen in the lumbar spine, although variances exist.
See *Kyphosis*

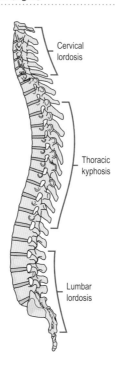

Cervical
lordosis

Thoracic
kyphosis

Lumbar
lordosis

Lordosis

Lower motor neurone (signs) These are factors that indicate that there may be
some damage to the structures described as the lower motor neurone. Signs
may include loss of the reflexes, marked wasting, no muscle tone and no
muscle activity.

Low-frequency current Electrotherapy term – an alternative name for pulsed
current. The problem is the lack of agreement as to how to define low,
medium and high. In clinical practice the frequency is usually from 1 Hz
to approximately 200 Hz (it must be less than 1 kHz or it becomes a medium
frequency current).

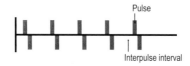

Pulse

Interpulse interval

Low frequency current

LTOT Common medical abbreviation – Long-term oxygen therapy.

Lumbar puncture A lumbar puncture is the insertion of a needle into the fluid within the spinal canal. It is used to analyze cerebro-spinal fluid. It is used in the diagnosis of many neurological conditions, e.g. in sub-arachnoid haemorrhage (SAH) it is said to be zanthrochromic if blood is present this confirms SAH and in multiple sclerosis it reveals local production of immunoglobulin within the central nervous system.

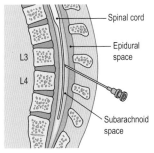

Spinal cord

Epidural space

L3

L4

Subarachnoid space

Lumbar puncture

Lumbar spine Made up of five vertebrae, commonly called the lower back.

Lumbosacral plexus See *Sacral plexus*

Lung function This is a measure of how well the lungs work. Assessment includes spirometry, arterial blood gases and measures of gas transfer and lung volumes.

Lung volume reduction surgery (LVRS) A procedure designed to improve respiratory function in patients with severe bullous emphysema. By excising the bullous tissue and shaping, the remaining lung expansion of the healthy lung and doming of the diaphragm can be achieved. This results in improved respiratory mechanics and symptomatic relief of dyspnoea (breathlessness). Patients should undergo a period of pulmonary rehabilitation preoperatively to maximize their respiratory function (Dyson 2003).

Lung volumes

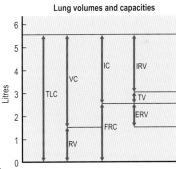

Lung volumes and capacities

Litres

IC

VC

IRV

TLC

TV

ERV

FRC

RV

Lung volumes
The total lung capacity can be divided into various volumes:

• Tidal volume (TV) is the volume of air moved into or out of the lungs during quiet breathing at rest.
• Inspiratory reserve volume (IRV) is the volume of air additional to TV that can be inspired during a maximum inspiration.
• Expiratory reserve volume (ERV) is the volume of air additional to TV that can be expired during a maximum expiration.
• Residual volume (RV) is the volume of air remaining in the lungs after a maximum expiration.

Lupus A systemic autoimmune disease. Individuals with lupus will produce antibodies to their own body tissues. The resultant inflammation can cause kidney damage, arthritis, pericarditis and vasculitis.

Lyme disease A bacterial disease. Infection occurs after the bite of an infected tick.

Lymphoedema Chronic and progressive swelling caused by a low output failure of the lymphatic system.

LYSIS The process of destroying cells.

Maitland symbols

Symbols

↕	Central postero-anterior pressure (PAs) with a Ⓛ inclination
↑	Central anteroposterior pressures (APs)
⌐•	Unilateral PAs on Ⓛ⤜ with a medial inclination
⌐•	Unilateral APs on the Ⓛ
←•—	Transverse pressure towards Ⓛ
↻	Rotation of head, thorax or pelvis towards Ⓛ
⌡	Lateral flexion towards Ⓛ
←•→	Longitudinal movement (state cephalad or caudad)
⌐↓	Unilateral PAs at angle of Ⓡ 2nd rib
⌐↓	Further laterally on Ⓡ 2nd rib
•⌐↑	Unilateral APs on Ⓡ
CT ↗	Cervical traction in flexion
CT ↑	Cervical traction in neutral (sitting)
IVCT ↑	Sitting
IVCT ↗	Lying
IVCT ↗ 10 3/0 15	Intermittent variable cervical traction in some degree of neck flexion, the strength of pull being 10 kg with a 3-second hold period, no rest period, for a treatment time lasting 15 minutes
LT	Lumbar traction
LT 30/15	Lumbar traction, the strength of pull being 30 kg for a treatment time of 15 minutes
LT crk 15/5	Lumbar traction with hips and knees flexed; 15 kg for 5 minutes
IVLT 50 0/0 10	Intermittent variable lumbar traction, the strength of pull being 50 kg, with no hold period and no rest period, for a treatment time lasting 10 minutes

Maitland grades

- Grade I – A small-amplitude movement near the starting position of the range out of resistance and used to treat pain.
- Grade II – A large-amplitude movement that carries well into the range. It can occupy any part of the range that is free of muscle spasm and resistance. Used commonly to treat pain.
- Grade III – A large-amplitude movement, but one that does move into muscle spasm and resistance. Used commonly to treat both pain and resistance.
- Grade IV – A small-amplitude movement stretching into muscle spasm and resistance. Used to treat end of range resistance.

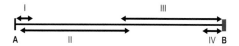

Grades in a normal range having a hard end-feel

Malignant The term that tends to be used with reference to cancer. Characterized by progressive and uncontrolled growth. Compare with benign, which means not dangerous to health or progressive.

Malignant melanoma A tumour that arises from the pigment-producing cells of the deeper layers of the skin. Melanoma is the leading cause of death attributable to skin lesions.

Mallet finger A common condition due to the rupture of the long extensor tendon of the finger, at its insertion into the base of the distal phalanx of the finger.

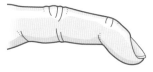

Mallet finger

Mal tracking patella Abnormal tracking of the patella (usually laterally) can be a cause of anterior knee pain and can be caused by abnormal foot or knee biome- chanics or soft-tissue length. For surgical management see *Lateral release*. As with all conditions, treatment depends on the cause but physiotherapy techniques include vastus medialis obliquus (VMO) exercises, taping, insoles if the foot is the primary cause of the problem or patellar mobilizations.

Mammogram A mammogram is an X-ray test that produces an image of breast tissue. Mammography is used to visualize normal and abnormal structures within the breasts.

Manipulation Maitland (2001) defines the term manipulation as all kinds of passive movement or, more specifically, as small-amplitude thrust tech- nique performed with speed not within control of the patient.

Mannitol A medication given to reduce brain swelling and raised intracranial pressure. It is also used to temporarily disrupt the blood–brain barrier prior to some forms of chemotherapy.

Manual guidance This is where a movement or task that is performed by an individual is helped by an external force, usually by a therapist as part of a treatment intervention, i.e. if there is weakness present the patient may require assistance to fulfil the goal of movement.

➕ Clinical note It is important to withdraw manual guidance as part of the re-learning process so that patients can re-educate their own movement.

Manual hyperinflation This is the intentional hyperinflation of the chest, usually by means of a handbagging circuit. This technique is used to facilitate the removal of secretions and reinflate areas of collapsed lung in the intubated patient.

Manual therapy This encompasses many therapeutic modalities including manipulation, mobilization and soft-tissue techniques.

MAOI Common medical abbreviation – Monoamine oxidase inhibitors. These are drugs that are used in the treatment of depression

Marburg's disease A form of multiple sclerosis.

March fracture A stress or fatigue fracture affecting the metatarsals in the foot.

Marfan's syndrome A hereditary condition that affects connective tissue. Symptoms and signs include tall lean body type, long extremities and abnormal joint mobility, aneurysms of the aorta may also occur Interestingly, some authorities believe that the pharaoh Akhenaten – father of Tut-ankh-amum, suffered from this condition in life. Some believe President Abraham Lincoln also had Marfan's syndrome.

Mark:space ratio Electrotherapy term – usually only used for pulsed ultrasound. See *On:off ratio*

Mastectomy The surgical removal of the entire breast, usually to treat serious breast disease, such as breast cancer.

Maximal voluntary torque (MVT) Maximal torque produced using a voluntary muscle contraction. Can be isometric (maximal voluntary isometric torque [MVIT]), isotonic or isokinetic. Used in a ratio with electrically initiated torque (EIT), but not reliable and so not recommended.

Maximum expiratory pressure (MEP) This is an effort-dependant measure of the maximal or peak static expiratory effort sustained for one second, measured in centimetres of water pressure using a breathing circuit with attached manometer and flanged mouthpiece. This is used as an index of global muscle weakness.

Maximum inspiratory pressure (MIP) This is an effort-dependant measure of the maximal or peak static inspiratory effort sustained for one second, measured in centimetres of water pressure using a breathing circuit with attached manometer and flanged mouthpiece. This is used as an index of global muscle strength.

Maximum voluntary ventilation (MVV) This is a measure of the ability to maximally sustain ventilation. The subject breathes as quickly and as deeply as possible over a 15-min period.

McKenzie approach The McKenzie approach of mechanical diagnosis and therapy was developed by New Zealand physiotherapist Robin McKenzie and is now used worldwide by clinicians and patients for the management of spinal and non-spinal musculoskeletal problems. During the history and physical examination, the symptomatic and mechanical responses to movement and postures are determined; the analysis includes repeated movements and sustained positions. An understanding of these responses allows classification into one of the mechanical syndromes: derangement, dysfunction or postural syndrome. Direction-specific exercises are then used to treat symptoms and restore function, with the emphasis always being on patient-generated forces to maximize patient independence. Management is dependent upon good patient education. Minimal therapeutic force is always used, but force progressions are introduced if there is failure to improve. A combination of exercise and therapist intervention is used if this is necessary to produce change. There are several textbooks that describe mechanical diagnosis and therapy in detail: *Lumbar Spine* (McKenzie 1981), *Cervical and Thoracic Spine* (McKenzie 1990), *Extremities* (McKenzie 2000) and *Lumbar Spine, 2nd edition* (McKenzie 2003). Also there are Treat Your Own Back/Neck booklets that are written specifically for patients. There is now a wealth of research that has been done to investigate components of the approach. This research has looked at mechanical diagnosis and therapy both as an assessment tool and as a treatment approach. For instance, the symptom response of centralization has consistently been associated with a good prognosis; the assessment system is reliable when used by those who are well trained; as an intervention it is equal to chiropractic manipulation and strength-training exercises. There is an international education programme available to qualified healthcare professionals. This has five sequential courses, a credentialing exam and a diploma programme.

Go to http://www.mckenziemdt.org and then to the research page. This contains a regularly updated annotated reference list of most relevant research, listed under a variety of headings.

MCL Common medical abbreviation – Medial collateral ligament usually refers to the collateral ligaments of the knee joint, but do not forget that there is also a medial collateral at the ankle and the elbow joint.

McMurray's test A test of the integrity of the menisci of the knee joint. A positive test occurs if pain is elicited or a snap or click of the joint will occur if the meniscus is torn.

Technique
Patient lies supine, with the knee flexed to 45°, hip flexed to 45°. Examiner braces lower leg, one hand holds ankle, other hand holds knee.

Medial meniscus assessment
Assess for pain on palpation. Palpate medial joint line with knee flexed. Assess for 'click' suggesting meniscus relocation. Apply valgus stress to flexed knee. Externally rotate leg (toes point outward). Slowly extend the knee while still in valgus.

Lateral meniscus assessment
Repeat above with varus stress and internal rotation.

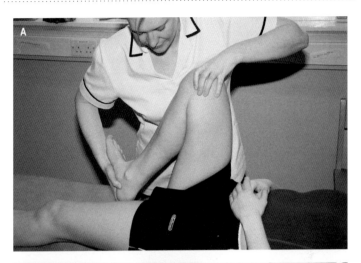

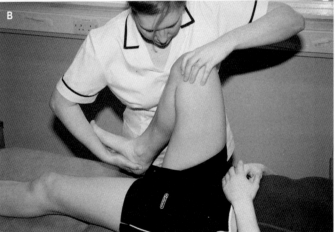

McMurray's test

Abnormal finding The examiner may be able to detect clicking or snapping sounds when performing this test, since there are various structures in the knee joint that may produce these signs, it is easy for this test to produce a false-positive result.

MDT Common medical abbreviation – Multidisciplinary team.

ME Common medical abbreviation – Myalgic encephalomyopathy.

Mean Research term – the average number in a set of values.

Mechanical ventilation See *Ventilators*

Mechanoreceptor A receptor that responds to mechanical pressure or distortion, e.g. touch receptors in the skin.

Meconium Dark-green material in the intestines at birth, which is the first stool that a baby passes.

Medial Nearer the midline.

Medial epicondylitis – also known as golfers elbow Inflammation of the tendons that insert at the medical epicondyle (of the humerus) at the elbow. Symptoms include pain on resisted wrist-joint flexion.

Median Research term – when values are arranged in order of magnitude, the median is the middle value for odd numbers of values and the average of the two middle values in the case of an even number of values.

Median nerve A large nerve, comprising segments from the cervical spine, that is involved in neural function of the upper limb. Commonly entrapped in the carpal tunnel of the wrist, resulting in carpal tunnel syndrome.

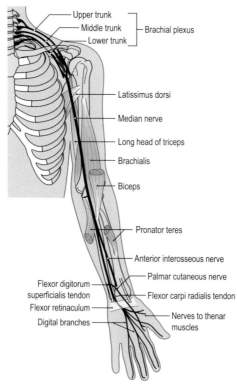

The course of the median nerve

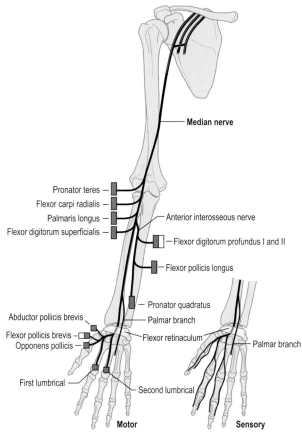

Muscles supplied by median nerve

Median plane A vertical plane passing through the centre of the body dividing it into left and right.

Median sternotomy The surgical incision that involves division of the sternum.

Medicalization The predominance or orthodoxy of a set of ideas, known as the biomedical model, for conceptualizing health and illness and a whole range of social phenomena, such as disability, bereavement and homosexuality. Processes that were once considered an ordinary part of life, such as childbirth, can thus become 'medicalized' and under the control of medical professionals.

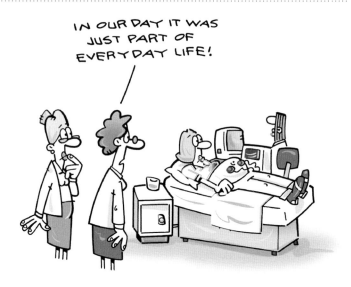

Medical research council (MRC) dyspnoea scale A measurement of breathlessness useful in providing an indication of exercise limitations.

Medium frequency current (MFAC) Electrotherapy term – an alternative name for alternating current in the frequency range of 1 kHz to 10 kHz. Bursts of pulses with a frequency of between 1 kHz and 10 kHz. Individual pulses may be sinusoidal, rectangular or triangular. See *Russian* and *interferential currents*. Russian has a frequency of 2.5 kHz and interferential typically 4 kHz or between 2 kHz and 10 kHz.

Medline An electronic database containing information relating to medicine and healthcare.

Mediastinum The space between the two pleural sacs in the thorax.

Medical devices All products, except medicines, used in healthcare for the diagnosis, prevention, monitoring or treatment of illness or disability.

Medicines and healthcare products regulatory agency (MHRA) The Executive Agency of the Department of Health protecting and promoting public health and patient safety by ensuring that medicines, healthcare products and medical equipment meet appropriate standards of safety, quality, performance and effectiveness and are used safely.

MEDLARS (Medical literature analysis retrieval system) This is the computer on which 'Medline' and 'AIDS Line' resides at the National Library of Medicine.

Meissner corpuscle Found in small elevations of the dermis that project up into the epidermis of glabrous skin, exclusively. These receptors respond to low-frequency vibration. They lie close to the surface of the skin and have small receptive fields, but adapt rapidly to stimuli.

Membrane attack complex A ring of complement fragments that has the ability to insert itself onto an invading cell and cause its destruction.

Memory A mental function that stores ideas, sensations and learned experiences for recall.

Meniere's disease Is an episodic disorder of the inner ear affecting balance and hearing, characterized by vertigo, dizziness and loss of hearing in one or both ears; tinnitus may also occur.

Meningioma These are slowly growing primary intracranial tumours arising from the arachnoid granulations. They are more common in women aged between 40 and 60 years old. They are usually benign, but a malignant form exists.

Meningitis Acute inflammation of the meninges, the membranes that cover the brain or spinal cord. It is usually caused by an infection. It can be viral or bacterial. The classical signs are fever, headache and neck stiffness. It can also cause photophobia and a skin rash. It is often preceded by an upper-respiratory-tract infection.

Meningocele A type of lesion seen in spina bifida, another form is myelomeningocele.

See *Spina bifida* and *Myelomeningocele*

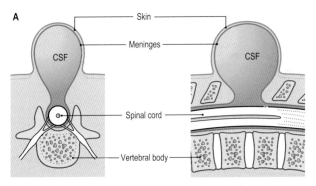

Types of spinal lesion in spina bifida. (**A**) Meningocele: no neural tissue outside the vertebral canal

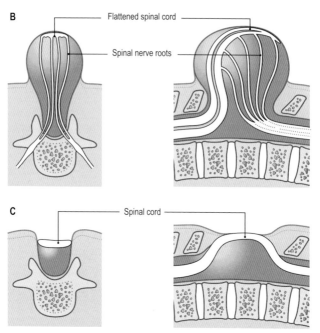

Types of spinal lesion in spina bifida. (**B**) Myelomeningocele: neural tissue and nerve roots may be outside the vertebral canal. There may be fatty tissue or a bony spur present. (**C**) Rachischisis: there is no sac and the neural tissue lies open on the surface as a flattened plaque. Redrawn from McCarthy GT 1992 Physical Disability in Childhood: An Interdisciplinary Approach to Management, Churchill Livingstone

Meningococcal meningitis An acute infectious disease affecting children and young adults, headache, vomiting, convulsions, neck photophobia, constipation, cutaneous sensitivity and a rash.

Meniscectomy Removal of a torn section (or complete) of meniscus. Usually performed arthroscopically.

Meniscus The menisci are fibrocartilaginous structures that function to increase the joint congruency (fitting together) of joint surfaces, act as shock absorbers, assist in joint lubrication and provide joint stabilization. Often damaged, particularly in the knee, when there is a rotational force.

Menopause Menopause is the cessation of menstruation. It has significant implications for a woman's health and quality of life and is, thus, of great relevance to the physiotherapist.

Biochemical and metabolic changes following menopause may cause distressing symptoms that can adversely affect quality of life (Brook 2003).

Mental illness Predominantly characterized as a mental pathology with disturbances of mental functioning, such as delusions, hallucinations, excessive elation or depression. The medical connotations of this term have been considered by some to be misleading or to serve the purposes of powerful groups within society. Social scientists have developed understandings of the causes of mental illnesses and of mental illness itself as social phenomena that set boundaries of what is deemed acceptable mental functioning in different cultures and societies and which regulates human conduct. People have, for example, been deemed mentally ill because of their political beliefs or because their behaviour violates a cultural norm.

Mental practice This is gaining in popularity as part of the rehabilitation process (and is also well used in the sporting arena). It is thought that if someone thinks about performing a task and mentally repeats the process in their head, it is sufficient to cause modulation of neural activity in the brain.

MEP Abbreviation for motor-evoked potential.

Meralgia paresthetica A compression neuropathy of the lateral cutaneous nerve of the thigh.

MESH Medical subject heading. Term used by National Library of Medicine.

Mesothelioma A rare malignant pleural disease, associated with previous asbestos exposure, unresponsive to all known interventions.

Meta-analysis A statistical technique for combining the results of a number of studies that address the same question and report on the same outcomes to produce a summary result. The aim is to derive more precise and clear information from a large data pool. A meta-analysis is thought more likely to reliably confirm or refute a hypothesis than the individual trials.

Metabolic acidosis May occur following ingestion of acids or generation of excess acid by the body.

Metabolic alkalosis Occurs following vomiting where $H+$ ions are lost.

Metaphysis The end of the actively growing diaphysis of a long bone below the epiphyseal plate.

Metastasis The transfer of disease from one organ to another not connected with it. It tends to be used in reference to malignant tumours.

Metered dose inhaler (MDI) A pressurized canister of aerosolixed drug for self-administration of exact doses. When used with a spacer device by lung-disease patients, lung deposition of pulmonary medication is markedly improved.

Microcephaly An abnormally small brain.

Microstreaming (cellular streaming) The phenomenon that occurs in certain electrotherapy modalities, in particular ultrasound. It is thought to affect cell membrane permeability and, therefore, affect tissue repair.

Microwave Electrotherapy term – an electromagnetic radiation with a frequency in the range 2.450 MHz to approximately 433 MHz. Currently most commonly used frequency 2.450 MHz, is the least effective for heating as **EMR** wavelength is inverse to penetration. Lower frequencies may become more commonly available leaving the higher ones for communications. Used for deep heating, but less frequently than ultrasound or **SWD**. Like SWD use, it is contraindicated within 3–5 m of a patient with an indwelling stimulator or pump and there is a risk of burns if used over indwelling metal implants. Risks common to all clinically used methods of heating are also relevant.

Micturition The process of urination.

Middle cerebral artery This is the largest branch of the internal carotid artery. This artery is a common site for occlusion by an embolus or thrombus in stroke.

Midline This is an imaginary line that runs through the centre of the body and thus gives a reference point for assessing the anterior–posterior and rotatory alignment of individual parts of the body, i.e. head, shoulders girdles and trunk.

Midline shift This term refers to a movement of the midline (see above) from the centre of the body.

> ✚ Clinical note Due to tonal changes following a stroke, it is common to see a midline shift. The shift is more commonly away from the hemiplegic side, but can occur towards the hemiplegic side.

> See *Pusher Syndrome*

Mind–body dualism A philosophical position that takes the view that the mind and the body are essentially distinct entities with separate realms of existence. This position lies at the ideological roots of contemporary orthodox medical practice, but is increasingly being challenged by the view that the mind and body are linked and influence each other. Excessive mental stress can, for example, lead to physical ill-health.

Minimal clinical important difference (MCID) (of outcome scores) A means of interpreting the score generated by an outcome measure. 'The smallest difference in score in the domain of interest which patients perceive as beneficial, and which would mandate, in the absence of troublesome side effects and excessive costs, a change in the patient's management' (Jaeschke et al. 1989).

Mitchell's osteotomy A distal osteotomy of the first metatarsal. It is commonly used in cases of hallux valgus.
The procedure entails:
- lateral displacement of the distal end of the first metatarsal
- slight shortening of the bone
- tightening of the medial soft tissues to correct the valgus angle at the first metatarsophalangeal joint.

Mitigating circumstances Circumstances offered by a student as a reason for poor performance in assessment procedures.

Mitochondrion The power plant of most cells of the body.

Mitral regurgitation Mitral regurgitation is the most common lesion of rheumatic heart disease. Changes in the chordae tendonae and papillary muscle of one or both cusps, or dilation of the valve ring, cause the valve to remain open during systole. Incomplete valve closure permits backflow of blood from the left ventricle to the left atrium during systole (Moore 2003).

Mitral stenosis A heart condition. Mitral stenosis is more common in women than men and the most frequent cause is rheumatic endocarditis. Scarring or fusion of the valve cusps, so that the valve opening becomes funnel shaped, causes mitral stenosis and calcification of the valve in middle age makes it more narrow and non-compliant (Moore 2003).

Mixed economy of welfare A means of describing the diversity of ways in which services are funded and delivered. This includes the statutory, voluntary and private sectors as well as informal care.

MMR Common medical abbreviation – Measles-mumps-rubella (vaccine).

MND An abbreviation of motor neurone disease.

Mobilization This is a passive movement performed in such a way that it can be controlled by the patient. This includes passive physiological movements and passive accessory movements through grades I–IV.

Rotation mobilizations

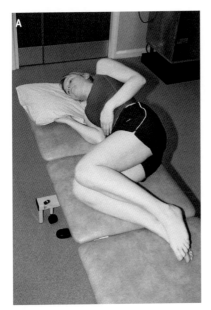

Patient position grade I

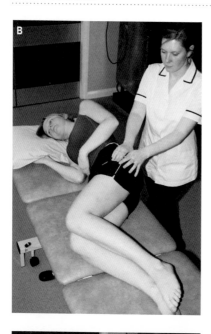

Demonstration of grade I technique

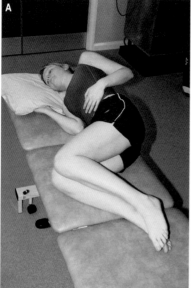

Patient position grade II

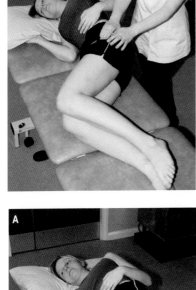

Demonstration of grade II technique

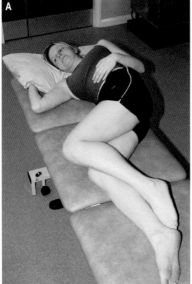

Patient position grade III

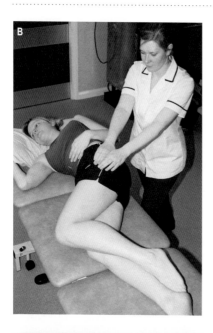

Demonstration of grade III technique

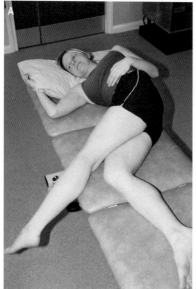

Patient position grade IV

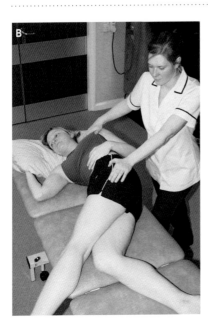

Demonstration of grade IV technique

Mode Research term – the mode is the value that occurs most often.

Modified Ashworth scale See *Ashworth scale*

Modified New York criteria Criteria for the diagnosis of ankylosing spondylitis (1984):

1. Low-back pain for at least 3 months, improved by exercise and not relieved by rest.
2. Limitation of lumbar spine movement in sagittal and frontal planes.
3. Chest expansion decreased relative to normal values for age and sex.
4. Bilateral sacroiliitis, grade 2–4.
5. Unilateral sacroiliitis, grade 3–4.

Modified Schober test See *Schober test*

Modulation Electrotherapy term – systematic variations in one or more characteristics of a current. For example: amplitude modulation occurs with crossed sinusoidal currents with quadripolar and premodulated interferential therapy (see interferential), the amplitude of successive pulses in each beat systematically increases to a peak and then decreases. The process repeats in the next beat (see *Interferential figure*). Some TENS machines offer frequency or pulse duration modulations or a combination of these to reduce adaptation to electrical stimulation.

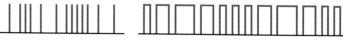

A Frequency modulated   **B** Pulse duration modulated

Monoparesis Paresis affecting a single limb or part of a limb.

Monophasic Electrotherapy term – a pulse with 1 phase.
See *Phase* and *HVPS*

Monteggia fracture Angulated fracture at the junction of the proximal and middle third of ulna accompanied by anterior dislocation of the radial head.

Morbidity The condition of being diseased or sick. Sometimes used to refer to complications.

Mortality To be subject to death. Though may be used to mean just 'death', i.e. mortality rate.

Mortality rate A measurement of the number of deaths per year in a population. For example, the infant mortality rate is the number of deaths in the first year of life per 1000 live births. Infant and child mortality rates are crude but useful indicators of poverty and development.

Morton's neuroma Painful swelling of one of the digital branches of the plantar nerves. Occurs usually at the bifurcation of the nerve as it lies between the two adjacent metatarsal heads. The most common site is between the third and fourth metatarsal heads.

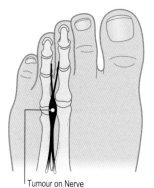

Tumour on Nerve

Morton's neuroma

Mossy fibre One of two fibre types (the other is a climbing fibre) carrying information to the cerebellar cortex.

Motivation A general term denoting the directing and regulation of goal-seeking and need-satisfying behaviour, thinking and emotions.

This is vitally important in the rehabilitation process and learning of skills. Motivation can be enhanced through achievement of goals and a positive learning environment.

⊕ Clinical note Motivation can be affected following brain injury due to factors such as poor memory, depression, cognitive and perceptual deficits.

Motor assessment scale This is an outcome measure used to assess gross motor function. It has a modified version called the Modified Motor Assessment Scale (MMAS). It was developed by J.H. Carr and R.B. Shepherd and so is used by neurological physiotherapists using the motor re-learning approach.

Motor control Being able to control the body movements in a meaningful and functional way.

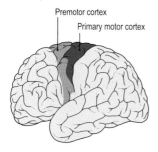

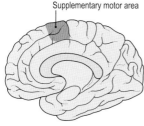

The three main motor areas of the cerebral cortex of the human brain. These locations are only approximate since the detailed neuroanatomical and neurophysiological studies that have been performed in monkeys have not been performed in humans

Motor cortex This is an area of the brain that contains the primary, premotor and supplementary motor areas.

Motor end plate The postsynaptic membrane at the neuromuscular junction.

Motor evoked potentials This is the stimulation of a nerve, the brain or spinal cord usually by an electrical (or magnetic) impulse and are recorded using EMG. Also abbreviated to MEP.

Motoricity index A measure of limb function with a maximum score of 100 for normal subjects. Used in neurological rehabilitation as a measure of function (impairment). Severe paralysis is defined as a score of 0–32, moderate as 33–64 and mild as 65–99.

Motor learning/relearning The attainment of functional movement skills based on experience and feedback on eventual outcome.

Motor neurone Nerves that supply the muscle. Each muscle is served by at least one motor nerve that contains hundreds of motor axons.

Motor neurone disease Commonly abbreviated to MND, this is a disease characterized by the progressive degeneration of anterior horn cells, corticospinal tracts and brain stem nuclei. Clinical features include loss of movement, pain, dyspnoea, dysarthria, dysphagia and other problems depending on the part of the nervous system affected. Sensation and cognitive functions remains intact.

See table below for more information.

Lesions in motor neurone disease and their related symptoms

Site of lesion	Type of lesion	Symptoms
	Upper neurone lesion – Pseudobulbar palsy	Tongue-spastic no fasciculation Speech-spastic and explosive dysarthria Dysphagia Increased reflexes Emotional lability and decreased control of expression
Medulla	Upper and lower motor neurone lesions	Dysarthria Dysphagia Wasting of the tongue Jaw jerk increased

(*Continued*)

Site of lesion	Type of lesion	Symptoms
	Lower motor neurone lesion – Bulbar palsy	Tongue-shrunken, wrinkled, fasciculation Speech-slurred Dysphagia Paralysis of diaphragm
Corticospinal tracts	Upper motor neurone lesion	Spastic weakness Stiffness Increased reflexes Extensor plantar responses
Anterior horn cells	Lower motor neurone lesion	Flaccid weakness Muscle wasting Muscle fasciculation

Motor neurone pool All the alpha motor neurones that supply the muscle fibres in an individual muscle.

Motor neurones α,β,γ.
See *Nerve fibre types*

Motor pathways These are descending pathways that arise from the brain and take movement signals primarily down to the neuronal pools in the spinal cord. The corticospinal tract is the principle route by which voluntary commands reach the motor neurones in the spinal cord.

Motor pattern generator These stored patterns of movement that are found in the cerebral cortex and brain stem.

Motor point The point on a muscle or muscle belly is the point where the supplying motor nerve enters. The usual guideline is at the junction of the upper and middle thirds of a muscle belly. The threshold for electrical stimulation at a motor point is lower than elsewhere in the muscle and is used clinically, the site of the active electrode when using unipolar stimulation technique and during strength–duration testing.

Motor unit The single alpha (α) motor neurone and the skeletal fibres that it supplies.
See *Innervation ratio*

Movement See *Active movement, Passive movement, Active assisted movement* and *Resisted movement*

Movement classification
Passive movement
A man falls asleep with his arm across a book; a friend arrives and lifts the sleeping man's arm to retrieve the book. This movement required no muscle action from the sleeping man and is, therefore, an example of passive movement.

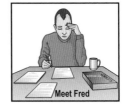
Meet Fred

Active assisted movement

A man is helped by his friend to dress and the friend helps him to lift his arm into his pullover. He does some of the work, but so does his friend; his own muscles did some, but not all of the work. This is, therefore, an example of active assisted movement.

Active movement

The man is now in the bathroom and reaches to grab the toothpaste. His own muscles controlled the movement completely. This is, therefore, and example of active movement.

Resisted movement

The man rushes down the hall; at the end of the hall a door sticks and he has to push it very hard. His muscles have to work against an external force. This is, therefore, an example of resisted movement.

Movement diagram A concept that is useful in manipulative therapy that allows the therapist to analyze their results on examination. Maitland states that a movement diagram is:

> ... a dynamic map representing the quality and quantity of passive movement perceived by the physiotherapist during their examination ... This will include the amount, behaviour and relationships of any abnormal physical findings present e.g. pain, resistance, spasm.

They have uses as self learning tools, teaching media and a means of communication. For further information the reader is advised to consult Maitland's *Vertebral manipulation* (2001). Examples of movement diagrams are provided below.

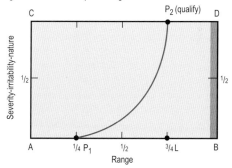

A Pain reaching a maximum at three-quarter range

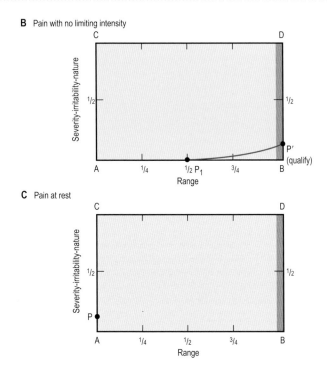

B Pain with no limiting intensity

C Pain at rest

Movement science approach This is also referred to as the motor relearning approach and was originally developed by Janet Carr and Roberta Shepherd in the early 1980s (Carr & Shepherd 1998). It is based on the model of motor learning and is used for the rehabilitation of patients following stroke.

MPG An abbreviation for motor pattern generators.

MRI (scanning) Commonly medical abbreviated – Magnetic resonance imaging. This type of scan is a radiographical technique, which uses magnetism and a computer to produce images. The MRI scanner is a tube surrounded by a giant circular magnet. The patient is placed on a moveable bed that can move in and out of the magnet. The magnet aligns the hydrogen atom's protons. They produce a faint signal, which is detected by the receiver portion of the MRI scanner. A computer processes the receiver information and an image is then produced.

MRSA Methicillin-resistant staphylococcus aureus, a bacteria that has developed resistance to many modern antibiotics. Acquisition appears now to be usually related to contact with the healthcare system (Johnstone et al. 2003).

MS Multiple sclerosis.

MUA Common medical abbreviation – Manipulation under anaesthesia.

If a person has limitation of movement that is caused by adhesions or other causes that cannot be rectified by conventional physiotherapy measure, it may be appropriate to give the person a light anaesthetic and then forcefully move the joint to regain movement, this is common following knee replacements or frozen shoulder, the role of physiotherapy is paramount after an MUA to maintain the range that the surgeon has attained.

Mucolytic agent An agent that liquifies mucous.

Mulligan concept

1. During assessment the therapist will identify one or more comparable signs as described by Maitland. These signs may be a loss of joint movement, pain associated with movement or pain associated with specific functional activities (i.e. lateral elbow pain with resisted wrist extension, adverse neural tension).

2. A passive accessory joint mobilization is applied following the principles of Kaltenborn (i.e. parallel or perpendicular to the joint plane). This accessory glide itself must be pain free.

3. The therapist must continuously monitor the patient's reaction to ensure no pain is recreated. Utilizing his/her knowledge of joint arthrology, a well-developed sense of tissue tension and clinical reasoning, the therapist investigates various combinations of parallel or perpendicular glides to find the correct treatment plane and grade of movement.

4. While sustaining the accessory glide, the patient is requested to perform the comparable sign. The comparable sign should now be significantly improved (i.e. increased range of motion and a significantly decreased, or better yet, absence of the original pain).

5. Failure to improve the comparable sign would indicate that the therapist has not found the correct contact point, treatment plane, grade or direction of mobilization, spinal segment or that the technique is not indicated.

6. The previously restricted and/or painful motion or activity is repeated by the patient while the therapist continues to maintain the appropriate accessory glide. Further gains are expected with repetition during a treatment session, typically involving three sets of ten repetitions.

7. Further gains may be realized through the application of passive overpressure at the end of available range. It is expected that this overpressure is again, pain-free.

Principles

In the application of manual therapy techniques, physiotherapists acknowledge that contraindications to treatment exist and should be respected at all times. Although always guided by the basic rule of never causing pain, therapist choosing to make use of SNAGS in the spine and MWMs in the extremities must still know and abide by the basic rules of application of manual-therapy techniques. Specific to the application of MWM and SNAGS in clinical practice, the some basic principles have been developed.

Self-treatment is often possible using MWM principles with adhesive tape and/or the patient providing the glide component of the MWM and the patient's own efforts to produce the active movement. Pain is always the guide. Successful MWM and SNAGS techniques should render the comparable sign painless while significantly improving function during the application of the technique. Sustained improvements are necessary to justify ongoing intervention.

Go to http://www.bmulligan.com/about/concept.html

With thanks to Brian R. Mulligan NZRP, Dip MT, FNZSP, MCTA and Jack Miller BSc(PT), Dip MT (NZ), FCAMT, MCTA.

Multidimensional health locus of control scale (Wallston et al. 1978)

Multidisciplinary Involving a number of disciplines/professions.

Multi-disciplinary team A team where a number of professionals and other workers undertake treatments and interventions relatively independently of each other with limited interaction. The team is headed by a leader and tends to be formal and hierarchical. Primary healthcare teams fall into this category where the general practitioner usually leads the team. Each team member is bound by his or her own professional education and beliefs, which may differ considerably from those of other members of the team. Patients and clients should be central in such teams.

Multifidus Deep lumbar spine muscle. Its primary function is to stabilize the lumbar spine.

Multi-infarct dementia This is caused by 'mini' strokes that lead to a progressive loss of function and can be worsened by the presence of hypertension and diabetes.

Multiple sclerosis This is a demyelinating disease of unknown cause that can lead to widespread degeneration of the central nervous system and progressive neurological deficits.

It is divided into:

- primary progressive – a steady progressive decline in function
- relapsing remitting – a history of 'attacks' with temporary periods of loss of function and then a recovery period back to previous level of ability. This may change over time to secondary progressive.
- secondary progressive – the disease will initially start off as 'relapsing remitting' and then move into a stage where the disease becomes progressive.

✪ Clinical note Multiple sclerosis is the most common cause of disability in young people. Clinical presentation can vary enormously depending on the sites of the lesions and include spasticity, ataxia, incontinence, altered vision and speech and swallowing difficulties.

Multiple systems atrophy This is a condition commonly confused with Parkinson's diseases where there is cell loss or gliosis in many sites. Patients with this condition, although rigid and with poverty of movement, do not respond to levodopa, whereas Parkinson's patients do improve with levodopa. Usually onset is around 50–60 years with death occurring within 6 years.

Multivariate analysis Research term – an analysis where the effects of many variables are considered.

Muscle fibre types See the table below.

Types of muscle fibre

Pure fibre type	1 (slow twitch)	1la (FTa) or fast twitch oxidative glycolytic (FTOG)	11x (Ftb)
Properties	Slow contracting	Suited to fast, repetitive,	Fast contracting,
	Slow fatiguing	low-intensity movement	Fatigue rapidly
	Reddish in colour	Recruited after type	Whitish colour
	Small diameter	1 fibres	Low myoglobin
	High oxidative	Fatigue resistant	Fibres large diameter
	capacity	(high numbers of	High glycolytic capacity
	Low glycolytic	mitochondria)	Low oxidative capacity
	capacity	Recover rapidly after	Suited to high-power
	Useful in maintain-	exercise	output recruited in
	ing posture		weight lifting

From Shamley D, McNeill G (eds) (In press) Clinical Physiology and Rehabilitation. Butterworth Heinemann, Oxford

Muscle imbalance Imbalanced muscle groups cause a wide variety of conditions, from joint wear-and-tear to arthritis and from tendonitis to sore muscles. All joints in the body are controlled by two or more groups of muscles. Usually one set of muscles stabilizes and supports the joint, while other adjoining muscle groups create movement. However, sometimes, one group becomes unusually strong and tight, while the opposite group weakens and becomes overstretched. This imbalance leads to poor joint control and abnormal biomechanics. If these faulty movement patterns repeat many times, tissues may begin to degenerate. Muscle imbalance techniques approach patients who present with movement dysfunction and its associated problems. Several classifications of imbalance have been suggested relating to muscles' structure, function and response to injury. Movement dysfunction may occur at both a segmental or local or single joint level and at a global level affecting many segments of a region.

Muscles can be thought of as either stabilizers or mobilizers. Stabilizer muscles are deep, with broad attachments and their role is postural and dynamic control. Mobilizer muscles are producers of force, they are more superficially situated and have long muscle bellies. In certain pathological states these two classifications of muscles change their recruitment patterns; this typically results in an alteration in function.

The muscle groups commonly affected by muscle imbalance

Muscles prone to tightness (mobilizers)	Muscles prone to weakness (stabilizers)
Sternocleidomastoid	Deep cervical flexors
Scalene muscles	Serratus anterior
Levator scapulae	Lower fibres trapezius
Pectoralis minor	Subscapularis
Upper trapezius	Transersus abdominis
Rhomboids	Gluteus medius and minimus
Erector spinae	Vastus medialis
Rectus abdominis	Psoas major
Hamstrings	Multifidus
Gracilis	
Vastus lateralis	
Tensor fascia latae	
Rectus femoris	
Quadratus lumborum	
Piriformis	
Gasrocnemius	

From Jull GA, Janda V 1987 Muscles and motor control in low back pain. In: Twomey LT, Taylor JR (eds) Physical Therapy of the Low Back. Churchill Livingstone, Edinburgh, pp. 253–278

Muscle pump The process whereby blood is squeezed from one valve to the next on its way back to the heart, physiotherapists often encounter people who have a deficient muscle pump, for example, after joint replacement surgery or immobility. This often results in oedema in the ankles.

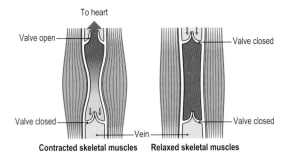

Contracted skeletal muscles   Relaxed skeletal muscles

Muscle spasm The state of a muscle being in contraction without the ability to release it voluntarily. It can occur locally in a muscle usually as a response to a soft tissue injury and in patients with neurological damage spasms can be more widespread, i.e. the whole leg or arm.

Muscle structure

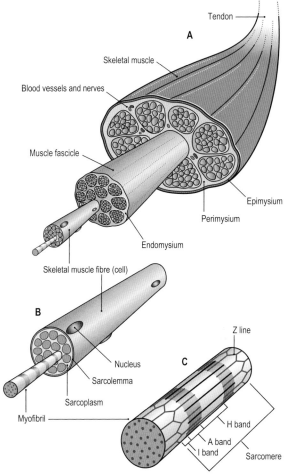

The parts of a muscle. The component parts of a voluntary muscle, from the functional units (myofibrils) to the epimysium which contains the whole muscle and is continuous with tendons of origin and insertion. (**A**) Muscle. (**B**) Muscle fibre (cell). (**C**) Myofibril

Muscle tone Muscle tone can be described as a state of readiness and is reliant upon viscoelastic properties of muscle as well as the presence of neural activity or force generated by skeletal muscle in the absence of conscious contraction.

Muscular atrophies These are the most common neuromuscular disease in childhood after Duchenne's muscular dystrophy. They are also called spinal muscular atrophies (SMA), which are a group of neurogenic disorders that affect the anterior horn cells in the spinal cord and lead to muscle weakness.

Muscular dystrophy A group of disorders characterized by progressive muscle weakness and loss of muscle tissue. See table below for more information.

Classification of some of the muscular dystrophies in relation to the genetic defect

Inheritance	Locus	Gene	Diagnosis	Onset
X-linked				
Short arm of X chromosome	Xp21.1 Xp21.2	Dystrophin Dystrophin	Duchenne dystrophy Becker dystrophy	3–5 years Childhood
Long arm of X chromosome	Xq28	Emerin	Emery-Dreifuss	Childhood
Abnormal recessive	Various	Various	Scapulohumeral Limb girdle 5 types 2A–E	Any age Early adult life
	6q2	Merosin	Congenital LAMA 2	Hypotonia at birth
	9q31–q33		Fukuyama	
Autosomal dominant	4q35		Fascioscapulohumeral Scapuloperoneal	Any age 2nd–5th decade
	5q22–q34		Limb girdle 1A LGMD 1B	Early adult life Early adult life
	14q11.2–q13 14q		Oculopharyngeal Distal	Adulthood Adulthood
	Chromosome 19	Myotonin protein kinase	Myotonic dystrophy	Adulthood, but can be congenital

Musculocutaneous nerve

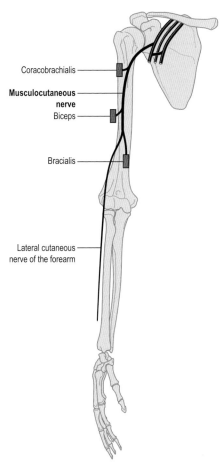

Coracobrachialis —

Musculocutaneous nerve

Biceps —

Bracialis —

Lateral cutaneous nerve of the forearm —

The muscles supplied by the musculocutaneous nerve

MWM Common medical abbreviation – Mobilization with movement.

Myalgia Pain felt within a muscle.

Myasthenia gravis A rare disorder that affects transmission of impulses at the neuromuscular junction. The main characteristics are weakness and fatigability of the limb, eye and other muscles, which is worsened on sustained or repeated movements and at the end of the day (Stokes 1998).

Myelin A fat-like substance that forms an insulating sheath around nerves in the central nervous system and the white matter in the brain. An intact myelin sheath is required for smooth nerve conduction.

○ Clinical note The myelin sheath is affected in multiple sclerosis.

Myelination The process of forming the covering, myelin, that surrounds nerve cell axons and white matter of the brain.

Myeloma A type of cancer that arises in plasma cells, a type of white blood cell.

Myelomeningocele This occurs where the posterior neural arch in the spine does not close during development. The spinal cord and roots protrude out of the bony defect and may lead to varying amounts of neurological damage and loss of function.

Myocardial infarction (MI) Common medical abbreviation – Myocardial infarction.

This is more commonly known as a heart attack. Most often caused by a thromobus or clot, there are various degrees ranging from those that cause immediate cessation of heart beat and death, to those that go undiagnosed.

Myoclonus Shock-like contractions of a muscle or a group of muscles.

Myofascial trigger point see trigger point Trigger points are localized hyperirritable spots located within skeletal muscle. They produce localized pain, referred pain and often accompany chronic musculoskeletal disorders. Repeated microtrauma may lead to the development of stress on muscle fibres and the formation of trigger points. Patients often have persistent pain that results in a decreased range of motion in the affected muscles. These include muscles used to maintain body posture, such as those in the neck, shoulders and pelvic girdle. Trigger points may also manifest as tension headache, tinnitus, temporomandibular joint pain, decreased range of motion in the legs and low back pain. On palpation of a trigger point, a nodule of muscle fibre of harder than normal consistency is often found (Alvarez & Rockwell 2002).

Myositis ossificans Ossification of a haematoma, secondary to trauma. If a haematoma does not fully resolve, calcification and subsequent ossification, can occur after approximately 3 weeks. Surgical intervention may then be necessary.

Myotome A muscle supplied by a particular nerve root level. See table below.

Myotomes

C1	Upper cervical flexion
C2	Upper cervical extension
C3	Cervical side flexion
C4	Shoulder shrug
C5	Shoulder abduction, external rotation
C6	Elbow flexion, wrist extension
C7	Elbow extension, wrist flexion
C8	Thumb extension, finger flexion
T1	Finger ab/dduction
L2	Hip flexion
L3	Knee extension
L4	Ankle dorsiflexion
L5	Great toe dorsiflexion (extension)
S1/2	Ankle plantarflexion, knee flexion
S-3 S-4	Rectal sphincter

N

NAD Common medical abbreviation – No abnormality detected.

NAG Common medical abbreviation – Natural apophyseal glide.

NAI Common medical abbreviation – Non-accidental injury.

Nail blanch test Test performed on the nail beds that is an indicator of tissue perfusion (the amount of blood flow to the tissues). Pressure is applied to the nail bed by the operator squeezing the nail until it turns white, indicating that the blood has been forced from the tissue (blanched). Once the tissue has blanched, the pressure is removed and the time it takes for blood to return to the tissue is measured as indicated by the return of a pink colour to the nail bed.

Nail pits The term for tiny depressions on the surface of the fingernails caused by defective nail formation seen commonly in people with psoriasis.

Narcolepsy A sleep disorder associated with excessive sleepiness during the daytime and disturbed night-time sleep.

Narcotic A substance that produces narcosis. Applied especially to drugs that have morphine-like actions.

Nasal flaring A sign of respiratory distress in infants.

Nasogastric feeding This is the process whereby a patient with swallowing difficulties following a neurological insult receives nutrition via a nasogastric tube (NG tube), which enters the body via the nasal passage and goes to the stomach.

○ Clinical note It is important to be aware that nasogastric tubes can become dislodged and feed is at risk of entering the lungs.

Nasopharyngeal Relating to the nasopharynx or the upper part of the throat behind the nose.

Nasopharyngeal suction See *Suction*

National health service (NHS) A state-funded and managed system of healthcare established in 1948. It aims to provide universal and comprehensive healthcare that is financed through general taxation and is free at the point of delivery. A system of charges were, however, introduced before 1950 and have gradually increased. The NHS changed considerably under the government of Margaret Thatcher, when the 'internal market' and a 'mixed economy of welfare' was introduced.

See *Internal market* and *Mixed economy of welfare*

National institute for clinical excellence (NICE) Go to http://www.nice.org.uk

NICE is the independent organization responsible for providing national guidance on treatments and care for those using the NHS in England and Wales. Its guidance is for healthcare professionals and patients and their carers, to help them make decisions about treatment and healthcare. NICE was established as a Special Health Authority in April 1999, to promote clinical excellence and the effective use of resources within the NHS. Once NICE guidance is published, health professionals are expected to take it fully into account when exercising their clinical judgement. Currently, NICE produces guidance in three areas of health:

1. The use of new and existing medicines and treatments within the NHS in England and Wales – technology appraisals.
2. The appropriate treatment and care of patients with specific diseases and conditions within the NHS in England and Wales – clinical guidelines.
3. Whether interventional procedures used for diagnosis or treatment are safe enough and work well enough for routine use – interventional procedures.

NICE also funds three enquiries that undertake research into the way patients are treated, to identify ways of improving the quality of care. (These investigations are known as Confidential Enquiries.) NICE guidance and recommendations are prepared by independent groups that include professionals working in the NHS and people who are familiar with the issues affecting patients and carers.

With thanks to Louise Fish, Senior Communications Manager, National Institute for Clinical Excellence.

National service framework (NSF) A government initiative that aims to provide the NHS with explicit standards and principles for the pattern and level of services required for a specific service or care group. Aiming to address the 'whole system of care', each sets out where care is best provided and the standard of care that patients should be offered in each of the settings. They provide 'a clear set of priorities against which local action can be framed' and seek to ensure that patients will get greater consistency in the availability and quality of services, right across the NHS (NHS 1998).

Nature See *SIN factors*

NBI Common medical abbreviation – No bony injury.

NBM Common medical abbreviation – Nil by mouth.

NDT See *Neurodevelopmental therapy*

Nebulizers Equipment used for putting medication into aerosol form for inhalation and deposition of the drug into the lung. Drugs administered via nebulizers include bronchodilators and some antibiotics (BTS 1997, European Respiratory Society Task Force 2001).

Necrosis Death of tissue.

Neer prosthesis A type of shoulder arthrolasty.

Neer classification A system of classification of fractures of the proximal humerus.

Neer classification

Group 1	Minimal displacement
Group 2	Anatomical neck fracture with less than 1cm displacement
Group 3	Displaced or angulated surgical neck
Group 4	Displaced fracture of greater tuberosity
Group 5	Fractures of the lesser tuberosity
Group 6	Fracture dislocations

Neglect See *Unilateral neglect*

Nelaton's line A line drawn from the anterior superior iliac spine to the ischial tuberosity, the greater trochanter should lie in this line, but in cases of the hip or femoral neck fracture, the trochanter lies above the line.

Neoplasm Abnormal growth of tissue, which may be benign or malignant.

Nephrectomy The removal of a kidney.

Nerve conduction test A nerve conduction test is an electrical test that is used to detect motor and sensory nerve impulse transmission. In this test, the nerve is electrically stimulated while a second electrode detects the downstream impulse.

Nerve fibre types

The major classifications of nerve fibres

Class	Myelination	Conduction velocity (m/s)	Diameter (µm)	Function
I (a & b)	+	70–120	12–20	Afferent from muscle spindles and tendon organs
II	+	25–70	4–12	Afferent from muscle spindles, touch and pressure
III	+	3–30	1–4	Afferent from cold and pain receptors
Aα	+	50–120	8–20	Efferent to extrafusal muscle fibres
Aβ	+	30–70	5–12	Efferent to intra- and extra-fusal fibres, skin afferents
Aγ	+	10–50	2–8	Efferent to intrafusal muscle fibres
Aδ	+	3–30	1–5	Afferent pain, cold
B	+	5–15	1–3	Preganglionic autonomic

(Continued)

Class	Myelination	Conduction velocity (m/s)	Diameter (μm)	Function
C (sometimes called IV)	–	<2	<1	Postganglionic autonomic, visceral and somatic afferents for pain and temperature sensation

Much of the confusion in fibre classification arises because there are two systems (I, II, III, IV and A, B, C) describing the same thing – the diameter and conduction velocity of the population of nerve fibres which extend from thick myelinated fibres at one extreme (group I or Aα or even simply α) to thin unmyelinated at the other extreme (group IV or C fibres). The major difference is that one focuses, but not exclusively, on afferent and the other on efferent fibres. The student should remember that, although the group I, II, III, IV system is usually used for muscle afferents and the Aα–δ, C system for motor nerves and skin afferents, both systems are based on fibre diameter and conduction velocity and are as equivalent as measuring length in millimetres or inches.

Nerve muscle interaction This term relates to the functional inter-relationship of the components of movement: muscles and nerves.

Neural mobilization Techniques by which neural tissues are 'moved', either by movement relative to their surroundings or by tension development.

Neural tension This term is interchangeably used when performing assessment of neural extensibility and mobility, but should be more aptly titled neural mobility.

Neural tube defect A type of birth defect that results from failure of the spinal cord or brain to develop normally. Spinal bifida is an example of one such disorder.

Neurilemma The outer sheath of a nerve fibre.

Neurodevelopmental therapy This is a common term used to describe an approach to the rehabilitation of neurological patients. The approach is based on principles derived from research into motor development and neurophysiology.

Neurodynamics The mobility of the nervous system is examined by procedures known as neurodynamic tests. These tests evaluate the mechanical responses for example neural movement such as gliding and physiological responses including blood flow within the nerve (intraneural), nerve impulses and axonal transport (Shacklock 1995).
   The testing procedures are outlined below.

Neurodynamic tests
Straight leg raise (SLR) – tests the sciatic nerve
Normal response would be pain, strong stretching feeling or tingling in the posterior thigh, knee, calf and foot. Sensitizing tests to differentiate nervous tissue from other tissues include:

* ankle dorsiflexion – sensitizes the tibial nerve
* ankle plantarflexion and forefoot inversion – sensitizes the common peroneal nerve
* hip adduction – sensitizes the sciatic nerve

- hip medial rotation – sensitizes the sciatic nerve
- passive neck flexion – sensitizes the meninges, spinal cord and sciatic nerve.

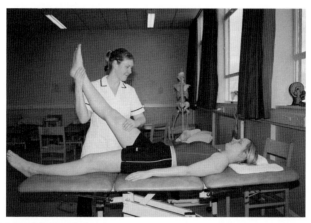

SLR 1 (Straight leg raise)

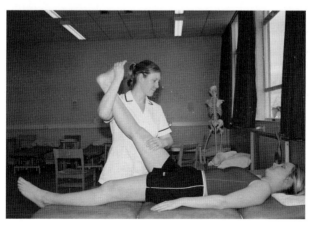

SLR 2

Prone knee bend (PKB) – tests the femoral nerve

Traditionally tested in prone position, however, this fails to differentiate between nervous tissue (femoral nerve) and the hip flexor muscles. Carrying out the test in side lying with the head and trunk flexed allows the cervical extension to be used as a desensitizing test.

A normal response would be full range of movement so that the heel approximates the buttock and is accompanied by a strong stretch on the anterior thigh.

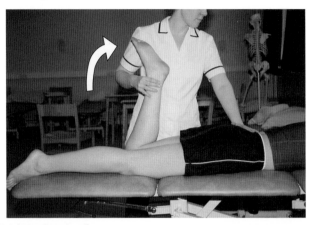

PKB 1 (Prone knee bend)

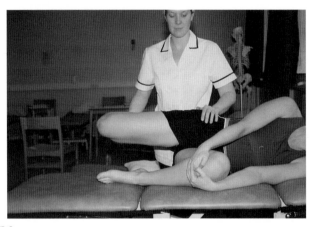

PKB 2

Passive neck flexion (PNF) – Tests the spinal cord, meninges of the lumbar spine and sciatic nerve

The test is performed supine and the patient's head is flexed passively by the clinician. A normal response would be a full, pain-free movement. Sensitizing tests include SLR and upper-limb neurodynamic tests.

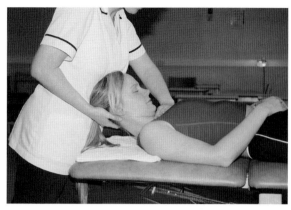

Passive neck flexion

The test evaluates all levels of the spine and should be incorporated in all cervical, thoracic and lumbar spine examinations. The test is performed in the sitting position and incorporates cervical, thoracic and lumbar flexion.
Sensitized by, e.g. knee extension and ankle dorsiflexion.

Slump test

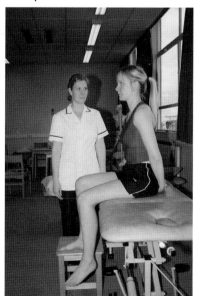

Slump test – starting position

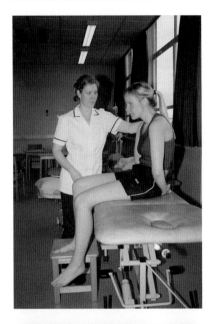

Slump test – slump position

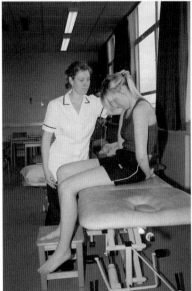

Slump with neck flexion

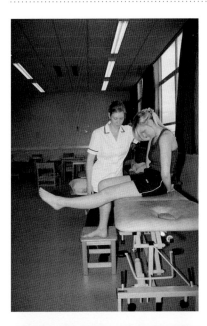

Slump with knee extension

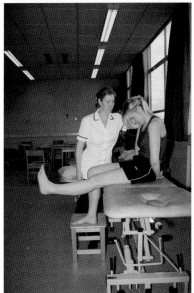

Slump with ankle dorsiflexion

Upper limb neural dynamic tests

There are four tests each biased towards a particular nerve and include:

1. Upper limb neurodynamic test 1, median nerve bias.

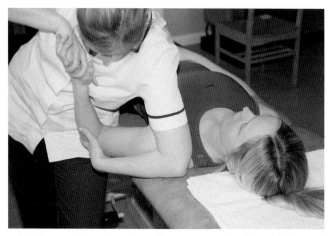

Upper limb neural dynamic test 1: median nerve bias – shoulder girdle depression

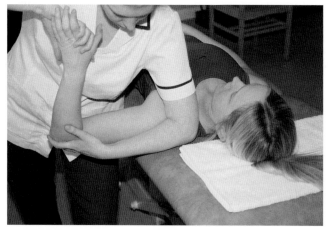

Shoulder joint abduction

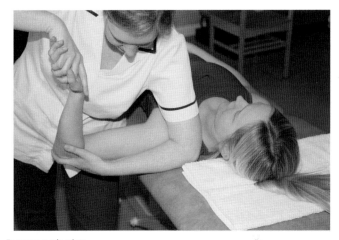

Forearm supination

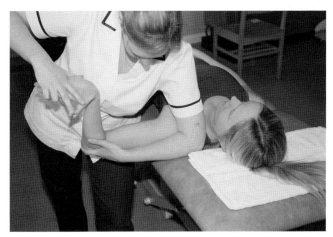

Shoulder joint lateral rotation

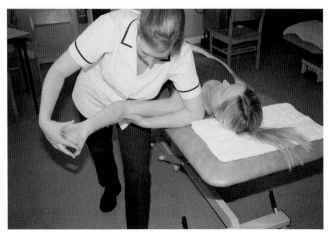

Elbow extension

This test consists of: shoulder girdle depression, shoulder joint abduction, forearm supination, wrist and finger extension, shoulder joint lateral rotation and elbow extension.

The sensitizing test involves cervical lateral flexion away from the symptomatic side and the desensitizing movement involves cervical lateral flexion towards the symptomatic side.

2. Upper limb neurodynamic test 2a, median nerve bias.

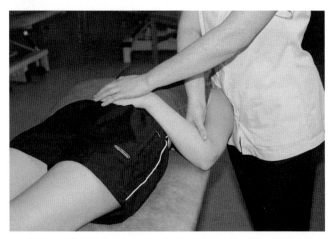

Upper limb neural dynamic test 2a: median nerve bias – shoulder girdle depression

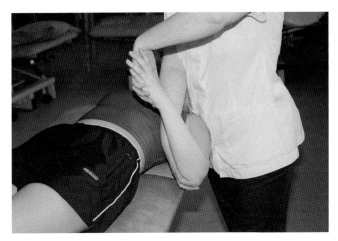

Shoulder joint abduction of 10°

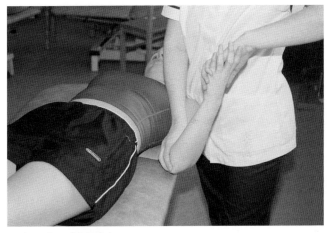

Lateral rotation of the whole arm

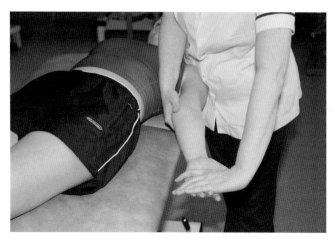

Elbow extension

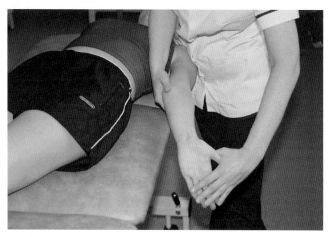

Wrist, finger and thumb extension

This test consists of: shoulder girdle depression, shoulder joint abduction of 10°, lateral rotation of the whole arm, elbow extension and wrist, finger and thumb extension.

The sensitizing test is cervical lateral flexion away from the symptomatic side or shoulder abduction. Desensitizing movement involves cervical lateral flexion towards the affected side or release of the shoulder girdle.

3. Upper limb neurodynamic test 2b, radial nerve bias.

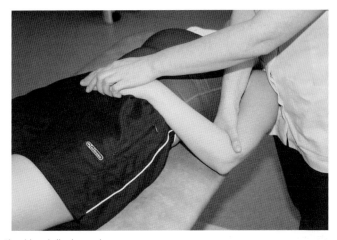

Shoulder girdle depression

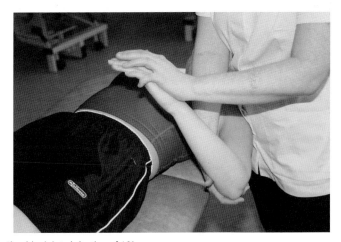

Shoulder joint abduction of 10°

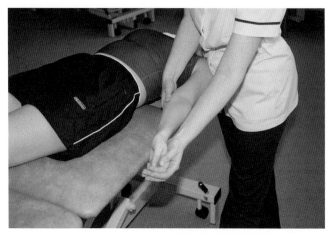

Medial rotation of the whole arm

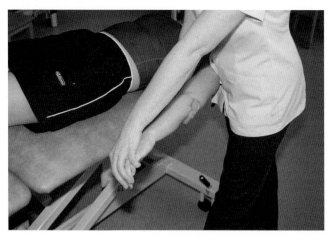

Elbow extension

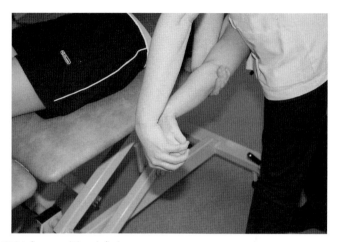

Wrist, finger and thumb flexion

This test consists of shoulder girdle depression, shoulder joint abduction of 10°, elbow extension, medial rotation of the whole arm, wrist, finger and thumb flexion.

The sensitizing test is cervical lateral flexion away from the symptomatic side and shoulder abduction. The desensitizing movement is cervical lateral flexion towards the symptomatic side or release of the shoulder girdle.

4. Upper limb neurodynamic test 3, ulnar nerve bias.

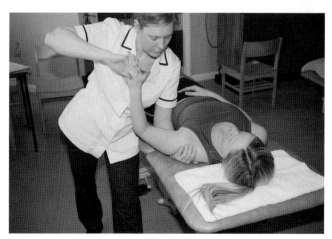

Upper limb neurodynamic test 3, ulnar nerve bias – shoulder girdle depression

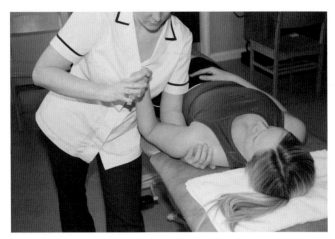

Wrist and finger extension

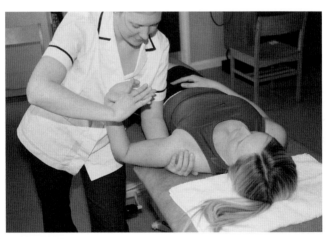

Forearm pronation

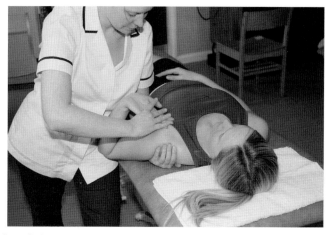

Elbow flexion

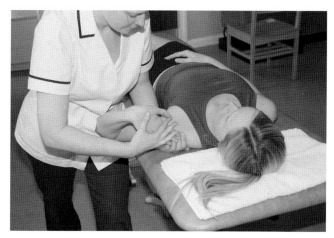

Shoulder lateral rotation

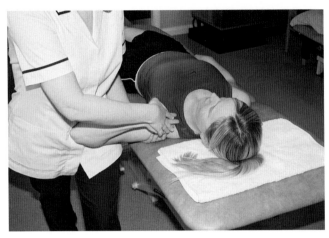

Shoulder abduction to 90°

This test consists of shoulder girdle depression, wrist and finger extension, forearm pronation, elbow flexion, lateral rotation of the shoulder and shoulder abduction of 90°.

The sensitizing test is cervical lateral flexion away from the symptomatic side and shoulder abduction. The desensitizing movement is cervical lateral flexion towards the symptomatic side or release of the shoulder girdle.

Neurofibromatosis See von Recklinghausen disease.

Neurogenic Of nerve origin, e.g. a person with sciatica as a result of nerve root irritation has pain that is neurogenic.

Neuroglia The supporting structure of the nervous system and consists of astrocytes, oligodendrocytes and microglia.

Neurolysis The release of a nerve from adhesions. Usually refers to a surgical procedure.

Neuromuscular disorders These are inherited or acquired disorders of muscle due to neuromuscular disease. They are characterized according to age of onset and site of defect.

Neuromuscular electrical stimulation (NMES) There are many clinical devices that deliver a form of electrical stimulation that aims to stimulate nerve and muscle. There is a degree of confusion in the terminology used, though NMES is probably the preferred generic term. Alternatives such as Chronic NMES (CNMES) imply that the stimulation is not a short-duration treatment rather than implying that it should be only employed for chronic lesions. NMES has been applied in many different clinical circumstances ranging from the reduction in spasticity in children with CNS lesions through to muscle strengthening in elite athletes, from electrically enhanced wound healing through to re-education of the skeletal muscles. It is probably most appropriate to describe the form of stimulation by virtue of the current being utilised (rather than using the name of a particular machine) – i.e. alternating, direct or pulsed. NMES can be used to achieve increases in muscle function for patients with significant atrophy, to prevent atrophy during immobilisation, as part of a neuromuscular re-education programme, to facilitate muscle balance, as part of a pelvic floor programme in incontinence. It has been used for patients with scoliosis as a means to facilitate correction. In neurology, NMES can be used to facilitate motor recovery and increase strength, to reduce the impact of shoulder subluxation after stroke and to help in spasticity management programmes.

Neuromuscular junction Also called the NM junction. This is a specialized system for the transmission of impulses from a motor nerve and a muscle to enable its contraction.

✚ Clinical note Myasthenia gravis is a disorder of the neuromuscular junction and the use of botulinum toxin in the treatment of focal spasticity acts at the level of the neuromuscular junction.

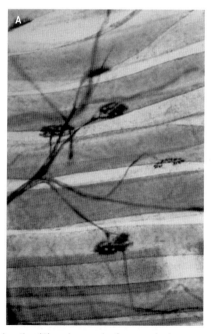

Neuromuscular junction (**A**) a micrograph of neuronal axis

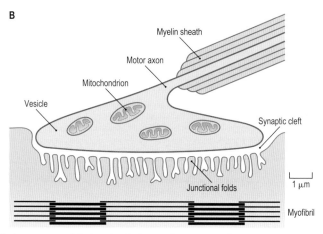

B

Myelin sheath

Motor axon

Mitochondrion

Vesicle

Synaptic cleft

1 μm

Junctional folds

Myofibril

(**B**) the structure of the junction is shown diagrammatically

Neuronal sprouting The process of nerve regrowth in response to injury or damage.

Neurone A nerve cell of the nervous system.

Neuropathy An abnormal and degenerative state of the nervous system. Certain states or diseases can cause a peripheral neuropathy marked by burning tingling sensations in the extremities, loss of deep tendon reflexes and decrease in sensitivity to touch stimulation, e.g. alcoholic and diabetic neuropathy.

Neuropharmacology Relates to the study of effects of drugs on the nervous system.

Neuroplasticity Functional changes in the central nervous system in response to demands from the internal or external environment.

⨁ Clinical note The evidence of neuroplastic changes occurring on magnetic resonance imaging scans has helped to show the benefit of therapy in the re-education of movement following brain injury.

Neuropraxia A measure of extent of peripheral nerve damage (Seddon's category; Type 1 Sunderland). A transient loss of nerve function following damage. Usual mechanism: prolonged compression, direct trauma or inflammation. Localized conduction block, no permanent damage to myelin sheath or axonal degeneration. Prognosis is good and recovery complete and usually takes 6–8 weeks. Example: cyclists palsy, compression of motor and sensory branches of ulnar nerve in Guyton's tunnel in hand.

Neurosurgery Surgery to the nervous system, usually the brain.

Neurotmesis A measure of extent of peripheral nerve damage (Seddon's category, Types 3, 4 & 5 Sunderland). Axonal disruption and damage to one or more layers of connective tissue in peripheral nerve. Usual mechanism: transection.

Followed by Wallerian degeneration of myelin sheath by day 7. Outcome: poor, may be improved with surgery, especially microsurgery.

Neurotransmitter A specific chemical agent that is released from pre-synaptic cells, travels across the synapse and leads to either excitation or inhibition of post-synaptic cells.

Neurotrophic Nutrition and maintenance of tissues as regulated by nervous influence.

Newton's laws
Newton's first law

If an object is at rest it will stay at rest and if it is moving with a constant speed in a straight line it will continue to do so; as long as no external force acts on it. In other words if an object is not experiencing the action of an external force it will either keep moving or not move at all.

This law expresses the concept of inertia. The inertia of a body can be described as being its reluctance to start moving or stop moving once it has started.

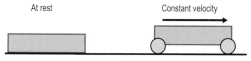

Newton's first law

Newton's second law

The rate of change of velocity is directly proportional to the applied, external force acting on the body and takes place in the direction of the force. Therefore forces can either cause an acceleration or deceleration of an object. **Acceleration** is usually defined as being positive and **Deceleration** as being negative.

$$F = ma$$

$$F = \text{applied force (N)}$$
$$m = \text{mass of body (kg)}$$
$$a = \text{acceleration of the body (m/s}^2)$$

Acceleration of an object with a constant Force

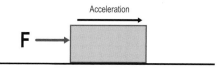

Therefore 1 N is that force which produces an acceleration of 1 (m/s^2) when it acts on a mass of 1 kg.

Newton's second law

Newton's third law

If the box shown in the diagram below exerts a force on the table top (action), then the table will exert an equal and opposite force on the box (reaction). This does not mean the forces cancel each other out, because they act on two different objects. The diagram below shows the forces acting on an object as it is resting on the ground.

The action of a force on the ground receives an equal and opposite reaction force. This is known as a ground reaction force (GRF) (Richards 2003).

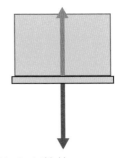

Newton's third law

NIDDM Common medical abbreviation – Non-insulin-dependent diabetes mellitus.

Nine-hole peg test This is a test to measure the dexterity and speed of the hand and upper limb. The equipment consist of a wooden base with nine holes and nine wooden pegs; a stopwatch is used to measure the time taken to place the pegs in the hole.

Nociceptive Relating to the process of pain transmission.

Nociceptor A peripheral nerve ending that transmits painful stimuli.

Node of ranvier The small constricted portions of the neurone's myelin sheath. These gaps are more permeable to potassium and sodium ions than the rest of the body. Consequently, they facilitate nerve impulse transmission.

NOF Common medical abbreviation – Neck of femur.

N-of-1 trials Research methodology in which a patient undergoes pairs of treatment periods organized so that one period involves the use of the experimental treatment and one period involves the use of an alternate or placebo therapy. If possible, blinding occurs and outcomes are monitored. Treatment periods are replicated until the clinician and patient are convinced that the treatments are definitely different or definitely not different.

Non-Hodgkin's lymphoma A group of lymphomas which differ in important ways from Hodgkin's disease.

Non-invasive ventilation (NIV) Non-invasive ventilation is often referred to as non-invasive positive pressure ventilation (NIPPV). Since negative pressure devices, volume ventilators and full-face masks are all used, this phrase is now considered ambiguous and inaccurate. The technique is now referred to in the UK as non-invasive ventilation or NIV (British Thoracic Society Guidelines 2002). It should be noted that the term NPPV (non-invasive positive pressure ventilation) is adopted throughout Europe in accordance with the International Consensus Guidelines document (2001/2). The earliest form of NIV was that of negative-pressure ventilation as provided by the tank and cuirass ventilators. Such devices were the mainstays of ventilatory support until the 1950s and were successfully used through both the polio epidemics of the 1930s and 1950s. Whilst proven to be reliable they are bulky (over 3 m long) and heavy (300 kg). The most commonly used negative-pressure ventilator today is the jacket ventilator, consisting of an impermeable nylon jacket suspended by a rigid chest piece that fits over the chest and abdomen. The chest and wrap ventilators are lightweight, but both must be connected to negative-pressure generators such as the NEV from Respironics. The development of negative-pressure ventilators is well described by Woollam (1976).

Negative-pressure ventilators work by intermittently applying a sub-atmospheric pressure to the chest wall and abdomen; this increases trans-pulmonary pressure and causes atmospheric pressure at the mouth to inflate the lungs. Expiration occurs passively by elastic recoil of the lung and chest wall, as pressure within the device rises to atmospheric levels. The technique has been successfully used in patients with chronic respiratory failure due to chest-wall deformity, neuromuscular diseases and central hypoventilation (BTS Guidelines 2001, Garay et al. 1981, Mehta & Hill 2001, Shapiro et al. 1992, Sullivan et al. 1981, Woollam 1976).

Indications for non-invasive ventilation
- As a trial of avoidance of intubation
- As a ceiling of treatment for patients deemed 'not for intubation'
- Acute exacerbations of COPD
- Hypoxic cardiogenic pulmonary oedema, unsuccessful with CPAP
- Acute/acute on chronic hypercaponic respiratory failure owing to neuromuscular or chest wall disease
- Decompensated OSA
- Trial in intensive therapy units/high-dependency units (ITU/HDU) with acute hypoxaemic pneumonia
- Trial with respiratory acidosis in acute bronchiectasis
- Facilitation of weaning from formal ventilation (BTS Guidelines 2002)
- Respiratory distress
- Where two or more of the following are present:
  - moderate to severe dyspnoea
  - use of accessory muscles
  - paradoxical breathing
  - pH < 7.35 with $PaCO_2$ > 6 kPa
  - respiratory rate ≥25 bpm (Kramer et al. 1995).

Non-invasive ventilation contraindications
- Recent facial or upper airway surgery
- Facial abnormalities (burns, trauma)
- Fixed upper airway obstruction
- Vomiting patient
- Undrained pneumothorax (BTS Guidelines 2002).

Considerations that require intubation facilities
- Unable to protect own airway
- Life-threatening hypoxaemia
- Severe comorbidity
- Bowel obstruction
- Upper gastrointestinal surgery
- Confusion/agitation
- Copious respiratory secretions (BTS Guidelines 2002).

Monitoring
Clinical considerations of patient status, comfort, breathing pattern, conscious level, heart and respiratory rate should all be evaluated. The use of blood gas analysis will be dictated by the clinical progress of the patient. BTS recommendations state they should be performed after 1–2 h of NIV and after 4–6 h if little improvement found on initial sampling. Intubation is then the recommendation if no improvements in pH and $PaCO_2$ is noted.

Oxygen saturation should be monitored and supplemental oxygen administered to maintain saturation between 85% and 90% or the patients' usual resting saturation. It should be remembered that these readings might be falsely reassuring in some patients.

Undesired changes in trends should be reported and acted upon immediately to ensure maximum management of the patient. Where intubation is deemed unsuitable, palliative management should commence.

Positive-pressure ventilators

NIV achieved through the application of positive airway pressure started to first appear with the use of continuous positive airway pressure (CPAP) for the treatment of obstructive sleep apnoea (Sullivan 1981). Garay et al. in 1981 realized that the use of nocturnal NIV could reverse the undesirable daytime blood-gas changes that were present in certain forms of chronic respiratory failure. As interfaces developed, the role of NIV was expanded to provide ventilatory support and today NIV can be used as an alternative to formal intubation for some patients. NIV ventilators have become specific tools for pressure-supported ventilation with NIV machines ranging from simple, e.g. the NIPPY1, to sophisticated, e.g. the Vision. The system should be selected appropriately for individual patient needs. However, there is a marked difference between the various manufacturers' pressure-targeted ventilators in coping with leak (particularly between ventilators normally used for invasive ventilation and those specifically built for NIV) (Metha et al. 2001). A pressure-controlled ventilator designed for NIV will deliver a variable flow to achieve pressure and, thus, ventilation. The BTS (2002) has stated that pressure-cycled ventilators are the most appropriate for NIV application. The International Consensus findings of 2001 state the choice of system should be dictated by the experience of the staff, the status and clinical requirements of the patient and the location of care.

Two categories of positive-pressure NIV exist. One is the application of a continuous-set pressure (CPAP), the other is the application of two different pressures or Bi-level ($B_iPAP^®$) (Concensus Conference 1999).

Continuous positive airways pressure (CPAP)

By applying one constant pressure to the airway regardless of patient effort, CPAP acts as a splinting device on the airways. As a result, extra air is always residual within the lungs, i.e. additional to the residual volume (RV). The beneficial effects of splinting the airways means that alveoli are held in a partially opened state, thus allowing more time for oxygen to diffuse across the alveolar capillary membrane. As a result, oxygenation is improved. The application of CPAP has the effect of increasing functional residual capacity (FRC), i.e. the amount of air remaining in the lung after a normal resting exhalation. This may result in improvements of collateral ventilation by recruiting additional alveoli from lesser dependent lung zones, so again helping with oxygenation. (It is easier to recruit an alveolus that is partly open than one that is totally collapsed). In some cases, the raised FRC may result in a more favourable position on the lung compliance curve. Again alveoli may be recruited and the overall work of breathing may be reduced.

Continuous positive airways pressure considerations
The patient may need help with the inspiratory effort required to maintain ventilation throughout the whole of the inspiratory phase. Where this is not applied, the patient may perceive CPAP to be a resistance to breathing out, so increasing expiratory effort. The application of a CPAP may be used to offset the disadvantages of PEEPi when present. This is further discussed with BiPAP, since CPAP does not offer ventilatory support, but is indicated more to correct hypoxaemia.

Continuous positive airways pressure complications
The residual air that is generated within the lungs causes an increase in intrathoracic pressure that may, in turn, affect the cardiovascular status of the patient, causing a squeeze effect on the thoracic vessels and subsequent possible reduction in cardiac output and blood pressure. The risk of barotrauma is also a possibility; particularly in the more at-risk patient, e.g. those with emphysematous or cystic lungs, who should be monitored closely. These patients are always susceptible to ruptured bulla even without the application of NIV – an ability to recognize the clinical signs and symptoms of a pneumothorax with appropriate action taken is essential. The clinician should have a high index of suspicion and monitor the patient appropriately to avoid missing early clinical signs and symptoms, as with any other treatment or intervention. Appropriate monitoring is essential to help detect such deleterious effects of application. Other interventions may also be required, e.g. insertion of nasogastric tube to reduce abdominal distension in the patient who swallows excessive amounts of air.

NB. increasing central venous pressure (CVP) reduces cerebral perfusion. Where this is likely to compromise a patient (e.g. head-injured patients) a 30° head-up tilt with the neck slightly flexed may help to prevent raising ICP.

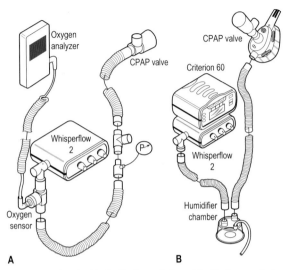

CPAP circuit. Reproduced with the kind permission of Profile Systems Ltd

Continuous positive airways pressure indications
- Type I failure
- Cardiac failure
- Non-distressed hypoxic patient
- OSA patients.

Also obesity, post operatively, weaning from intubated ventilatory support, avoidance of intubation in pneumocystis pneumonia in AIDS patients, post-thoracic trauma, rib fractures, contusion or where restrictive ventilatory patterns occur, e.g. pancreatitis.

Continuous positive airways pressure cautions
- Absence of atelectasis as cause for hypoxaemia
- Emphysematous bullae/other lung cysts
- Chronic obstructive pulmonary disease (COPD)
- Raised intracranial pressure
- Undrained pneumothorax
- Low CO states.

Bi-level positive airway pressure (B$_i$PAP®)

This provides two levels of respiratory support: expiratory positive airway pressure (EPAP), which acts as a splint similar to CPAP, and inspiratory positive airway pressure, which reduces the work of breathing, resulting in a larger tidal volume for the same amount of patient effort, thus facilitating the removal of carbon dioxide.

EPAP	IPAP
Maintains the airways in an 'open state'	Supports inspiratory effort, so reducing the work of breathing
Improves alveolar gas exchange	Improves tidal volume
Improves oxygenation	Improves CO_2 removal
Increases lung volume (FRC)	
Overcomes intrinsic PEEP	

Non-maleficence An ethical principle that dictates that we should avoid doing harm to others.

Non-parametric test Research term – a statistical test that is less sensitive than a parametric test, but that can be used on nominal and ordinal data. Non-parametric tests can be used on data that do not possess normal distribution. See *Normal distribution*

Non-steroidal anti-inflammatory drugs (NSAIDs) Medication that produces antipyretic, analgesic and, most importantly, anti-inflammatory effects. They act by modifying the complex chemical process that mediates inflammation in musculoskeletal conditions. Many have side effects including their effects on gastric mucosa.

   ○ Clinical point There are a great number of NSAIDs on the market now, physiotherapists will come across them frequently.

Normal distribution Research term – data that are spread out in a bell-shaped curve, e.g. the size of people's feet, a few people have small feet, a few have large feet but most people will be in the centre.

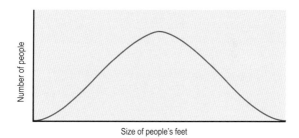

Normal distribution chart

Normality A dominant shared expectation of behaviour and personal characteristics that defines what is considered culturally desirable and appropriate.

Normalization A principle that has played a major role in the move from institutional to community living for people with learning difficulties. When originally conceived, the prime focus was the right of people with learning difficulties to live and to be assisted to live socially valued lives of their own choosing within the community. As it has developed, the principle has been subject to much criticism, particularly as an attempt to 'normalize' people by imposing traditional, middle-class standards of behaviour.

See *Social role valorization*

Normal movement analysis Normal movement is a learned attribute through experience and practice based on a background of activity that arises from the integration of sensori-motor skills for the execution of efficient function. Analysis of normal movement is based upon in depth knowledge of how people move, and thus enables deviations from the norm to be recognized. It is important to acknowledge that there is a wide variation in the range of how people move and normal varies with the individual.

Normal movement approach This term relates to the adoption of the analysis of normal movement as a basis to recognize deviations from the norm on which to formulate a plan for treatment intervention. This term is sometimes associated with the Bobath Concept.

Normative play Play exhibited by children that is child led, with no intrinsic goals. It is spontaneous and pleasurable compared with therapeutic play, which is professional led with specific goals to achieve.

NOS The National Osteoporosis Society. Go to www.nos.org.uk

Nottingham health profile A measure mainly used to measure perceived health status in population surveys. It is self-report and is aimed at measuring generic quality of life. It was developed on populations with disabilities and it may be more appropriately used in this group than on healthy normals; the latter tend to have an inability to demonstrate responsiveness in this measure (Hunt and McKenna 1991).

Nucleus pulposus Semi-gelatinous substance contained within the annulus fibrosus of the intervertebral disc. Internal derangement of the disc may result in leakage of the nucleus pulposus through the breached annular fibres.

It is made up from mainly Type 11 collagen, it is hydrophilic (water loving) and is kept in check by the annulus. It does not possess any nerve endings.

See *Annulus fibrosus*

Number needed to treat (NNT) The number of patients who, on average, must be treated to prevent a single occurrence of the outcome of interest. It is the inverse of the absolute risk reduction (ARR):

$$NNT = 1/ARR$$

Null hypothesis Research term – the proposal that there is no difference between groups. A typical study aims to reject the null hypothesis.

NWB Common medical abbreviation – Non-weight bearing.

Nystagmus An involuntary oscillation (back and forth movements) of one or both eyes in a horizontal, vertical, rotatory or mixed direction. It can result from retinal or labyrinthine disease or disorders of the cerebellum or part of the brain stem.

O

OA Common medical abbreviation – Osteoarthritis.

Ober's test A test that determines the extensibility of the iliotibial band. Performed with the person in side lying with the hip fully laterally rotated and the knee joint in unlocked extension.

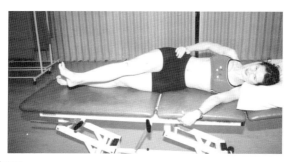

Ober's test

Normal finding The uppermost leg should be able to drop (adduct) to the plinth.

Abnormal finding The leg cannot drop to the plinth.

Objectivity A state of mind that is not influenced by personal feelings, opinions or prejudices. The notion of objectivity has been contested on the grounds that all human activity is dependent on subjective processes. For example, 'objective' research is influenced by factors relating to culture and history including what is considered worth researching:

> It is by the aid of non-objective mental operations that we switch to being 'objective'. Non-objective changes bring into view the objective world. (Laing RD 1983 The voice of experience. Penguin Books. Harmondsworth.)

Obstructive lung disease This is characterized by obstruction to airflow and may be diagnosed on spirometric testing.
See *COPD* and *Spirometry*

Obstructive Sleep Apnoea Hypopnoea Syndrome (OSAHS) This is a disorder characterized by excessive daytime sleepiness with irregular breathing during sleep. As sleep ensues, the sufferer loses muscle tone in the upper pharynx resulting in loss of airway patency and airway narrowing with flow limitation. Inspiratory effort is increased to offset this narrowing with a transient arousal from deep sleep to lighter sleep or wakefulness. This is often repeated many times throughout the night resulting in poor sleep quality through repeated fragmentation. The clinical features of OSAHS include: impaired concentration, excessive daytime sleepiness, apnoeas and choking episodes during sleep (witnessed by partners), snoring, irritability and changes in personality, and reduced libido. Diagnostic procedures include full polysomnography, overnight pulse oximetry and electro-encephalography, with severity calculated using the Apnoea Hypopnoea Index (AHI). Disease management includes behavioural interventions, e.g. sleep hygiene, smoking cessation, weight control, non-surgical interventions (e.g. CPAP, intra-oral devices and pharmacological interventions) and surgical intervention (e.g. uvulopalatopharyngoplasty [UPPP]). See SIGN guidelines (2003) for full details available from www.sign.ac.uk

Other useful websites: www.sleep-apnoea-trust.org; www.sleepapnea.org; www.users.cloud9.net/~thorpy

Obturator nerve   See *Femoral nerve*

OCC   Common medical abbreviation – Occasional.

Occupational diseases   Diseases due to factors encountered during the course of a person's employment, for example, asbestosis.

Odontoid process   The peg-like process on the upper surface of the axis, which articulates with the atlas.

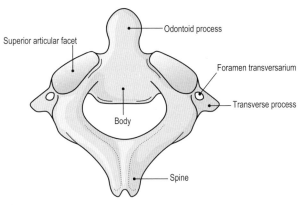

The axis

OE (X2)   Common medical abbreviation – Objective examination or on examination.

Oedema   An accumulation of excess tissue fluid.

Ohm's law   Electrotherapy term:

$$V = IR$$

where V is the voltage (volts) in the circuit, I is the current (amps) and R is the resistance (ohms).

Used to calculate changes in circuits with direct current. For an alternating current see an electrical engineering textbook.

Oligodendrocytes   Myelin-producing cells in the central nervous system.

One-tailed hypothesis   Research term – implies a direction to a predicted change, e.g. group A will score higher than group B. Whereas a two-tailed hypothesis implies a difference, but no direction to the change, e.g. group A will have a different score than group B.

On:off ratio   Electrotherapy term – the time for which current (or another pulsed output such as ultrasound or SWD) flows and is off in a complete cycle, measured in s or ms usually. Can be used as a ratio or to calculate duty cycle.

Ontology   Research term – the study of the fundamental categories of what sorts or kinds of things may exist. For example, propositions, facts, numbers, causal connections, ethical values, forces, substances, spiritual beings and purposes.

It is also the branch of metaphysics concerned with the fundamental categories of things.

Open fracture – also known as compound fracture   There is a communication between the fracture and the outside environment. These types of fractures occur when the bone end or some other object has pierced the skin. These fractures are an additional cause for concern because of the possibility of introduction of microorganisms leading to bone infection, i.e. osteomyelitis.

See *Closed fracture* and *Fracture classification*

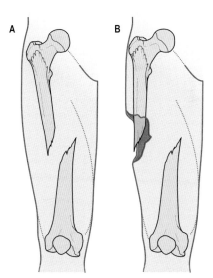

(**A**) Closed fracture; (**B**) An open fracture with contamination

Open kinematic chains See *Kinetic chain exercise*

These terms refer to chains of joints. For instance, the shoulder, elbow and wrist form a chain of three upper extremity joints. In open chain-joint movements, the proximal joint member is fixed or stable while the distal member moves. Reaching to grasp an object in space, or kicking a ball are examples of open chain movements.

Opportunistic infection An infection in an immune compromised person caused by an organism that does not usually cause disease in healthy people. Many of these organisms are carried in a latent state by virtually everyone and only cause disease when given the opportunity of a damaged immune system.

Oppression See *Internal oppression*

Opsonization The part of the immune response whereby antigens are coated in another substance so making it more open to phagocytosis.

Optic neuritis This is caused by a lesion to the optic nerve and can cause a loss of vision and eye movement may be painful.

  ✪ Clinical note This is a common early sign in multiple sclerosis and is caused by demyelination of the optic nerve. It may also be called retrobulbar neuritis.

Oral high frequency oscillation This refers to the application of high frequency vibrations (applied either externally via a high frequency chest wall compressor or internally via devices such as the flutter) to the airways to facilitate sputum clearance. The rapid vibratory movements of small volumes of air within the airways results in the enhancement of cough and mucus clearance.

Ordinal data Research term – refers to a scale where the numbers are ranked, but not necessarily with equal distances between each category.

Orientation This term relates to the awareness of a person to time, place and person. Orientation may become altered following brain injury or disease.

ORIF Common medical abbreviation – Open reduction internal fixation.

Surgical intervention by applying a plate and screws to the fracture is known as open reduction and internal fixation, often abbreviated to ORIF.

Advantages
• Permits a detailed inspection and accurate surgical assessment of the site of injury and procedure to be undertaken.

Disadvantages
• Surgery inevitably causes additional trauma and potential exposure to microorganisms.
• Can convert a closed fracture into an open fracture.
• Requires surgery with all its sequelae and potential complications. Ironically, rigid fixation may remove the stimulus for callus formation. The implants may be removed 12–18 months in the future or if they start to become a problem, e.g. the screws may become an irritant.

They will be removed in the young, as whilst they are in place bone will not grow and respond to stress normally, because some of the stresses are taken by the implants themselves.

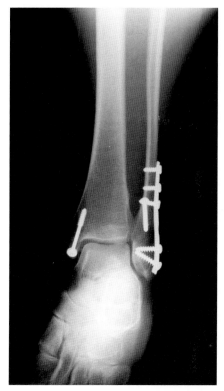

Open reduction internal fixation – X-ray – fracture of the tibia/fibula

Orofacial movements This relates to movements of the face and mouth and problems can occur in this area following brain injury or after Bell's palsy.

⊕ Clinical note The restoration of orofacial function should be of paramount importance for the physiotherapist and speech and language therapist. Problems in this area can lead to an inability to close the lips, move food around in the mouth and thus eating can become embarrassing for the patient. If eye closure is a problem then eye care is crucial and the eyelid may require temporary stitching for protection.

Oropharynx This is the area at the back of the throat extending from the uvula to the epiglottis and tongue base.

Orthopnoea This is the presence of dyspnoea in a lying position and is common in cardiac-failure patients. It is thought to occur as a result of pulmonary vascular congestion caused by the inability of the left ventricle to cope with the sudden increase in venous return, which occurs when reclining. Another cause of orthopnoea is diaphragmatic weakness or paralysis.

Orthosis An external device that is fitted to a body part, e.g. an ankle foot orthosis, which assists/maintains or prevents a movement by the application of external forces.

Osgood-Schlatter's disease Traction epiphysitis of the tibial tubercle, commonly seen in adolescents. It usually manifests itself as pain on direct pressure and contraction of the quadriceps muscle group, e.g. landing on the leg, jumping or squatting. There is often a noticeable lump, with X-rays showing some separation of the apophysis.

Osteitis pubis Inflammatory reaction in the pubic symphysis.

Osteoarthritis Often described as degenerative joint disease (DJD) it covers a variety of signs and symptoms, including osteophyte formation, stiffness and deformity (e.g. Heberben's nodes) and pain. There are two main types – primary and secondary.

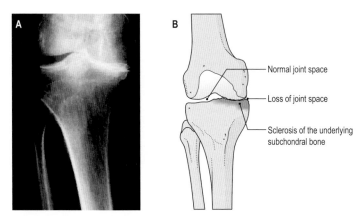

(**A**) X-ray: Osteoarthritis of the medial compartment of the knee; (**B**) Osteoarthritis of the medial compartment of the knee

Primary osteoarthritis

There is no obvious cause, it is due to an intrinsic alteration of the articular tissues themselves. It affects joints in a classical pattern and is common in post-menopausal women who typically exhibit Heberden's and Bouchard's nodes. The joints commonly affected by primary OA are shown in the figures below.

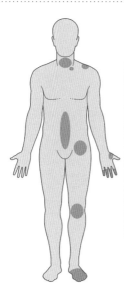

- Intervertebral joints and facet joints particularly in the lower cervical and lower lumbar areas.
- Distal interphalangeal joints of the fingers.
- Metatarsophalangeal joints of the big toe.
- 1st Carpometacarpal joint of the thumb.
- Temperomandibular joints.
- Sternoclavicular joint, acromioclavicular joint.
- Hip joint.
- Knee joint including patello-femoral joint.

Primary OA is not common in the wrists, shoulders, or ankles.

Joints commonly affected by primary OA

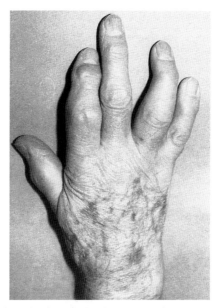

Heberden's and Bouchard's nodes in primary osteoarthritis

Secondary osteoarthritis

Arises as a consequence of another condition. The causes of secondary OA can be divided into one of the following four categories: metabolic, anatomic, traumatic or inflammatory. OA appears to be more common in people with a previous injury or fracture to a particular joint (Coggon et al. 2001). Repeated minor trauma may lead to micro fractures and subsequent OA. Occupational factors are thought to be important in the development of secondary OA. Miners knees are at risk, as are tailors first carpometacarpal and metacarpophalangeal joints, as are the elbows and shoulders of pneumatic drill operators. Joint infection puts a joint at risk of OA, as does deformity, for example, following fractures that cause biomechanical anomalies or direct cartilage damage if the fracture included the articular surface. The relationship between obesity and OA is complex and still not fully understood. Being overweight is linked to development of OA in some joints but not in others. There is a correlation between high body mass index and knee OA, which may be due to varus deformities in obese persons (Sharma et al. 2000), but the correlation is less strong between obesity and OA of the hip and with generalized OA (Sturmer et al. 2000). Being overweight may result is premature muscle fatigue, which in turn leads to abnormal kinematics and the subsequent development of OA. The relationship seems to be much stronger in women. Increased load across the joints clearly plays a role, but hormonal abnormalities associated with obesity may also be to blame, as suggested by an increase, albeit modest, in hand OA in obese women.

Clinical features of osteoarthritis (OA) related to pathology

Clinical feature	Pathology
Pain	Multiple causes and presentations multi factorial Causes of pain in OA are discussed later in this chapter
Heat/redness	Can not always be detected, especially in the deeper joints such as the hip joint Superficial joints, however, such as the knee joint can become warm to palpation signifying active inflammation
Joint effusions/swelling	Effusion = swelling confined to a synovial cavity Swelling is a more general term
Muscle spasm	A protective mechanism, movement causes pain so the body attempts to stop movement, but spasm often occurs out of all proportion to the underlying pathological cause Prolonged spasm causes pain due to metabolite accumulation and fatigue in itself and it may limit joint movement It may also interfere with sleep Adaptive shortening of muscles may also occur, e.g. hamstrings if the knee is held in flexion for prolonged periods
Stiffness (articular gelling)	Stiffness refers to the impairment of quality of movement not quantity Stiffness is present after rest and takes a little time to wear off with movement

Clinical feature	Pathology
	It may be due to loss of joint lubrication, chronic oedema in the periarticular structures, swelling of the articular cartilage, or possibly the accumulation of hyaluronate in the capsule and synovium
Loss of movement	Due to adaptive soft tissue shortening or lengthening, alteration of joint contour, or osteophytes
Radiographic findings: 1. Loss of joint space 2. Sclerosis 3. Altered bone end shape 4. Osteophytes Muscle atrophy	X-ray changes may not correlate with pain or disability levels The term joint space is a misnomer, hyaline cartilage is invisible on X-ray so only appears as a space (see figure of the X-ray appearance of OA of the medial compartment of the knee) Either through disuse or because of pain inhibition, muscles become weak, often on the aspect of the joint that is opposite to contractures, e.g. the hip extensors in cases of hip flexion deformity
Joint enlargement	Chronic oedema of synovial membrane and capsule makes the joint appear large Osteophytes and chronic effusions also contribute Muscle atrophy may also make the joint look bigger, for example, affecting the vastus medialis
Crepitus	From mild creaking (which may also indicate synovitis), to loud cracking sounds in advanced disease The flaked cartilage and eburnated bone ends grate against each other with a characteristic sound on movement
Joint instability	Loss of proprioception and loss of ligamentous control and the loss of negative pressure within the joints as a result of effusions all contribute to joint instability in OA
Loss of function and deformity	A combination of all the above clinical features Each joint adopts a characteristic deformity or restriction of movements known as the capsular pattern

Osteoblast The cells that are responsible for building bone.
How to remember: osteo**B**lasts **B**uild bone, osteo**C**lasts **C**hew bone.

Osteochondritis dissecans A fragment of cartilage and subchondral bone that becomes detached, either partially or completely, from the bone underneath. Common in the knee joint.

Osteoclast The cells that are responsible for bone resorption.

Osteogenesis impefecta (brittle bone disease) Go to www.brittlebone.org

Osteomalacia Involves softening of the bones caused by a deficiency of vitamin D, or problems with the metabolism of this vitamin.

Osteophyte Outgrowth of bone, seen in osteoarthritis, usually in reaction to pathological processes within or at a joint. Often formed as a result of traction on the bony margin.

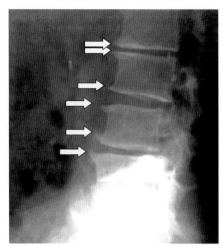

Lateral X-ray of the lumbar spine of a 55-year-old male with lumbar spondylosis. Arrows indicate anterior osteophytes

Osteoporosis A progressive skeletal disorder, characterised by low bone mass and microarchitectural deterioration of bone tissue, leading to a consequent increase in bone fragility, and susceptibility to fracture (WHO 1991).

Osteoporosis risk factors for women

A lack of oestrogen, caused by:

- an early menopause (before the age of 45)
- an early hysterectomy (before the age of 45), particularly when both ovaries are removed by oophrectomy
- missing periods for 6 months or more (excluding pregnancy) as a result of over exercising or over dieting.

Osteoporosis risk factors for men

- Low levels of testosterone (hypogonadism).

Osteoporosis risk factors for men and women

- Long-term use of high dose corticosteroid tablets (for conditions such as rheumatoid arthritis and asthma)
- Close family history of osteoporosis (maternal or paternal), particularly with history of a maternal hip fracture
- Medical conditions such as Cushing's syndrome, liver and thyroid problems
- Malabsorption problems (coeliac disease, Crohn's disease, intestinal diseases or gastric surgery)
- Long-term immobility

- Heavy alcohol consumption and smoking
- Poor diet
- Low body weight in proportion to height (Carne 2003).

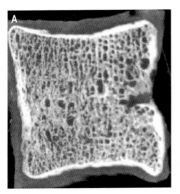 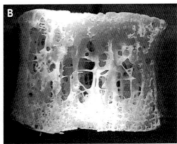

(**A**) Normal vertebra; (**B**) Osteoporotic vertebra

Osteotomy An operation to cut across a bone usually done to realign a joint.

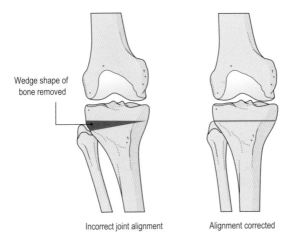

Wedge shape of
bone removed

Incorrect joint alignment   Alignment corrected

Osteotomy

Oswestry standing frame This is a standing frame, originally designed to help
people with spinal injury independently stand. They are now widely used in
neurological rehabilitation, but due to manual handling regulations, unless

the patient is able to assist with the manoeuvre from sit to stand, they have limited use.

O Clinical note Many standing frames are now being fitted or designed with motors to gradually move the patient from sitting to standing.

Outcome measures A test or scale that aims to record information about a particular attribute(s) of interest. Prior to use, the measure should be evaluated to appraise the extent to which it is valid for the intended use, can be reliably used, is sufficiently responsive, acceptable to the intended users, feasible for use in the intended setting, the results interpretable and sufficiently user-friendly.

The use of outcome measures (see *Motor Assessment Scale* and *Ashworth Scale*) promotes the standardization of objective measurement and evaluation of practice. Outcome measures should have key qualities of:

- reliability
- validity
- responsiveness.

Outrigger A type of splint used commonly after tendon or joint replacement in the hand and wrist.

Over pressure This is a passive pressure applied to the end of a joint's active range when pain free. A movement cannot be classed as normal unless the range is pain free actively and passively and with the addition of passive overpressure at the limit of the active range. The recording of a normal movement in relation to its range, quality and symptom response is recommended as $\sqrt{\sqrt{}}$ (Maitland 2001, p.124).

Oxford scale (The) A relatively quick and easy-to-use scale that is used widely in clinical practice. However, it is not very objective, functional or sensitive to change since the movements resisted are concentric contractions and the spaces between the grades are not linear:

0 – no contraction

1 – flicker of contraction only, movement of the joint does not occur

2 – movement is only possible with gravity counterbalanced

3 – movement against gravity is possible

4 – movement against resistance is possible

5 – normal functional movement is possible.

Oximetry Oximeters are used to measure the oxygen saturation of haemoglobin. This is done using an oximeter, a photoelectric device specially designed for this purpose. An ear oximeter is attached while a finger oximeter is attached to a finger. The concept of infrared light absorption provides the basis for measurement. The advantages are that constant monitoring of oxygen saturation can be performed non-invasively. However, many factors may impair accuracy, e.g. poor peripheral tissue perfusion, optical interference and excessive patient movement.

Oxygen debt The phenomenon that occurs after prolonged exercise where there has been a large 'dipping into' the metabolic reserves, this must be 'repaid' after exercise.

Oxygen saturation (SaO$_2$) The percentage of haemoglobin saturated with oxygen.

Oxygen therapy Oxygen therapy plays a vital role in the management of hypoxaemia and respiratory failure. It is a potent drug with associated potential hazards of use, e.g. fire, oxygen toxicity (which can occur if breathing $>60\%$ O$_2$ for >48 h), progression to ARDS carries a high mortality and absorption atelectasis while patients' responses to its administration are varied. One hospital survey found 21% of O$_2$ prescriptions were inappropriate and 85% of patients were inadequately supervised. Similar studies in GP surgeries show inadequate prescribing of the drug. Safety and effectiveness may be achieved with prescription of flow rate, delivery system, duration and monitoring of such treatment (Bateman & Leach 1998).

The amount of oxygen in the arterial blood (i.e. the oxygen content) is the vital factor for patient well-being, since this, in conjunction with cardiac output, determines oxygen delivery (i.e. the amount of oxygen delivered to the tissues per unit time). This in turn, is dependant upon blood flow to the tissues (i.e. the cardiac output) and the amount of oxygen contained in that blood (i.e. the arterial oxygen content).

Oxygen is carried in combination with haemoglobin (Hb) and dissolved in plasma. Its oxygen capacity and its percent saturation with oxygen determine the amount carried by Hb, while the volume in solution depends on the partial pressure of oxygen.

'Normally' oxygen consumption is around 250 ml min^{-1} (utilizing only one-quarter of the oxygen available), so providing a safety margin should oxygen consumption increase or delivery falls, e.g. during exercise. The normal value for arterial PO$_2$ is 11–15 KPa in adults, but this value falls steadily with age (probably due to increasing ventilation–perfusion [V/Q] inequalities).

Oxygen therapy should be aimed at correcting arterial hypoxaemia. When tissue hypoxia occurs **without** arterial hypoxaemia, treatment should address the underlying cause (e.g. cardiac failure). Treatment should be administration of a high enough concentration of oxygen to establish a PaO$_2$ greater than 8 kPa. Accuracy of delivery is vitally important when managing chronic lung patients (North-West Oxygen Group 2001). A fixed performance device (such as a Venturi) assures delivery of a stated concentration, while normal variables, such as rate and depth of breathing, equipment and peak inspiratory flow demands, will affect the concentrations delivered by the low flow devices (such as MC masks and nasal cannulae) resulting in delivery of anything between 24% and 90% oxygen concentrations.

Acutely, oxygen dosages may be critical. Inadequate oxygenation results in more deaths and disability than can be justified by the relatively small risks associated with higher doses (Bateman & Leach 1998).

Extra vigilance should be used when administering oxygen to the patient with high PaCO$_2$ and hypoxia (see *Hyperbaric oxygen*). A recent publication provides guidance on safe oxygen administration for the chronic-obstructive-pulmonary-disease patient (North West Guidelines 2001).

Oxyhaemoglobin dissociation curve This curve is obtained when the saturation of Hb with oxygen is plotted against the PaO_2 forming an S-shaped curve (i.e. the curve demonstrates the relationship of Hb saturation with changes in the arterial partial pressure of oxygen). The flat upper portion of the curve where there are minor changes in PaO_2 demonstrates Hbs large affinity for O_2 and represents the arterial circulation. Below a PaO_2 of ~8 kPa (the normal functioning level of tissues) the curve sharply steepens and Hb saturation with oxygen falls, since Hb affinity for O_2 is reduced, so O_2 is readily given up to the tissues.

In chronic lung disease patients presenting with Type II respiratory failure, it is recommended that O_2 be titrated to achieve and maintain an oxygen saturation of 90%, as there is no clinical gain to be obtained from a higher saturation, whereas overoxygenation in the hypoxic drive patient, may result in a worsening of acidosis.

PA Common medical abbreviation – Postero anterior.

Pacemaker Implanted stimulator to control cardiac function. Output may alter in proximity to high-intensity radio-frequency radiation such as SWD or MW. See *SWD* and *MW*
Ensure patients with pacemaker of any type are not within 3–5 m of such equipment if operating.

PACI Common medical abbreviation – Partial anterior cerebral infarction. Patients with this type of stroke are at high risk of further strokes.

Pacinian corpuscles Rapidly adapting mechanoreceptors. Pacinian corpuscles contain an afferent nerve fibre surrounded by a capsule. They are sensitive to high-frequency stimuli, such as vibration.

PaCO$_2$ This refers to the partial pressure of carbon dioxide within the arterial blood. The normal range is 4.5–6.0 kilo Pascals (kPa).

Paget's disease This is a disease of bone that initially results in the excessive resorption of bone followed by the replacement of normal bone marrow with fibrous and vascular tissue. It is a metabolic bone disease that involves bone destruction and regrowth that result in deformity. The cause of Paget's disease is unknown.

Painful arc The term that describes pain in a certain part of a movement, it usually refers to shoulder abduction, typically pain occurs in the middle of

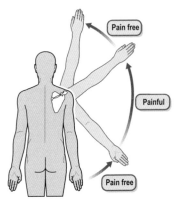

the range but inner and outer ranges are pain free. Pain is usually caused by impingement of the supraspinatus tendon under the acromion process.

Pain-gate theory The pain-gate theory was initially proposed in 1965 by Melzack and Wall based on the fact that small-diameter nerve fibres carry pain stimuli through a 'gate mechanism', but larger-diameter nerve fibres going through the same gate can inhibit the transmission of the smaller nerves carrying the pain signal. It is this interruption of C-fibre-mediated pain pathways by Aβ fibres that is now known as the pain-gate theory. Chemicals released as a response to the pain stimuli also influence whether the gate is open or closed for the brain to receive the pain signal. This led to the theory that the pain signals can be interfered with by stimulating the periphery of the pain site, the appropriate signal-carrying nerves at the spinal cord, or particular corresponding areas in the brain stem or cerebral cortex.

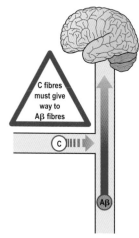

Pain-gate theory

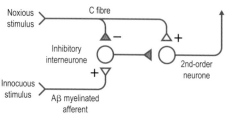

A model of the 'gating' of pain

○ Clinical point This concept is of great importance to physiotherapists since we spend so much effort on trying to relieve pain. The 'pain-gate' may be closed by stimulating mechanoreceptors, which enables the relief of pain through massage ice packs and deep transverse frictions. Acupuncture and electrical analgesia (TENS) may also stimulate release of opioids, thereby inhibiting the transmission of pain signals.

PAIVMs Common medical abbreviation – Passive accessory intervertebral movements.

These are passive intervertebral movements and are oscillatory accessory movements graded I–IV and used to assess and treat vertebral symptoms such as pain, resistance and spasm.

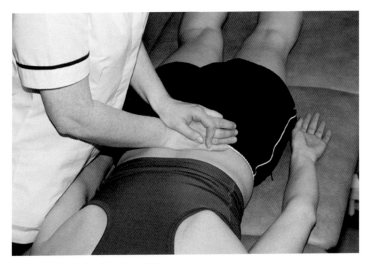

PA central lumbar spine using pisiform grip

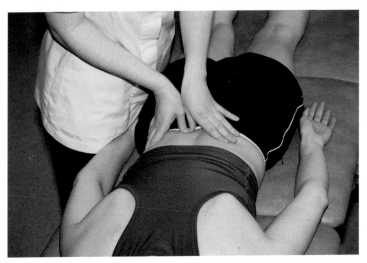

Unilateral lumbar spine

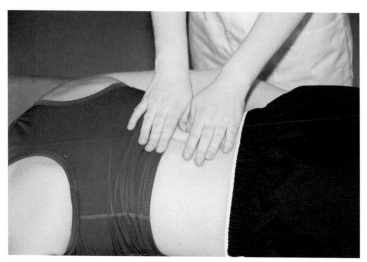

Transverse lower thoracic spine

These are passive physiological intervertebral movements and are oscillatory physiological movements graded I–IV and are used to assess and treat vertebral symptoms, such as pain, resistance and spasm.

Palate – cleft An opening in the roof of the mouth, due to a failure of the palatal shelves to fuse during development in the uterus.

Palliative care Palliative care is an approach that improves the quality of life of patients and their families who are facing a life-threatening illness. Palliative care:

- provides pain relief
- intends neither to hasten or postpone death
- integrates the psychological and spiritual aspects of patient care
- offers a support system to help patients live as actively as possible until their death
- offers a support system to help the family cope during the patient's illness, including bereavement counselling, if indicated.
  World Health Organization (WHO) definition of palliative care (2002).

Palpation To examine medically by touch.

Panniculitis An inflammatory reaction of the subcutaneous fat tissues.

Pannus Granulation tissue which is derived from synovial tissue, overgrows the articular surface of the joint in rheumatoid arthritis and is associated with its subsequent breakdown.

Paradoxical breathing A change in breathing pattern that results from loss of chest-wall integrity or gross-muscle weakness/failure. The chest is pulled in during inspiration and moves out on expiration, e.g. flail segment.

Parameters Electrotherapy term – the variables that describe precisely the settings used. Ultrasound parameters include: frequency, BNR, size and ERA of applicator, intensity (SATA, SATP), duration and frequency of treatments, continuous or pulsed, location and size of area treated, brand and model of machine. Electrical stimulation parameters depend on if the current is pulsed, alternating or direct, generally they include: frequency, pulse duration and shape, intensity, duration and frequency of treatments, electrode size and location. Laser parameters include: frequency, type of laser, J/cm^2 applied, size and location of treatment area, which applicator and method, duration and frequency of treatments, etc. SWD parameters include: if capacitive or magnetic field method, pulsed (PSWD) or continuous (CSWD), duration and frequency of treatments, size and location of electrodes or coil. UVR parameters include: which lamp, distance from skin, duration and date of treatment, etc. Ice, superficial heating parameters include: method used and duration and frequency of treatments.

Parametric test Research term – a type of statistical test that is more sensitive and robust than a non-parametric test. In order to be able to carry out a parametric test on your data, the data must be interval/ratio and should, ideally, be normally distributed.
See *Normal distribution*

Paraparesis Weakness or partial loss of movement and or sensation in the lower half of the body following damage to the spinal cord in the thoracic, lumbar or sacral regions.

Paraplegia The loss of movement and or sensory function in the lower half of the body, usually as a result of damage to the spinal cord in the thoracic, lumbar or sacral regions.

Parasympathetic nervous system See *Autonomic nervous system*
One of the two divisions of the vertebrate autonomic nervous system.

Paresthesia Abnormal sensations: numbness, tingling, burning.

Parkinson's disease A degenerative disease of unknown origin that occurs in the latter half of life and involves the substantia nigra of the brain. It is characterized by slow movements, a resting tremor, rigidity and postural instability.

✚ Clinical note Parkinson's disease is always progressive, although the rate of deterioration varies. It is important to try to maintain movements of extension and rotation, as posture generally becomes dominated by flexion, there is a tendency to stoop and gait becomes festinating (short shuffling steps).

Parkinsonian syndrome This is a term used to describe a group of degenerative brain disorders where slowness of movement, facial musculature immobility, rigidity, tremor and a festinating gait may be seen and may be referred to as 'Parkinsonism'.

Pars interarticularis The segment of bone between the superior and inferior articular facets, especially in the lumbar spine.

Parturition The end of labour where the foetus is expelled from the uterus.

Passive accessory intervertebral movements (PAIVMs) Investigation of accessory gliding movements occurring in a joint.

Passive insufficiency The inability of a two joint muscle to fully stretch simultaneously across two joints, e.g. the hamstrings cannot stretch across hip and knee joints at the same time or gastrocnemius cannot permit full dorsiflexion if the knee is fully extended.

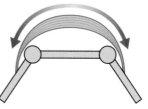

Passive insufficiency

Passive movement A movement which is performed by a force, which can be another person or a machine, i.e. continuous passive movement machine (CPM), but does not require voluntary activity of the patients own muscles.

The uses for passive movements are listed below:

• maintain integrity of joint and soft tissues
• promotion of synovial sweep over articular cartilage, thus nutrition
• maintain existing range of movement
• minimize risk of joint contractures (full range needed)
• maintain elasticity of soft tissues
• assist circulation if performed quickly (stimulation of the muscle pump)
• pain inhibition (movement can act as an analgesic)
• relaxation
• promote circulation, therefore, healing
• preserve memory of normal movement patterns
• psychological.

Passive neck flexion (PNF) See *Neurodynamics*

Patella The largest sesamoid bone in the body.

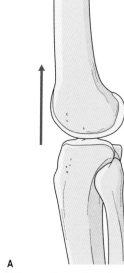

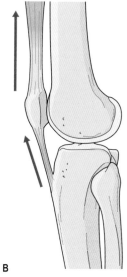

A

Without a patella when the quadriceps
contracted they would not be at a good
mechanical advantage

B

The angle of attack of the patella tendon
is altered by the patella making knee extension
more efficient

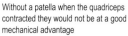

(**A**) Knee without a patella; (**B**) knee with a patella

Patella alta Refers to an abnormally high patella in relation to the femur; it
   may result in subluxation and dislocation of patella.

Patella baja An abnormally low patella.

Patellar dislocation/subluxation Instability of the patello-femoral joint,
   whereby the patella usually dislocates laterally.

Patellar tap test A test to determine the presence of an effusion at the knee
   joint. It is performed with the patient in the supine position. Any excess
   fluid is squeezed out of the suprapatellar pouch by sliding the index finger
   and thumb from 15 cm above the knee to the level of the upper border of the
   patella. Then place the tips of the thumb and three fingers of the free hand
   squarely on the patella and jerk it quickly downwards.

   Abnormal finding A 'click' sound indicates the presence of effusion. Note the test
   will be negative if the effusion is gross and tense, e.g. a haemarthrosis of the knee
   (blood within the joint) following an anterior cruciate rupture.

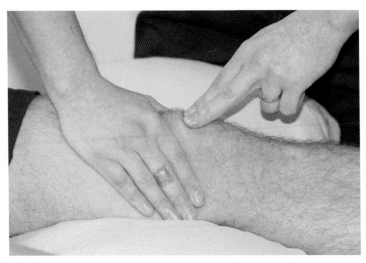

Patellar tap test

Patellar tendinitis Inflammatory condition of the patellar ligament.

Patellectomy Surgical removal of the patella.

Patello femoral joint See *Mal tracking patella*
  The joint between the posterior of the patella and the femur, the patella should track up and down in the channel between the condyles, if it does not it is known as a mal tracking patella.

Pathogenesis The natural evolution of a disease process in the body without intervention, i.e. without treatment. Description of the development of a particular disease.

Pathological fracture A fracture that has occurred because the normal architecture of a bone had been compromised by a disease, commonest examples are bone tumours either primary or secondary or osteoporosis.

Paternalism A condescending relationship where one person is thought to be superior to the other as in the traditional relationship between a father and his children. The professional–patient relationship has been criticized on the grounds of being paternalistic.

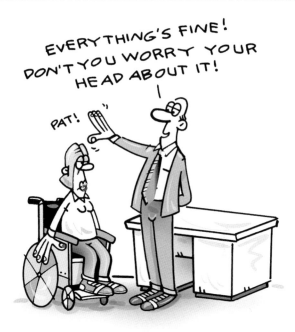

Patient-centred medicine An approach to medicine where the views, opinions and values of patients and clients are central. The professional relinquishes control so that power within the relationship can be shared.

Patient's charter A document that was introduced into the NHS in 1991 as a way of increasing patient involvement and control. It has been criticized for concentrating on procedural matters (for example, how to complain) rather than on patients' rights.

PCA (X2) Common medical abbreviation – Posterior communicating artery or Patient controlled analgesia.

Posterior communicating artery is a branch of the basilar artery that supplies the occipital cortex and the inferior part of the temporal lobe. It can be affected in stroke, resulting in a homonymous hemianopia on the opposite side.

PE Common medical abbreviation – Pulmonary embolism.

Peak expiratory flow rate – also known as peak flow The maximum flow at the outset of forced expiration. The peak expiratory flow rate is a measure of how quickly a person can exhale the air in the lungs. It is a useful test of airway function, which is commonly affected by diseases such as asthma or chronic obstructive pulmonary disease (COPD). In these lung diseases, air flow during exhalation is decreased by narrowing or blockage of the airways. The severity of asthma of COPD can change with time and peak expiratory flow monitoring is used by many patients to monitor their lung function over time.

Peak torque Measure of isokinetic performance, whereby the maximum 'torque' is achieved.

Pectus carinatum – also known as pigeon chest An anterior protrusion of the sternum, often seen in children with asthma.

Pectus excavatum – also known as funnel chest An inward depression of the sternum.

PEEP (Positive End Expiratory Pressure) This is the application of positive airway pressure at the end of expiration. This acts as a splinting pressure on the airways, thus holding them open. By doing so, functional residual capacity is raised and oxygenation improved.

See *NIV*

Peer review The academic process where work is scrutinized by eminent members of the same profession who make a judgement as to whether it is worthy of publication.

PEME Common medical abbreviation – Pulsed electromagnetic energy.

How does pulsed short wave work? A light hearted but useful explanation for patients.

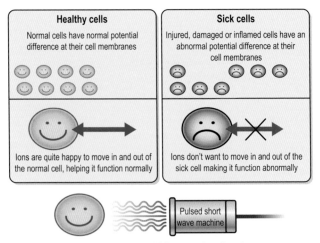

Pulsed short wave returns potential difference at the cell membrane
to normal thus turning it happy again so function returns back to what it
should be so the cell can repair, divide, whatever they need to do.

Penetration depth Electrotherapy term – the depth at which 37% of energy applied to an object or body remains (i.e. 63% of applied energy has been absorbed). The extent of absorption of energy by successively deeper levels of body tissue is an exponential function. The actual value will depend on the type and intensity of the energy (e.g. if ultrasound, cold, laser or infrared) and on the type and arrangement of tissue and other structures through which it passes. For example, ultrasound at a frequency of 1 MHz has a greater penetration depth than 3 MHz ultrasound. This is why 3 MHz frequency ultrasound is often chosen to treat superficial tissues and 1 MHz frequency if deeper. To ensure energy reaches deeper tissues the general principles are: use a lower frequency ultrasound (e.g. 0.8–1 MHz) and a higher intensity so sufficient energy is available at depth.

PEP mask Positive expiratory pressure mask. This is a mask device used to deliver positive expiratory pressure to facilitate the clearance of pulmonary secretions as first demonstrated by Falk et al. (1984).

Perception This is the ability to process and interpret sensory information.

   ◯ Clinical note Perceptual problems can follow brain injury and require careful assessment by the multidisciplinary team, especially the occupational therapist and psychologist. If problems are mild and not diagnosed they may cause problems with recovery of function.

Perch sitting This is when someone sits, with feet flat on the floor, on the edge of a high stool (called a perching stool) that has a slightly downward angulated seat that helps to attain/maintain the pelvis in a position of anterior tilt and thus encourages extensor activity in the upper body.

   ◯ Clinical note Patients can be sat on a perching stool whilst carrying out activities of daily living and thus maximize the therapeutic effect.

Percutaneous Applied through the skin directly to the subcutaneous tissues (e.g. some bone stimulators have an external power source with the current passing through wires that penetrate the skin; an electromyography needle is used percutaneously. This means it is passed through the skin directly to the motor unit being examined).

Perianal abscess An abscess that forms adjacent to the anal opening.

Pericarditis Inflammation of the pericardium.

Pericardium The membrane that lines the heart.

Perimysium The connective tissue sheath that surrounds a muscle and sends divisions between the bundles of muscular fibres.
   See *Muscle structure*

Periostitis Inflammatory condition at the border of muscular attachment and bone. Commonly seen in the lower leg, known in this case as 'shin splints'.

Peripheral nervous system This relates to the structures of the nervous system, i.e. nerves that do not include the brain and spinal cord.

PERLA Common medical abbreviation – Pupils equal reacting to light and accommodating.

Peroneal tendon subluxation Occurs commonly after an inversion injury, whereby there may be a shallow peroneal groove that predisposes to the subluxation or dislocation. The patient will often complain of a 'popping' sound or a 'snapping' sensation behind the lateral malleolus.

Personal development The planned process whereby an individual develops skills and knowledge that is beneficial to themselves and their career.

Personality An amalgam of an individual's characteristics and traits whereby he or she is recognized as being unique.

Personal tutor A member of academic staff allocated to a student to monitor their progress. This may be in an academic or pastoral capacity.

Perthe's disease Avascular necrosis of the femoral head, usually more common in boys than girls and occurring between 3 and 12 years of age. It usually results in a flattened femoral head.

Pes anserinus bursitis Inflammation of the bursa between the medial collateral ligament insertion and the 'pes' muscle group consisting of sartorius, gracilis and semitendinosus.

Pes cavus Foot deformity characterized by an increased elevation of the medial longitudinal arch of the foot.

Pes planus Characterized by a lowering of the medial longitudinal arch of the foot. Also known as 'pronated feet'.

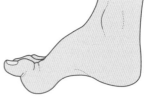

Pes cavus

PET scan Common medical abbreviation – Positron emission tomography.
This is like a computerized tomography (CT) scan (see *CAT scan*), but utilizes positron emitting radioisotopes. It can be used to show regional blood flow and oxygenation in the brain.

PFJ Common medical abbreviation – Patello femoral joint.

PFTs Common medical abbreviation – Pulmonary function tests.

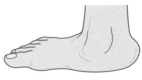

Pes planus

pH A term used to describe the acidity or alkalinity of a solution. It directly measures the hydrogen concentration of a solution. If the pH is below 7, the solution is acidic, if above 7 it is alkaline.

Phalen's test A test for carpal tunnel syndrome, whereby the wrists are held in a flexed position for one minute. If symptoms of paresethesia are reproduced in the fingers, the test is positive.

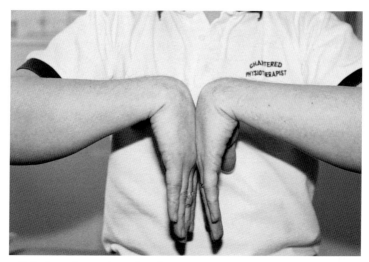

Phalen's test for carpal tunnel syndrome

Phantom limb The sensation that the amputated part of the body is still present.

Phases Electrotherapy term – a biphasic pulse has two phases and a monophasic has one phase. Illustrations of a phase indicate the rate of application of charge (slope and shape), the amount of charge applied (area of each phase) and the duration of each phase (duration).

Phenol block An injection of phenol into a particular nerve. It is sometimes used in the management of severe spasticity. The affect is permanent and so the decision to use this modality should only be undertaken after assessment from a specialist multidisciplinary team.

⨁ Clinical note If used to help control lower-limb spasticity, the patient should no longer have bowel and bladder function.

Phenomenology Research term – the study of the lived experiences of people, i.e. a description of the appearance of things, disregarding any account of their origin, explanation or causes.

Phenylketonuria A condition that manifests itself with microcephaly (small brain) and learning difficulties.

Phonophoresis The term used to describe the process of administration of a drug by means of ultrasound waves. There is still debate, but some evidence that this technique can deliver increased concentrations of certain anti-inflammatory drugs.

Phrenic nerves The nerves supplying innervation to the diaphragm arising from cervical root levels 3, 4 and 5. Where this is disrupted, diaphragmatic pacing may be indicated (i.e. the electrical stimulation of the diaphragm to illicit a contraction and sustain breathing).

Physiotherapy A healthcare profession concerned with human function and movement and maximizing potential. It uses physical approaches to promote, maintain and restore physical, psychological and social well-being, taking account of variations in health status. It is science-based, committed to extending, applying, evaluating and reviewing the evidence that underpin and informs its practice and delivery. The exercise of clinical judgement and informed interpretation is at its core (Chartered Society of Physiotherapy 2000).

PID (X2) Common medical abbreviation – Pelvic inflammatory disease or prolapsed inter vertebral disc.

Piedellos sign A test for the amount of movement at the sacro iliac joint. The seated patient is asked to flex forwards. The physiotherapist palpates the PSIS (sacral dimples) bilaterally.

Normal finding Both of the sacral dimples (PSIS) should move equally towards the head.

Abnormal finding Excessive rising of one side indicates hypomobility at that sacroiliac joint.

Piezoelectric effect Electrotherapy term – passing a rapidly alternating current through a crystal produces rapid mechanical vibrations of the crystal. This is a reversed piezoelectric effect, used for ultrasound production.

Pilot study Research term – a small-scale 'test' run of the proposed larger research study under the same conditions, useful as a means of ironing out problems before the study starts.

Piriformis syndrome Piriformis is implicated in the irritation of the sciatic nerve, as it passes through or underneath the muscle. Often accompanied by deep buttock pain.

Pituitary adenoma This is a tumour of the pituitary gland, often arising from the anterior part of the gland. They are usually benign.

Pivot shift test This is a test for anterolateral instability of the knee joint, with the foot in medial rotation and the knee in 30° of flexion, a valgus stress is applied to the knee whilst simultaneously extending it.

Abnormal finding A 'clunk' indicates a positive test and suggests anterior cruciate ligament (ACL) pathology.

Placebo A substance or procedure, with no known medicinal properties, which may modify or eliminate symptoms of illness if the patient and the health professional believe it will do so. The context in which it is administered may also be an important aspect of the placebo effect.

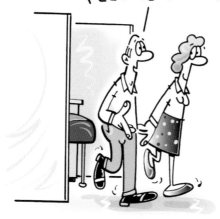

SHE'S ONLY ASSESSED ME BUT I'M ALREADY FEELING BETTER!

Plagiarism Where the (academic) work of others is used without proper acknowledgement, a serious academic offence.

Plantar fasciitis Also sometimes known as painful heel syndrome. Its main symptom is pain at the attachment of the plantar fascia to the medial tubercle of the calcaneum. Morning pain is predominant and may be aggravated by running or jogging. May be due to biomechanical abnormalities or as sequelae of other conditions such as ankylosing spondylitis.

Plantar response See *Babinski reflex*

Plantar wart A wart on the sole, often painful; commonly caused by the human papilloma virus.

Plaque A term used to describe areas with loss of myelin and the hardening of tissue in multiple sclerosis, or the fatty deposits that line the arteries in peripheral vascular disease.

Plasma The liquid (non-cellular) component of blood.

Plasmapheresis This is where a patient's plasma is removed and treated to remove antibodies thought to be attacking the myelin sheath.

○ Clinical note This process may be used in the treatment of Guillain–Barre syndrome (GBS).

Plaster of Paris (POP) This is a plaster-impregnated bandage that can be moulded to the part when wet, and subsequently sets. The standard method of external splinting is still plaster of Paris. Synthetic materials are now used for splinting some fractures because of their light weight and waterproof qualities. Custom-made lightweight thermoplastics can be moulded to the limb and re-moulded if swelling or atrophy cause changes in the limb contour. Some synthetic casting materials, however, are less malleable and cannot be moulded as effectively as plaster of Paris. They can occasionally cause allergies. A plaster saw is needed to remove a cast, this special tool has an oscillating blade that will cut through the hard cast without damaging the skin.

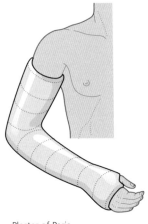

Plaster of Paris

Advantages of plaster of Paris

- No surgery or its complications
- No infection risk
- Quick to apply
- Rapid patient discharge
- Cheap, relatively easy to apply if trained
- New lightweight casts are an alternative
- Radio translucent (bones can be X-rayed through the cast)
- May absorb fluids or bleeding. The extent of bleeding can be traced on the cast itself and monitored daily
- Can be moulded for several minutes before hardening.

Disadvantages of plaster of Paris

- It may not be possible to reduce the fracture correctly or maintain reduction
- May require surgery at a later date
- Plaster needs removal/or windowing (removal of a piece of the cast) to inspect the skin
- May need removal in case of increased swelling or reapplication once swelling has subsided
- Smelly if it gets wet
- Heavy
- May crack
- May rub the skin and cause sores
- Medical advice should be sought if any of the following occur to a limb that is in plaster of Paris or similar splint:
  - pale or blue coloration of the skin on the injured part
  - numbness, tingling, or throbbing of the injured part

- inability to move the fingers or toes
- excessive pain in the injured part
- swelling, bulging or puffiness around the edges of the cast
- a foul smell from under the cast
- if it becomes loose and slides around.

Plasticity The ability to change.
 See *Neuroplasticity*

Platypnoea Shortness of breath in the upright position.

Pleura A thin layer of tissue covering the lungs (visceral pleura) and inner surface of the chest wall and mediastinum (parietal pleura). Although given different names, this constitutes a single continuous lining.

Pleural effusion This is an abnormal collection of fluid in the pleural space, the cause of which facilitates categorization. Increased production of pleural fluid or obstruction or blockage of drainage can cause accumulation of pleural fluid. Causes include para pneumonic, viral, malignancy, connective tissue diseases, lymphatic obstruction and many more. Clinical features vary with the size and onset, e.g. small effusions may have no symptoms while larger ones may be accompanied with dyspnoea and, if infective, cause pleuritic-type pain followed by fluid accumulation. Malignant effusions are often blood stained, while a turbid, fluid-associated post-bacterial pneumonia is termed empyema (pus-filled pleural fluid). Investigative procedures include chest radiology, pleural fluid aspiration and biopsy, thoracic ultrasound and video-assisted thoracoscopic (VATS) biopsy. Management of effusions is determined by the cause, so may involve no intervention, analgesics, antibiotics, chest drainage or surgical interventions.

Pleural pressure This is the negative pressure within the pleural space. It is fundamental in keeping the lung inflated and is more negative at the apex than the base (in the upright position). Disruption of the pleurae, e.g. trauma and pneumothorax cause an increase in pleural pressure to above atmosphere and will result in lung compression and collapse.

Pleural rub A creaking sound that is heard during auscultation, it signifies inflammation of the pleura.

Pleural space This is the potential space between the two pleurae. It is filled with a thin layer of serous fluid, which allows the pleural surfaces to glide easily over each other throughout the breathing cycle, while permitting chest wall forces to be transmitted to the lungs. Interruption of this space (e.g. chest trauma) can result in the separation of the two pleural surfaces when the parietal pleura will remain against the chest wall, while the visceral pleura and lung is displaced inward, away from the chest wall, e.g. pneumothorax.

Pleurectomy Removal of the parietal pleura of the lung.

Pleurisy Inflammation of the pleura, with subsequent pain. This usually results from a viral infection but has been generalized to any condition causing pleural pain, e.g. pneumonia. The pain is increased by deep breathing, coughing and chest movement. The pleural surfaces, roughened by inflammation, rub together with each breath and may produce a rough, grating sound called a 'friction rub'. This can be heard with the stethoscope.

Pleurodesis This is the fusion of the pleural surfaces. It may be performed where pneumothorax is persistent, or to prevent recurrence of pleural fluid formation.

Plexus The term for a gathering of inter-connected ventral rami that are best thought of as junction boxes, the main plexuses of the body are shown below.

Plica A synovial fold that is occasionally found in the knee joint, which may become pathological and painful, the most common plicae are the mediopatellar plica and the suprapatellar plica.

Plyometric exercise These employ an eccentric muscle contraction that is quickly followed by a concentric muscle contraction. Plyometric exercises often involve a jumping movement. For example, skipping, bounding, lunges.

PMH Common medical abbreviation – Past medical history.

PMR Common medical abbreviation – Polymyalgia rheumatica.

Pneumonia This is inflammation of the lung parenchyma, usually as a result of infection that can be either bacterial or viral, but may occasionally be fungal or parasitic. Pneumonia is classified into its causative group, i.e. either hospital- or community-acquired pneumonia (but was previously classified according to the site of infection as either 'lobar' or 'broncho').

The clinical features usually present as a rapid onset of pyrexia, cough (initially unproductive) and pleuritic chest pain, with rapid shallow breathing and possibly cyanosis. The affected portion of lung will often display features of consolidation radiologically, with bronchial breath sounds and dullness to percussion being common findings. Sputum and blood cultures should be obtained as soon as possible. Close monitoring of

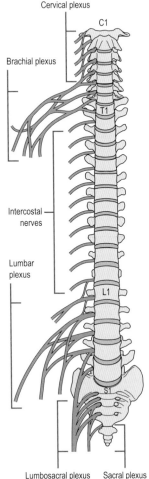

Cervical plexus

C1

Brachial plexus

T1

Intercostal nerves

Lumbar plexus

L1

S1

Lumbosacral plexus   Sacral plexus

The major somatic nerve plexuses of the body

these patients is required as severe pneumonia carries a significant risk of mortality (BTS 2001, 2002).

Pneumoconiosis An occupational or environmental lung disease caused by the repeated inhalation of inorganic dusts, e.g. coal miners lung.

Pneumomediastinum This is the collection of air in the mediastinum and may be indicative of barotrauma or oesophageal rupture (less commonly).

Pneumonectomy The surgical removal of a whole lung.

Pneumonia Is an inflammation of the lungs caused by a bacterial, viral or fungal infection.

Pneumonitis This is inflammation of the lung.

Pneumothorax This is the presence of air in the pleural space, which may occur either spontaneously (as with spontaneous rupture of a bulla) or on induction (e.g. through surgical intervention, resulting from trauma or as a complication of subclavian line insertion).

Pneumothorax usually presents as a sudden onset of pleuritic chest pain accompanied by shortness of breath and can be confirmed with chest radiology. Where the pneumothorax is small, there may be no symptoms, while those with underlying pulmonary disease or encountering a larger pneumothorax, may experience respiratory distress. Occasionally, a tension pneumothorax may develop (i.e. the pneumothorax is large enough to cause mediastinal shift away from the affected lung causing collapse of the heart as well as the lung). This will require immediate emergency medical intervention. (See BTS guidelines 1993 for further information.)

PNF Common medical abbreviation – Proprioceptive neuromuscular facilitation.

Polarity Electrotherapy term – the charge on a conductor, positive (anode) or negative (cathode).

Polycystic ovarian disease A gynaecological condition characterized by multiple ovarian cysts.

Polycythaemia An increase in the number of red blood cells. This is associated with chronic pulmonary disease. In response to chronic hypoxaemic states, more red blood cells are produced to raise the oxygen-carrying capacity of the blood. However, polycythaemic patients carry an increased risk of cor pulmonale and pulmonary embolus.

Polymyositis A type of acquired muscle disease.

Polypharmacy The use of excessive medications or use of unnecessary drugs by a person.

POMR Common medical abbreviation – Problem-oriented medical records.

POP Common medical abbreviation – Plaster of Paris.

Population Research term – every person who satisfies inclusion criteria for the study about to be performed.

Pores of Kohn Interconnecting ventilation channels between the alveoli (collateral ventilation channels).

Porphyria A condition characterized by abnormalities of porphyrin metabolism and results in the excretion of large quantities of porphyrins in the urine. Some cases can result in severe light sensitivity, reddish-brown urine and teeth, mutilation of the nose, ears, eyelids and fingers and an excess of body hair. Not surprising, therefore, that some people think that this disease is the basis of the vampire legend.

Positioning This is a term used to describe the active therapeutic management of the effect of different positions on the tonal influences on the body and limbs, e.g. supine is dominated by extensor tone and thus the therapist may break up this position by the use of wedges (see *Wedge*) to introduce an element of flexion.

○ Clinical note It is important to assess each individual for their optimal therapeutic positions and ensure that all members of the multidisciplinary team reinforce postures during the 24-h period.

Positive discrimination See *Affirmative action*

Positive supporting reaction (PSR) This is a term used by Magnus in 1926, to describe a response whereby the leg turns into a stiff pillar. A pattern of plantarflexion and inversion in the foot complex is seen when the patient attempts to weight bear through the affected leg.

○ Clinical note The presence of a positive supporting reaction can lead to soft tissue shortening in the foot and affected leg and can interfere with functional activities, such as walking and sit to stand. A local injection of botulinum toxin can be used to good short-term effect whilst manual techniques can work towards gaining length in shortened muscle groups (Magnus 1926).

Positivist research paradigm This philosophy assumes an objective measurable world.

Posterior Nearer the back of the body.

Posterior (AP) draw test Tests the integrity of the posterior cruciate ligament. The patient is supine. The therapist sits on the patient's foot to stabilize the leg and grasps around the posterior aspect of the proximal tibia and pushes the tibia backwards.

Abnormal finding Excessive translation of the tibia posteriorly. Compare this to the other side.

NB. A 'sag sign' is observed with the patient in crook lying whereby the tibia appears to be posteriorly displaced in relation to the femur, this may give the false impression that the patient has a rupture of the anterior cruciate ligament (ACL) since when a PA test is performed a considerable amount of movement may be noted, but this is due to the tibia returning to its resting position.

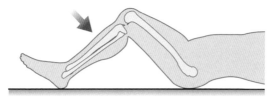

AP draw test

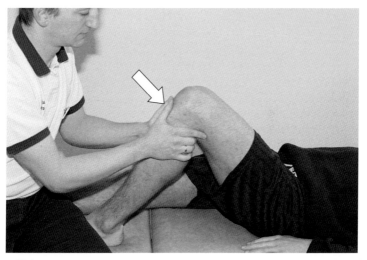

AP draw test

Posterior cruciate ligament (PCL) One of two major stabilizing and propiocep-
tive ligaments in the knee, the PCL primarily restrains posterior movement
of the tibia on the femur but has other functions including proprioception.
To test for a rupture see *Posterior (AP) draw test*

See *ACL* for illustration of anterior and posterior cruciate ligaments.

Posterior-fossa lesions This term relates to damage or injury that occurs to
the brain in the region of the posterior fossa.

   ○ Clinical note Ataxia is commonly seen following lesions in this area.

Postgraduate The term used to describe work, levels or students at a level
after the award of an honours degree.

Post hoc analysis Research term – analysis conducted after the results are
available that were not defined before the start of the trial. Such analyses
have weaknesses in that they are particularly prone to false-positive claims
or type I error.

Postpartum After childbirth or after delivery.

Post-traumatic amnesia (PTA) This relates to the period of time between a brain injury and the point at which the functions concerned with memory are determined to have been restored. It is a permanent memory loss and tends to reflect the severity of the damage.

Postural adjustments These are slight, spontaneous and often small movements that occur in the body, to allow the better execution of another body part, i.e. when reaching with the arm, postural adjustments occur in the trunk. These reactions require information from the vestibular and proprioceptive systems.

Postural drainage This is the therapeutic use of gravity-assisted patient positioning to facilitate the removal of excessive pulmonary secretions. It may be used in conjunction with other techniques such as chest percussion, thoracic expansion exercises and IPPB.

Postural hypotension A low blood pressure that only emerges upon the adoption of a particular posture by a person.

Postural sets This is a term primarily used by Bobath-trained therapists to describe a patient's posture that takes into account the influence of tone on the posture, e.g. unsupported sitting is a 'mixed postural set' as it has both elements of flexion and extension, whereas the postural set of supine is dominated by extension.

This term can also be found in the literature to describe adaptations of posture or adjustments that precede and accompany a movement (Bobath 1990).

Postural tremor A pathological tremor (3 to 5 Hz) that occurs when the body or limb is working against gravity.

Posture This relates to the position of the body or body part in relation to space or another object or body part. A good posture (Edwards 2002) is said to be the attitude of the body that facilitates maximum efficiency of a specific activity without causing damage to the body.

See *Flat back* and *Sway back*

Potential difference Electrotherapy term – also called electromotive force and measured in volts (V).

Pott's fracture Fracture of the lower end of the fibula and of the medial malleolus, with outward displacement of the foot.

Poverty Lack of material resources that is often associated with lack of social and emotional resources. It means less to spend on food, housing, clothes, transport, holidays and other human and social needs. When people are poor compared with others in the same society they are said to be in 'relative poverty' as they cannot engage fully in the society of which they are a part. Poverty, in terms of lack of social and emotional resources is not necessarily associated with wealth. There are formal government definitions of poverty (in terms of material resources) for the purposes of collecting statistics and providing financial benefits.

Power A central concept within the social sciences, defined in different ways by different theorists. It is generally seen as a feature of all social life and interpersonal relationships and is central to understanding inequality. Those who have power have authority and influence over others. They possess and can accumulate valued resources such as wealth and property. Power is an important dimension of professional–patient/client relationships with services defined, planned and delivered by professionals.

Power Electrotherapy context – the rate of energy flow or dissipation, measured in watts (W). Concept applied clinically to uses of electrical stimulation and laser. For example, P (power, watts) = VI or P = I^{2}R where V = voltage [V], I = current [A] and R = resistance [Ω].
  See *Energy*

PPAM aid (pneumatic post-amputation mobility aid) A device used in rehabilitation of people post amputation.

PR Common medical abbreviation – Per rectum.

Prednisolone A form of steroid medication that is commonly seen in clinical practice.

Prejudice Literally means to pre-judge. It usually refers to an attitude of hostility towards a person or a group. People may, for example, be prejudiced against old people. Prejudices can, however, be positive.

Preload Force applied to resting muscle to stretch it to initial length. In heart, preload corresponds to end-diastolic filling pressure.

Prepatellar bursitis Lying between the anterior surface of the patella and the skin, this is the most commonly injured bursa at the knee. When inflamed, it is known as 'housemaid's knee'.

Presentation The term usually used to describe the process whereby information is given to a group by one of its members, as in a student presentation. It may be assessed as part of a course.

Preventative medicine Interventions which are designed to prevent disease from occurring or to detect disease at an early stage. Genetic screening and routine mammograms are examples of preventative medicine.

Primary care Front-line care for people in need of medical or social assistance. Primary-care workers include general practitioners, physiotherapists, social workers, opticians, dentists and pharmacists. The telephone service, NHS Direct, is another example of a primary-care service where advice is given on medical matters by nurses.

Primary healthcare team Health workers who are usually based at a GP surgery or health centre who provide health services in the community. They comprise a wide spectrum of professionals including physiotherapists, who have increasingly becoming a part of primary care.

Primary osteoarthritis See *Osteoarthritis*

Primary referencing The gold standard of referencing where the source is the original piece of published work.

Primary research Study generating original data rather than analyzing data from existing studies (which is called secondary research).

PRN Common medical abbreviation – As needed (pro re nata).

Problem-based learning (PBL) A system which promotes learning by using problems encountered in clinical practice as a means of providing context and motivation.

Profession A work organization with a number of characteristics, which include a central regulatory body, a code of conduct, management and control of knowledge and expertise and control of numbers, selection and training of those entering the profession. Professions can be viewed as motivated by altruism, as self-interested monopolies, or as 'agents of the state' whose function is to control 'deviant' behaviour.

Professional–patient relationship Can be conceived as a power relationship through which social problems are conceived and defined, by professionals, as the needs and problems of patients and clients. The relationship also allows professionals to define solutions to these problems. The professional–patient relationship has come under considerable criticism and now a 'patient-centred' approach is frequently advocated that allows patients and clients more power and control.

See *Patient-centred medicine*

Professional socialization A process by which those becoming members of a profession internalize the norms, values and dominant ideologies of that profession.

Prognosis A probable course or outcome of a disease. Prognostic factors are patient or disease characteristics that influence the course. Good prognosis is associated with low rate of undesirable outcomes; poor prognosis is associated with a high rate of undesirable outcomes.

Pronation Movement of the forearm so that the hand faces downwards. Also applies to the foot in which the sole faces down.

Prone A term used to describe the position of a person laying flat on their abdomen, facing the supporting surface.

Prone knee bend (PKB) See *Neurodynamics*

Prone-standing This is a position of half standing, where a high plinth carefully supports the trunk, head and upper limbs. The hips are generally at an angle of 90°, but this is dependent on the individual patient.

○ Clinical note This position can be used when treating neurological patients. It is a useful position in that the weight of the upper body is supported by the plinth and thus allowing the therapist to concentrate on the pelvis and legs.

Proprietary name The brand name given by the manufacturer to a drug or device it produces.

Proprioception The feedback mechanism that enables us to have awareness of our position in space or the position of a limb. It is essential for balance and normal function and is achieved by a variety of means.

There are many receptors within joints, muscles and the skin that continually convey information to the central nervous system (CNS). Using this information, we continually make subconscious and conscious modifications to how we move, allowing us to carry out normal functional activities. Each receptor supplies a different type of information, e.g. joint pressure, joint acceleration/deceleration and joint velocity. When the receptors are stimulated through movement or other forces, they act as transducers and convert this mechanical deformation into an electrical impulse. This sensory impulse then passes onto the CNS triggering the appropriate motor response.

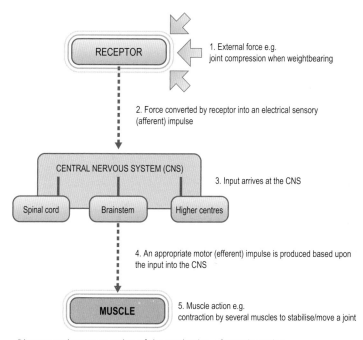

Diagrammatic representation of the mechanism of proprioception

When walking upon uneven ground the muscles of the foot and ankle continually have to adjust in order to keep the body upright and prevent a fall. The peronei and anterior tibials, for example, will be continually controlling the movement of the foot and ankle, responding to constant positional changes. Proprioception is a continuous process occurring at different levels of the CNS at the same time.

Consider all the potential tasks that you might undertake whilst walking, e.g. carrying a rucksack, using a walking pole, walking the dog. All of these tasks will be bombarding the CNS with all sorts of afferent information. Imagine if the responses to this information were all at the conscious level, it would be a slow walk. This is a key point to understand when rehabilitating a patient with a proprioceptive deficit – many actions need to function at a subconscious level.

From Mason D, Kilmurray S 2003 In: Porter S (ed.) Tidy's physiotherapy, 13th edn. Elsevier Ltd., Edinburgh.

✚ Clinical note Patients with poor or absent proprioception tend to rely heavily on another sense (often vision) and often have to look at their feet when walking to compensate. They will, therefore, have difficulty moving around in the dark.

Proprioceptive neuromuscular facilitation (PNF) This technique utilizes the properties of proprioception that respond to pressure and stretch and was developed as a therapeutic approach for the re-education of movement. It involves the use of resistance and facilitation of movements in recognized mass patterns of spiral or diagonal movements, along with the use of stretch, repetition and verbal commands.

Prostaglandin Potent substance found in many tissues produced in response to trauma. They may affect blood pressure and metabolism and smooth muscle activity.

Prosthesis An appliance used to replace an absent part of the body.

Protective deformity The posture adopted by a person in an attempt to minimize their discomfort, pain or disability. An example may be seen in chronic back pain where a person may adopt a shifted spinal posture.
This is often subconscious.

Protective spasm Muscle spasm often occurs following injury, trauma or pain. It is the body's attempt to stop movement, unfortunately the spasm is often out of all proportion to the initial injury. Patient stating 'my back locked up', for example, or, worse still, spasm may become a perpetuation that becomes the overriding problem. This is one reason why a hot pack or massage may be so dramatically effective in relieving pain and facilitating movement.

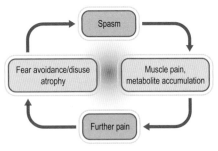

Protective spasm

Protocol The standard process that is used over and over to ensure that an experiment (or similar activity) is conducted in the same way each time.

Proximal Nearer to the axial skeleton.

Pruritus Itching, an unpleasant sensation that provokes the desire to rub or scratch the skin to obtain relief.

Pseudo-bulbar palsy Features are due to the degeneration of corticobulbar pathways to motor nuclei of the cranial nerves V, VII, X, XI and XII.

⊕ Clinical note Patients present with apparent weakness when chewing and making facial expressions and can be emotionally labile (cry a lot or laugh). This condition can be seen in motor neuron disease.

Pseudomonas aeruginosa A species of rod-shaped bacteria commonly isolated from clinical specimens (wound, burn and urinary-tract infections).

Psoriasis A common chronic condition characterized by the presence of rounded, erythematous, dry patches covered by greyish white scales, which tend to occur on the extensor surfaces of the body.

Psychology The study of the mental processes and behaviour of humans and animals.

Ptosis Drooping of an eyelid.

PU Common medical abbreviation – Passed urine.

Pubic symphysis The anterior joint of the pelvis.
See *Symphysis pubis*

Puerperium Describes the first 6 weeks post delivery. Some body systems return to the non-pregnant state and other changes are initiated, e.g. lactation. Within this period, the uterus involutes (returns to its pre-pregnant size and position). As the site of the placenta heals and the endometrium regenerates, the woman experiences a discharge (lochia), initially bloody, for up to 8 weeks (Brook et al. 2003).

Pulmonary embolism (PE) This is a blood clot within the pulmonary circulation, which can be fatal (approximately 20 000 hospital deaths occur in the UK each year from PE). Predispositions to this can include trauma, recent surgery, immobility, smoking, malignant disease and pregnancy, to name but a few. The size of the clot is of clinical significance since when 25% of the pulmonary circulation is obstructed, cardiac function is impaired. Clot size, patient age and existing pulmonary co-morbidities and the general health will all impact upon outcome. Clinical presentation is non-specific since signs and symptoms include dyspnoea, pain, echocardiogram (ECG) changes, peripheral oedema tachycardia and cyanosis. Investigations include ECG, chest X-ray, arterial blood gases, V/Q scanning, angiography, spiral computerized tomography (CT) scan and D-dimer tests, though some of these are useful only in excluding the diagnosis of PE. Treatment regimes include: oxygen therapy, analgesia, anticoagulation therapy, thrombolysis and pulmonary embolectomy (though this is rarely performed and requires specialist input from a thoracic surgeon). About 10% of PEs are rapidly fatal and an additional 5% cause death later, despite diagnosis and treatment.

There is approximately 50% resolution of PE after 1 month of treatment and perfusion eventually returns to normal in two-thirds of patients (Kearon 2003).

Pulmonary fibrosis Chronic inflammation and fibrosis of the alveolar walls, with steadily progressive shortness of breath resulting finally in death from oxygen lack or right-heart failure.

Pulmonary oedema Fluid accumulation within the alveoli. Hydrostatic pulmonary oedema occurs when there is a rise in the hydrostatic pressure of the lung interstitium resulting in a flooding of alveolar spaces. Non-hydrostatic pulmonary oedema involves the disruption of epithelial and endothelial barriers inducing a systemic inflammatory response associated with widespread microvascular injury including the lungs (e.g. ARDS). This is associated with increased total lung water despite a normal hydrostatic pressure. Often results from the ineffective pump function of the heart.

Pulse Electrotherapy context – the interrupted flow of current. Basic unit of both pulsed and alternating currents. Needs additional information from the following list:

- Type: monophasic (i.e. the pulse has one phase only, for example, HVPS {high-voltage pulsed stimulation}, interrupted galvanic) or biphasic (i.e. there are two phases per pulse, for example, output of most motor stimulators)
- Symmetrical/asymmetrical: biphasic and both phases are same or different shapes
- Shape of phase: can be rectangular, triangular, sinusoidal, sawtooth, for example
- Balanced/unbalanced: biphasic and balanced if the charge in each phase is equal, unbalanced if greater in one phase
- Duration: usually measured in μs or ms
- Frequency: number per second (hertz, Hz).

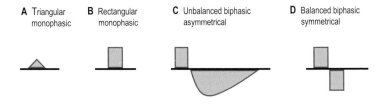

A Triangular monophasic   **B** Rectangular monophasic   **C** Unbalanced biphasic asymmetrical   **D** Balanced biphasic symmetrical

Pulsed current Electrotherapy term – one of three recognized categories of therapeutic currents (pulsed, direct and alternating currents). A series of pulses separated by interpulse intervals. The pulse duration varies, ranging from μs to ms, and the pulse may be monophasic (e.g. HVPS {high-voltage pulsed stimulation}) or biphasic (typical sensory and motor stimulation currents). The distinguishing feature is that a pulsed current has an interval between

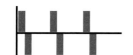

Pulses separated by interpulse intervals

successive pulses (interpulse interval). A frequency of 50 Hz, for example, means 50 separate pulses per second.

See *Pulse* for more characteristics

Pulse duration (width) Electrotherapy term – the time for which a pulse continues, one complete cycle of current flow. Usually measured in μs or ms. Incorrectly referred to as 'width' as is a measure of time, not a spatial dimension. Pulse duration, together with intensity, indicates which types of nerve fibre are most likely to be stimulated and hence the probable level of comfort and type of response to stimulation.

Pulses

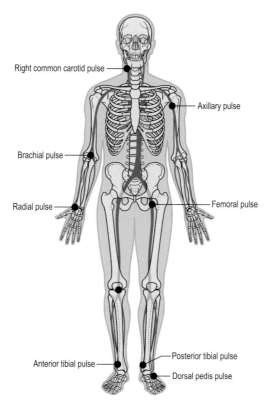

Pulse points

Right common carotid pulse

Axillary pulse

Brachial pulse

Radial pulse

Femoral pulse

Anterior tibial pulse

Posterior tibial pulse

Dorsal pedis pulse

Pulsus alternans An abnormal pulse associated with left-sided heart failure, felt as a bounding, followed by weak pulses.

Pulsus paradoxus (Paradoxical pulse) A weak pulse occurring through spontaneous inspiration. It is associated with both cardiac and respiratory problems, e.g. where there is restriction of the pumping action of the myocardium and acute obstructive pulmonary disorders, e.g. asthma.

Pump handle Movement.
   See *Rib movement*

Purchaser/provider split This refers to the split between the purchasing and the provision of health and social care services. Before the NHS and Community Care Act (1990) statutory health and social care agencies typically purchased and provided services for their patients and clients. For example, social services purchased and provided residential and day-care facilities for older people. Services are now purchased from a wide variety of agencies some of which are from the private and voluntary sectors. Many hospital services, such as cleaning and laundry, are 'contracted out' to private companies and GPs may purchase services for their patients from nearby hospitals who compete for contracts.
   See *Internal market*

Purkinje cell These are large neurons found in the cerebellar cortex, giving rise to efferent axons and provide the only output from the cerebellar cortex.

Purkinje fibres An extensive network of branching fibres, that play an important role in the conduction of electrical impulses through the heart.

Purposive sampling Research term – sampling that is done with a particular group in mind, for example, if you wanted to undertake a survey of reasons of non-attendance in physiotherapy departments, you would use a purposive sample, there is no point in doing a randomized sample of attendees and non-attendees if your research question is looking at non-attendees only.

Pursed lip breathing (PLB) Breathing through tightly pursed lips, which results in the generation of a backpressure so avoiding compression of collapsible lung segments (i.e. the equal pressure point is moved towards the mouth). The emphysematous patient often automatically adopts this breathing in times of extreme dyspnoea.

Pusher syndrome This is a term used to describe patients, normally people who have had a severe stroke, who have a tendency to push towards their hemiplegic side and resist attempts to correct their posture towards midline. They tend to extend their unaffected arm and leg pushing them over, but their perception is that they are falling to their good side.

   ✚ Clinical note This presentation is often accompanied by cognitive and perceptual problems.

P value Research term – the probability of a finding occurring by chance alone given that the null hypothesis is actually true. A P value <0.05 is often considered significant.

PVS Common medical abbreviation – Persistent vegetative state.
   See *Vegetative state*

P wave The portion seen on an echocardiogram (ECG) trace that is due to depolarization of the atria.

See *ECG*

PWB Common medical abbreviation – Partial weight bearing.

Px Common medical abbreviation – Prescribing.

Pyarthrosis The terms for pus within a joint.

Pyogenic Producing pus.

Pyramidal tract – also known as Corticospinal tract This is the main route by which voluntary commands reach the motor neurones in the spinal cord. Originating in the motor cortex it goes through the internal capsule to the white matter then travelling to the target motor neurones in the spinal cord.

✚ Clinical note Patients with pure pyramidal loss present with diminished fine finger control and difficulty in isolating finger movements.

See *Corticospinal tract*

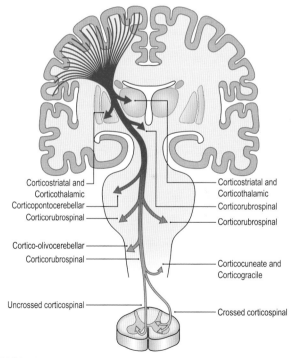

The Pyramidal tract

Pyrexia Rise in body temperature frequently caused by infection.

Q

QAA Quality Assurance Agency – the body responsible for assuring academic standards in Higher Education by inspection and report; also for producing professional 'benchmark' statements.

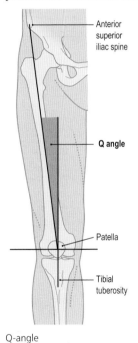

Anterior superior iliac spine

Q angle

Patella

Tibial tuberosity

Q-angle

Q-angle The direction of the pull of the quadriceps – as measured by a line drawn from the anterior superior iliac spine (ASIS), through the centre of the patella and intersecting a line to the tibial tuberosity. The average angle for females is 15.8° ± 4.5° and for males is 11.2° ± 3.0°. Abnormal Q angles are thought to predispose to anterior knee pain and other syndromes.

QD Common medical abbreviation – Every day.

QID Common medical abbreviation – Four times per day.

QOD Common medical abbreviation – Every other day.
  See *ECG*

Q (PERFUSION) Blood flow as determined by cardiac output.

QRS complex Part of an echocardiogram.
  See *Cardiac cycle*

Quadraparesis Weakness of all four limbs.

Quadriceps Large muscle located at front of thigh, made up of rectus femoris, vastus medialis, vastus lateralis and vastus intermedius.

Quadriplegia Paralysis of all four limbs.

Qualitative research Research term – research not based on numbers, useful for assessing opinions attitudes, feelings, etc.

  NB. Qualitative research is now widespread in healthcare as we begin to realize that humans are more than a collection of atoms that can be measured objectively (the reductionist para-digm), neither qualitative or quantitative methods are better than the other, it is merely a question of which is the right tool for the right job.

Quality adjusted life years (QALY) A measurement that has been used to prior-itize medical treatment. It attempts to provide an objective estimate of the costs and benefits of medical intervention. The basic measure is one year of healthy life as a result of medical treatment multiplied by an assessment of the quality of life on a scale from 0 to 1. The costs per QALY can then be measured and those with the lowest costs are given priority. There are many ethical problems with this measure as it may discriminate against people needing expensive treatment and may misjudge the quality of life possible when a person is ill or disabled.

These are quotations from disabled people:

Being disabled is not the end of things but rather is the start of some-thing else, a way forward. (Barlow JH and Williams B 1999 'I Now Feel That I'm Not Just a Bit of Left Luggage': the experiences of older women with arthritis attending a personal independence course. Disability and Society, 14: 1, 53–64.)

I am never going to be able to conform to society's requirements and I am thrilled because I am blissfully released from all that crap. That's the liberation of disfigurement. (Shakespeare T, Gillespie-Sells K and Davies D 1996 The Sexual Politics of Disability. Cassell. London.)

I cannot wish that I had never contracted ME, because it has made me a different person, a person I am glad to be, would not want to miss being and could not relinquish even if I were cured. (Wendell S 1996 The Rejected Body: feminist philosophical perspectives on disability. Routledge. London.)

Quality of life measures Measures that are usually based on self report and determine the quality as defined by the measure of the person's life. A broad measure usually covering domains related to physical, mental (emotional and cognitive), social, and role functioning as well as the individuals per-ception of their own well-being.

Quantative research Research term – research that is based upon numbers.

Quasi-market See *Internal market*

Questionnaire A common format to obtain research data from a population, there are various way of administering questionnaires such as postal, tele-phone questionnaires, etc. Each has its advantages and disadvantages. Questionnaire design needs careful planning and thought. The points below should assist in designing a questionnaire.

Student tips on questionnaire design:

• The first priority is to assess whether a questionnaire is the correct research tool for your chosen research question. If it is, how will you ensure validity and reliability, i.e. is there already a validated questionnaire in existence?

- A questionnaire must:
    - undergo an adequate pilot stage
    - have a brief introduction and cover page
    - be clear and easy to understand by the respondents, e.g. avoid jargon that will not be understood
    - be formatted and presented professionally with accurate grammar
    - avoid bias
    - explain the rationale behind asking the questions
    - consist of non-judgemental phrases
    - present the questions succinctly
    - guarantee confidentiality and anonymity to the respondent
    - have serial numbers ascribed
    - have page numbers
    - have a return address
    - have neatly formatted coding boxes
    - only include essential questions
    - indicate what respondents should do next at the end
    - include informed consent form, or details of ethical approval obtained if necessary.

Quiet breathing This is normal resting tidal breathing.

Q wave The initial deflection of the QRS complex when such deflection is negative (downward).

RA Common medical abbreviation – Rheumatoid arthritis.

Racism The unequal treatment and institutional discrimination experienced by groups of people on the basis of physical or other characteristics socially defined as denoting a particular race or ethnic minority.

Radial nerve The radial nerve controls wrist and finger extension and has a sensory supply to the back of the hand.

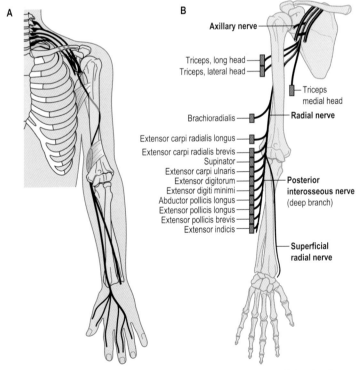

(**A**) The course of the radial nerve; (**B**) muscles supplied by the radial and axillary nerves

Radial nerve palsy This nerve can be injured, especially on the outside of the arm above the elbow, either by direct trauma, prolonged pressure, or mid-shaft humerus fractures. This commonly results is a wrist drop.

Radial tear A type of meniscal tear seen in the knee joint.
See *Bucket handle tear*

Radiculopathy Damage or inflammation of the peripheral nerves and spinal roots, accompanied by weakness and numbness.

Radius and ulna The two bones of the forearm.

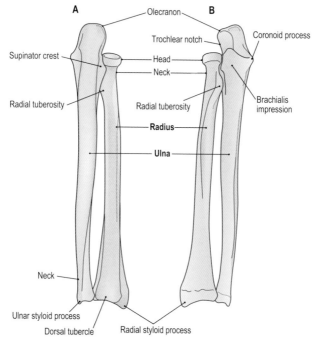

Bones of the forearm: (**A**) posterior view; (**B**) anterior view

Rales Old name for crackles upon stethoscope auscultation.

Ramp Electrotherapy context – the rate of change in amplitude of a series of bursts of pulses. Ramp up means the amplitude is increasing and ramp down, decreasing.

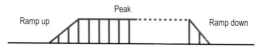

Ramp

Randomization Research term – the process by which every member of a population has an equal chance of being included in the sample.

Randomized controlled trial (RCT) Research term – an experiment in which the researcher randomly assigns some patients to at least one manoeuvre and other patients to a placebo. When properly done, an RCT can be used to determine cause and effect.

Range of motion See *Joint range of motion*

Ranges of joint motion Typical normal values.

Shoulder		Hip	
Flexion	0–165°	Flexion	120°
Extension	60°	Extension	10–20°
Abduction	0–180°	Abduction	45°
Internal rotation	70°	Adduction	25°
External rotation	90°	Internal rotation	45°
		External rotation	45°
Elbow		**Knee**	
Flexion	150°	Flexion	135°
Pronation	75°	Extension	0–5°
Supination	80°	Internal rotation	(hyperextension)
		External rotation	30°
			40°
Wrist		**Ankle**	
Flexion	80°	Dorsiflexion	20°
Extension	70°	Plantarflexion	50°
Ulnar deviation	30°		
Radial deviation	20°		
Thumb		**Subtalar**	
CMC Flexion	15°	Inversion	35°
CMC Extension	20°	Eversion	15°
CMC Abduction	70°		
Finger			
MCP flexion	90°		
PIP flexion	100°		
DIP flexion	80–90°		

Ratio data Research term – continuous data where both differences and ratios are interpretable. Ratio data has a natural zero. A good example is birth weight in kg.

RBC Common medical abbreviation – Red blood cell.

Reading week The term used to describe a period of time given to students to study away from the university.

Reciprocal inhibition Activation of a motor nerve to a muscle is usually accompanied by inhibition of antagonist muscles acting at that joint. So, for example, if the person is contracting their biceps then their triceps would be reciprocally inhibited.

Reciprocal innervation The interplay between opposing muscle groups allowing dynamic co-contraction for postural stability and controlled movements for function.

Reciprocal lengthening As a set of muscles work concentrically, the opposite muscles have to lengthen to allow movement otherwise we would never move anywhere!

Reciprocal shortening As a set of muscles work eccentrically, the opposite muscles have to 'gather up the slack', but the muscle is not actively contracting, there is some cross bridge formation.

Red flag See *Flags*

Reduction Putting a fracture or dislocation back in correct alignment the term is also used to describe the relocation of a dislocated prosthetic joint.

Reductionist paradigm Research term – the belief that measurement and quantification of phenomena can be replicated by an independent observer. The fragmentation of a phenomenon into its constituent parts.

Reduction of fractures This means to realign into the normal or as near normal anatomical position as possible. Reduction of a fracture may be either open or closed.

Closed reduction means that no surgical intervention is used; the fracture is manipulated by hand under local or general anaesthesia.

Open reduction means that the area has been surgically opened and reduced. Reduction may not always be necessary even when there is some displacement, e.g. fractures of the clavicle may heal with a bump that may only be a problem in the cosmetic sense.

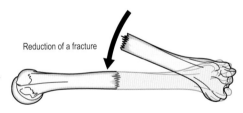

Reduction of a fracture

Reference The clear indication in a piece of work that a source is from another persons work.

Secondary referencing (citation)

Where the source of material is taken from a reference used in another piece of work, i.e. without going to the original primary reference. This is unwise in academic assignments.

Reflective practice The capacity of a practitioner or professional to think, talk or write about an aspect of his or her practice and to review the interaction with clients, patients or other participants. The purpose of such reflection is to develop or enhance practitioner skills and competence and produce practitioner knowledge that is grounded in practice.

Reflex An automatic reaction to some form of stimulus.

Deep-tendon reflex

All muscles have a deep-tendon reflex, when the muscle or tendon is briskly hit, a reflex contraction occurs. These are monosynaptic reflexes that test the integrity of the nervous system.

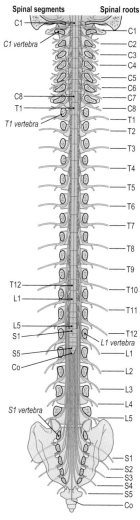

Nerve roots and the spine

Analysis of reflex behaviours

- Hypoactive/diminished reflex – this could indicate problems with compression of a nerve root.
- Hyperactive/increased reflex – this could indicate an upper motor neurone component.

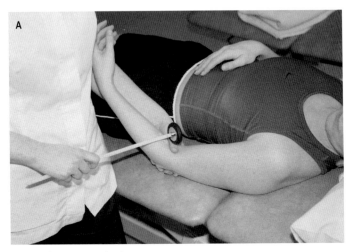

Biceps reflex C5/6 root level

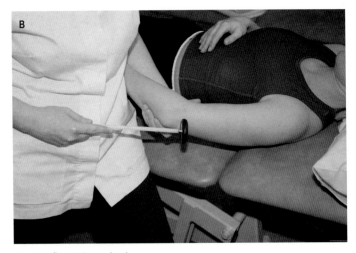

Triceps reflex C7/8 root level

Reflex disturbance cannot be used as complete evidence of abnormality of the nervous system, but should be used along with other objective neurological findings. See the figure below for an illustration of common tendon reflexes.

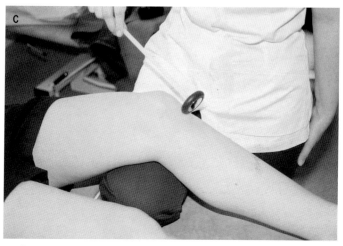

Patellar tendon reflex L3/4 root level

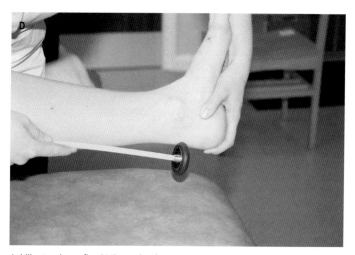

Achilles tendon reflex S1/2 root level

Reflex arc Consists of an afferent and an efferent part joined by a monosynaptic connection in the spinal cord. Stimulation of the reflex results in a muscle contraction. For example, tapping the quadriceps tendon leads to a knee jerk due to contraction of the quadriceps.

Reflex sympathetic dystrophy (RSD) Now normally described as complex regional pain syndrome. Caused by an abnormal sympathetic reflex, giving rise to a response that is out of proportion to and inconsistent with the injury. Quite variable with regard to signs and symptoms, with treatment ranging from sympathetic block, to TENS, to physiotherapy.

See *Shoulder-hand syndrome*

Refractory period The period following an action potential (AP) when the responsiveness of nerve to stimulation is non-existent or reduced. In the immediate period (absolute refractory period) no response is possible irrespective of the intensity of the stimulus. Immediately after this (relative refractory period), the nerve remains less excitable than prior to the action potential but, with a sufficiently high stimulus may respond. The clinical implication is that with alternating current (e.g. Russian), if at a sufficiently high intensity more than one action potential per burst may occur. If no further stimulation occurs the nerve reverts to the pre AP resting state.

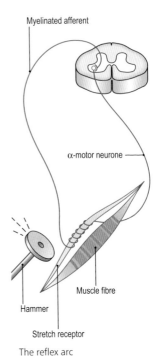

Myelinated afferent

α-motor neurone

Muscle fibre

Hammer

Stretch receptor

The reflex arc

Registration The requirement for all health professions who work in the NHS, including physiotherapists, to be on the register of the HPC as a means of protecting the public.

Regression Research term – statistical techniques that are concerned with predicting one variable by knowing others. Regression is used to answer such questions as 'how well can we predict the values of one variable, (such as survival) by knowing the value of another (such as treatment technique)?

Rehabilitation A goal-orientated and time-limited process aimed at enabling a person to maximize their physical, mental and social functioning. It can aim at recovering function or compensating for functional loss, or at providing the patient with tools to deal with their change in function.

Reiter's syndrome A reactive arthritis usually made of the triad of urethritis, conjunctivitis and arthritis. Any peripheral joint may be involved, usually joints of the lower limb, with a synovitis that is often intense and asymmetrical. Achilles tendinitis is very common, as are tendon sheath or tendon conditions.

Relaxin A hormone released during pregnancy, it replaces the collagen in target areas with a modified form, which has greater pliability and extensibility. It also is thought to have a softening effect on connective tissue, i.e. pelvic floor and abdominal fascia, increasing their extensibility. The symphysis pubis and sacroiliac joints are particularly affected to allow for the birth of the baby. This ligamentous laxity may continue for 6 months postpartum.

○ Clinical point This has obvious implications for physiotherapists, and relaxin may be one of the reasons that low back pain is common during pregnancy.

Reliability Research term – the repeatability of a study.
  A clinical example would be that measuring knee flexion with a very small goniometer is not reliable since there are many potential sources of error in positioning of the goniometer arms and also in the differences between one test and the next (intra rater reliability) and between the different physiotherapists performing the same test (inter rater reliability).

Research The active process of inquiry into an area or subject.

Research ethics committee An independent committee that scrutinizes proposals for research to ensure they are ethically acceptable.

Research into practice Where the validated results of a piece of *academic* research are used to change or modify existing accepted practice (e.g. clinical or educational).

Research question Research term – the question contains the population, the manoeuvre, the study population and the outcomes. The research question should specify one measurable outcome, in addition to all conditions and any other important variables.

Residual volume (RV) This is the air remaining in the lungs at the end of a forced expiration. This lung volume can only be measured in the lung function laboratory by means of body box plethysmography or gas transfer tests (it cannot be measured with simple spirometry).

Resisted movement A movement performed that overcomes an additional resistance in addition to the weight of the body part itself, for example, an arm curl with a 5 kg weight is a resisted exercise.

Respiration This is the exchange of metabolic gases (oxygen and carbon dioxide). External respiration involves the movement of oxygen from the air to the lung and carbon dioxide from the lung to the outside environment. Internal respiration involves the movement of oxygen from the arteriole to the tissues and carbon dioxide from the tissues to the blood vessel for transport back to the lung.

Respiratory acidosis A drop in pH of the blood and raised PCO_2, seen commonly in chronic lung disease where CO_2 cannot be removed effectively, therefore, making the blood plasma more acidic.

Respiratory alkalosis Results when a person removes too much CO_2 from their blood, raising its pH it may occur in states of anxiety.

Respiratory failure (RF) This is a common medical condition that occurs when the lungs fail to oxygenate arterial blood adequately (Type I RF) and/or fail to prevent undue CO_2 retention (Type II RF). While no absolute diagnostic values for arterial PO_2 and PCO_2 have been defined, values generally quoted are a PaO_2 of less than 8.0 kilo Pascals (kPa), and a $PaCO_2$ of greater than 6.0 kPa (West JB 1977 Pulmonary gas exchange. Int Rev Physiol 14: 83–106). However, the significance of such values is dependent upon a number of factors pertinent to the individual history and the normal variables.

While various physical signs and symptoms such as breathlessness, dyspnoea, cyanosis, agitation and the use of accessory muscles, frequently accompany respiratory failure, they are not diagnostic of the condition. Arterial blood gas tensions must, therefore, be measured to make the diagnosis.

Respite care Services for ill or disabled people that are primarily designed to give carers a rest. Care may be provided within institutions or within the person's own home. It has been argued that access to respite care should be the right of all carers. Others argue that respite care demeans ill and disabled people by viewing them as a burden and by failing to resource more appropriate forms of assistance.

Responsiveness (of a measure) The extent to which a measurement instrument detects clinically important changes over time. These changes are often defined in terms of how significant they are to patients. There is no single agreed method for expressing an instrument's responsiveness.

Resting splint A splint that is used during night time or when a person is at rest to preserve normal joint alignments or alleviate pain/prevent deformity.

Restrictive lung disease This is where the total lung capacity (the expansion of the lung) is limited. Such diseases occur with: disorders of the lung itself, e.g. pulmonary fibrosis; pleural disease, e.g. pneumothorax and mesothelioma; neuromuscular disease, e.g. muscular dystrophy and phrenic nerve palsy; chest-wall disease, e.g. pectus excavatum and ankylosing spondylitis and with subdiaphragmatic conditions, e.g. obesity and ascites. Its diagnosis is facilitated with simple spirometric measures where possible.
See *Spirometry*

Reticular formation This extends throughout the brain stem; it is associated with levels of arousal, motivational and effective responses to stimuli, autonomic reflex responses including breathing and locomotion.

Reticulospinal tract A branch of the nervous system that arises in the reticular formation and have projections into axial and proximal muscles.

Retinaculum Anatomical term for a net of tissue that binds down tendons, they occur in the wrist and the foot.

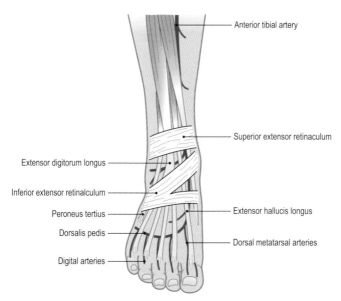

Anterior tibial artery

Superior extensor retinaculum

Extensor digitorum longus

Inferior extensor retinalculum

Peroneus tertius

Dorsalis pedis

Digital arteries

Extensor hallucis longus

Dorsal metatarsal arteries

Retinaculae in the ankle

Retrograde amnesia Being unable to remember an event that happened prior to a brain injury.

Retrolisthesis Posterior slippage of one vertebra on another.
See *Spondylolisthesis*

Rhabdomyolysis Excretion of myoglobin in the urine, it results from muscle degeneration.

Rheobase Electrotherapy term – a measure applied to a strength–duration graph to evaluate peripheral nerve function. Is defined as the intensity of current required for a minimally perceptible response (motor or sensory, depending on the test) using a monophasic pulse with a duration of 100 ms and a frequency of approximately 1 Hz. Normal values vary whether constant current or constant voltage stimulator used (reading in current or voltage depending on the equipment). See textbook for normal values.

Rheumatoid arthritis (RA) Inflammatory disease affecting synovial joints and connective tissues. Commonly seen in the upper cervical spine, with loosening of the transverse ligament of the dens, leading to a subluxation of the atlantoaxial joint. Many deformities are characteristically seen in the person with rheumatoid arthritis (RA). Management of RA is now being revolutionized by biologic therapies.

Rheumatoid factor Rheumatoid factor is an antibody that is measurable in the blood. Rheumatoid factor is actually an antibody that can bind to other antibodies.

Rhomberg test This is a test for distinguishing between sensory and cerebellar ataxia. The person is asked to stand with heels together first with their eyes open and then with their eyes shut. If they show excessive sway or lose their balance only when their eyes are closed this indicates proprioceptive loss.

Rhonchi A whistling or vibration/sound heard on auscultation of the chest when the air channels are partially obstructed.

Rib movement During respiration the ribs are thought of as having two different types of movements, these are called pump handle which increases the AP diameter of the chest and bucket handle movements, which increase the lateral diameter of the thorax.

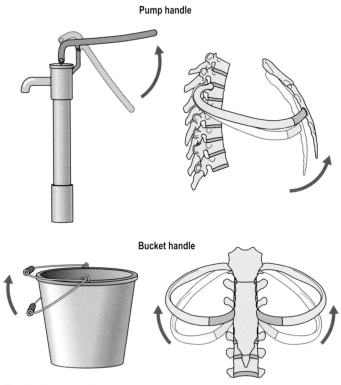

Pump handle

Bucket handle

Chest wall movement

RICE (Rest ice compression elevation) Acute injury management, to prevent inflammatory processes to go uncontrolled and to speed up the recovery process by eliminating swelling.

See *Cryotherapy*

Righting reactions Automatic reactions occur in response to alteration of body alignment, aiming to maintain and restore the head position in midline and with a normal relationship to the trunk and limbs. These can be seen in the developing infant, but are not normally able to be distinguished from equilibrium reactions in the adult.

Rights An umbrella term covering entitlements and privileges enjoyed on the basis of being a human being (human rights) or a citizen (civil rights) though the two are not entirely discrete. Human rights can include freedom of thought conscience and religion and freedom of peaceful assembly and association. Civil rights are recognized as belonging to all individuals within a society and can be upheld by appeal to the law. Rights play an important, though contested, role in political life, such as the conflicting claims to the right to life and the right of women to choose in relation to abortion.

Rigidity A neurological phenomenon where there is increased resistance to a slow passive movement, it is not velocity-dependent unlike spasticity. The table below provides more information about spasticity and rigidity.

Comparisons of spasticity and rigidity

	Spasticity	**Rigidity**
Pattern of muscle involvement	Upper limb flexors: lower limb extensors	Flexors and extensors equally
Nature of tone	Velocity-dependent increase in tone; 'clasp-knife'	Constant throughout movement; 'lead pip'
Tendon reflexes	Increased	Normal
Pathophysiology	Increased spinal stretch reflex gain	Increased long-latency component of stretch reflex
Clinical significance	Upper motor neurone (pyramidal) sign	Extrapyramidal sign

⊕ Clinical note Cogwheel rigidity is seen in Parkinson's disease and decerebrate and decorticate rigidity are seen following head injury.

Rivermede motor assessment A test of motor function following stroke. The items are organized in a hierarchy based on the assumption that recovery occurs in a pattern. It is quite extensive and so can take time to undertake but can be easily carried out in the clinical environment and is hence in widespread use.

Role A key concept in sociological theory. It focuses on the social expectations associated with particular statuses or social positions.

Role conflict A situation that occurs when the expectations of two or more roles conflict. Role conflict may occur, for example, when the expectations of paid employment conflict with the expectations of the role of carer. Role conflict can cause anxiety.

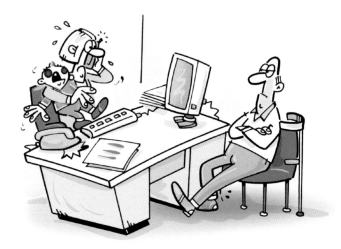

Role conflict

Rollator frame This is like a Zimmer frame only it has wheels on the front to enable it to be pushed forwards rather than lifted.

⊕ Clinical note This frame is sometimes preferable to the Zimmer frame as it allows for a more normal reciprocal pattern of walking, and greater velocity.

Rotation Movement about the long axis and requires a co-ordinated response between flexion and extension.

⊕ Clinical note Impaired rotation is often seen in patients where there is any muscular shortening or imbalance. Loss of rotation in the trunk is usually noted in walking by the absence of arm swing.

Rotator cuff Made up of four muscles: subscapularis, supraspinatus, infraspinatus and teres minor. Their tendons converge to form a 'cuff' over the shoulder joint, on their way to attaching from the scapula to the humerus. One of its major functions is to control and produce rotation of the shoulder. They may be considered as dynamic ligaments, continually changing their relative tensions to maintain the stability of the humeral head.

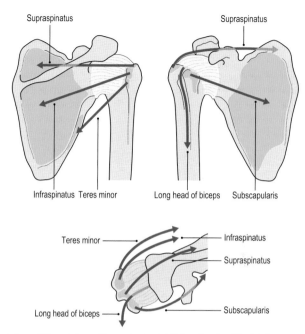

The action of the rotator cuff muscles in stabilizing the shoulder joint

RS Common medical abbreviation – Respiratory system.

RSD Common medical abbreviation – Reflex sympathetic dystrophy.

RSI Common medical abbreviation – Repetitive strain injury.

RTA Common medical abbreviation – Road traffic accident.

Ruffini end organs Subcutaneous sensors that respond to stretching of the skin.

Rule of nines See *Burns*

Rules of professional conduct Rules of Professional Conduct were endorsed at the very first council meeting of the Chartered Society of Physiotherapists (CSP) in 1895 (Barclay J 1994 In Good Hands: History of the Chartered Society of Physiotherapy, 1984–94. Butterworth-Heinemann) and have been revised and updated at intervals since. Rules of Professional Conduct set out a framework for the ethical, moral and legal basis of the profession, providing statements of the conduct expected of chartered physiotherapists and students. The current Rules (go to www.csp.org.uk) set out a number of principles, the basis for all of which is to safeguard patients. They include requirements that physiotherapists:

- respect the dignity and individual sensibilities of every patient
- work safely and competently

- ensure the confidentiality of patient information
- report circumstances that might otherwise put patients at risk
- do not exploit patients
- act in a way that reflects credit on the profession and does not cause offence to patients.

Although the Society has had Rules of Professional Conduct since its inception, Standards of Physiotherapy Practice were not published until 1990. These provide statements about the practical application of the ethical principles set out in the Rules. The third edition (CSP 2000) has evolved to place more emphasis than in earlier editions on practitioners:

- involving patients in decision making
- being fully abreast of the evidence of effectiveness in order to inform patients and offer the most effective interventions
- evaluating their practice and measuring a patient's health gain as a result of treatment.

Russian current Electrotherapy term – a name used to indicate an alternating current with a pulse frequency of 2.5 kHz (carrier frequency), sinusoidal, triangular or rectangular pulses and a burst frequency of 50 Hz, used for motor stimulation. Burst duration is typically 10 ms (interburst interval = 10 ms), but can be less, especially if aim is to reduce the rate of fatigue in the muscles being stimulated. Name of current due to use by Kots in Russia to train elite athletes prior to the Montreal Olympic games in 1976.

See *Alternating current*

Rx Common medical abbreviation – Treatment.

SAB Common medical abbreviation – Sub acromial bursa.

Sacral plexus (Lumbosacral plexus) The collection of nerves that lead on to the formation of the major nerves in the lower limb.

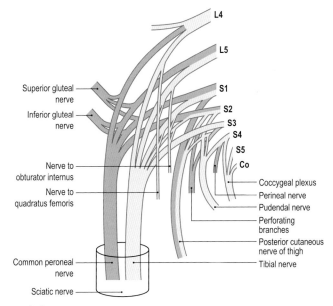

The sacral plexus

Sacro-iliac joint (SIJ) Partly fibrous and partly a synovial joint formed between the medial surface of the ilium and the lateral aspect of the upper sacral vertebrae. Comprising and surrounded by very strong ligamentous structures. The major function is to transmit body weight, but does have a role in movement. There is probably a small amount of rotation that occurs at this joint.

The SIJ can be affected by various conditions including trauma, biomechanical mal-alignment, hormonal changes or inflammatory joint disease such as ankylosing spondylitis.

Sagittal plane The plane that divides the body into left and right portions.

Sag sign The phenomenon observed in a person who has a ruptured posterior cruciate ligament, in crook lying the tibia sags posteriorly in comparison to the unaffected leg.

Sah Common medical abbreviation – Sub-arachnoid haemorrhage.
This is where bleeding occurs in the sub-arachnoid space which is the space between the arachnoid mater and pia mater in the brain. Cerebral aneurysms and arterio-venous malformations are cited as causes of SAH. Patients often require neurosurgical intervention and may have a neurological deficit that requires management by the multidisciplinary team.

Salbutamol (Ventolin) A drug used as a vasodilator in asthma.

Saltatory conduction The term that describes the transmission of a nerve impulse along myelinated nerves. Action potentials are generated at intervals along the nerve, as shown below. This results in a faster transmission than if the sheath were continuous.

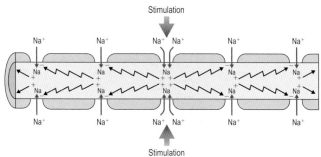

Saltatory conduction

Sample Research term – the individuals who satisfied the inclusion criteria and who actually entered the research study.

Sarcoidosis A granulomatous disease of unknown origin affecting many organs, but most commonly the skin, lungs and eyes. The diseased organs contain collections of nodules consisting of epithelioid cells (similar to TB but without a necrotic centre). The respiratory presentation is common in young adults and, while the disease is often symptom limiting, 90% will recover with no treatment, 10% may run a relapsing or chronic course. A monitoring period may be pursued initially to await spontaneous recovery but where this does not occur, corticosteroids may be used if deteriorating lung function is observed. See *Interstitial lung disease*. The respiratory symptoms are those of cough and dyspnoea, with >25% of patients being accidentally diagnosed through abnormal radiological findings. Features of the respiratory manifestations include hilar lymphadenopathy (enlarged hilar lymph nodes), pulmonary opacities and irreversible pulmonary fibrosis. Investigations will reveal a restrictive lung disorder with low lung volumes and reduced transfer factor. Where histological evidence is sought, transbronchial biopsy may be performed.

Owing to the multi-organ involvement of the disease, the non-respiratory manifestations include uveitis (inflammation of the eye chamber), hepato-splenomegaly, myocarditis (inflammation of the myocardium), erythema nodosum (raised and red skin lesions), meningitis, hypercalcaemia and lethargy.

Sarcolemma The plasma membrane surrounding a muscle cell.

Sarcomeres These are subunits of myofibrils containing organized thick and thin filaments bounded by Z lines.
See *Muscle structure*

Sarcoplasmic reticulum Smooth endoplasmic reticulum of muscle fibres; calcium store, which is released and sequestered during and after contractions.

SC Common medical abbreviation – Sub cuticular.

Scaphoid fracture Common following a fall onto the outstretched hand. A fracture of the scaphoid bone in the carpus of the hand is sometimes difficult to detect on initial X-ray and requires repeat X-ray in a couple of weeks to confirm. Often, if the fracture involves the proximal third of the scaphoid, there is a high risk of non-union and threat of avascular necrosis, due to the poor blood supply.

Scapula The shoulder blade, braced away from the chest wall by the clavicle and acting as a mobile platform for the movements of the upper limb, it is thin in its central portion (hold one up to the light and see) and thick along its medial and lateral borders where powerful muscles attach.

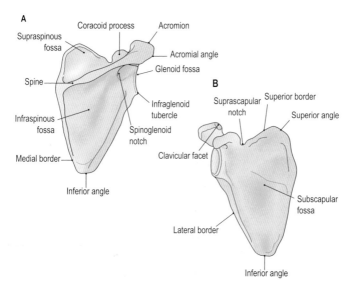

The right scapula: **(A)** posterior view; **(B)** anterior view

Scapulo-humeral rhythm The movements of clavicular rotation, scapular gilding, scapular rotation and gleno-humeral elevation, during movement of the shoulder complex.

Scarf test This tests for problems at the acromio clavicular joint (ACJ).

    The test is performed by forced cross body adduction in 90° flexion, pain at the extreme of motion indicates ACJ pathology.

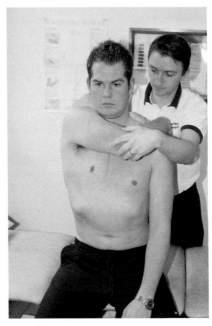

Scarf test for ACJ pathology

Scheuermann's disease Osteochondrosis of the vertebral epiphyses in adolescents.

    It consists of wedging of the vertebrae, Schmorl's nodes or endplate irregularity and narrowing of the intervertebral disc spaces. Its aetiology is not clear. Scheuermann's disease commonly affects the lower thoracic and upper lumbar spine. It usually begins at puberty and males and females are equally affected. The condition results in a thoracic kyphosis and half of those affected show a scoliosis as well.

Schmorl's node The phenomenon of sequestration or breaking off of part of a disc and its herniation into the vertebral body or movement up and down the spinal canal. Sometimes described as fractured end plates, often large

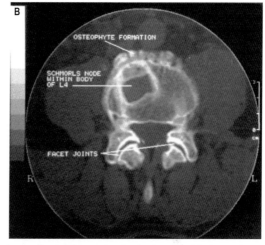

(A) Lumbar spondylosis at L4 level; (B) Scan showing lumbar spondylosis at L4 level

enough to allow the nucleus pulposus to extrude into the vertebral body. Often a feature of lower thoracic and/or thoracolumbar spines.

See *End plate, Sheuermann's disease* and *Sequestered disc*

Schober's test A measure of lumbar flexion. Draw a line at L4/5 junction, make a mark 10 cm above this line and 5 cm below it, the patient bends forwards with the knees slightly flexed. The therapist holds the end of the tape measure on the upper mark and measure between the two marks. Any increase beyond 15 cm is the lumbar flexion (see figure).

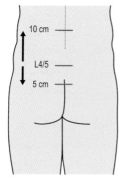
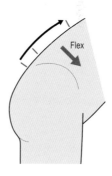

Schober's test

Schwann cell The cell that sends out a covering of myelin to wrap around myelinated nerves.

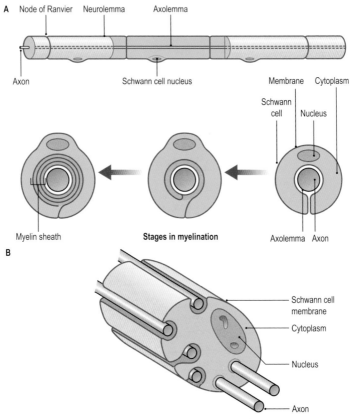

A
Node of Ranvier   Neurolemma   Axolemma
Axon   Schwann cell nucleus
Membrane   Cytoplasm
Schwann cell   Nucleus
Axolemma   Axon
Myelin sheath   **Stages in myelination**
B
Schwann cell membrane
Cytoplasm
Nucleus
Axon

(**A**) A myelinated axon in the peripheral nervous system; (**B**) The relationship between unmyelinated axons and Schwann cells

Sciatica Pain in the distribution of the sciatic nerve or its branches that is caused by direct pressure or irritation. It does not include referred pain derived from spinal joints, ligaments or muscles.

Sciatic nerve The large nerve that runs down the posterior of the leg, it splits into tibial and common peroneal nerves.

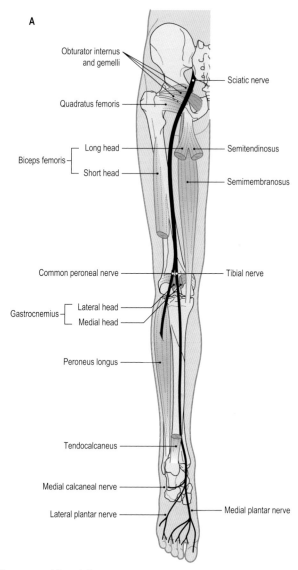

A

Obturator internus
and gemelli

Sciatic nerve

Quadratus femoris

Long head

Biceps femoris

Semitendinosus

Short head

Semimembranosus

Common peroneal nerve

Tibial nerve

Lateral head

Gastrocnemius

Medial head

Peroneus longus

Tendocalcaneus

Medial calcaneal nerve

Lateral plantar nerve

Medial plantar nerve

(A) The course of the sciatic nerve

B

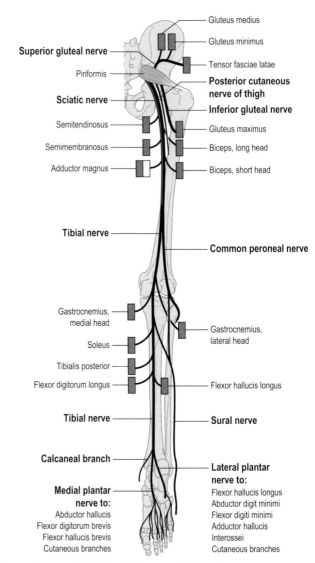

Gluteus medius

Gluteus minimus

Superior gluteal nerve

Tensor fasciae latae

Piriformis

Posterior cutaneous nerve of thigh

Sciatic nerve

Inferior gluteal nerve

Semitendinosus

Gluteus maximus

Semimembranosus

Biceps, long head

Adductor magnus

Biceps, short head

Tibial nerve

Common peroneal nerve

Gastrocnemius, medial head

Gastrocnemius, lateral head

Soleus

Tibialis posterior

Flexor digitorum longus

Flexor hallucis longus

Tibial nerve

Sural nerve

Calcaneal branch

Lateral plantar nerve to:

Medial plantar nerve to:

Flexor hallucis longus
Abductor digit minimi
Flexor digiti minimi
Adductor hallucis
Interossei
Cutaneous branches

Abductor hallucis
Flexor digitorum brevis
Flexor hallucis brevis
Cutaneous branches

(B) The muscles supplied by the sciatic nerve and its branches

Sciatic nerve stretch See *Lasegues test/sign*
A test of the mobility of the nerve roots and dura mater that lines them.

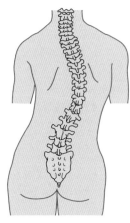

Scoliosis

Scoliosis A lateral curvature of the spinal column. The cause may be structural, compensatory or protective. In structural scoliosis, there is a vertebral rotation associated with the lateral curvature, with both the curve and the rotation being accentuated in forward flexion.

SDH Common medical abbreviation – Subdural haematoma.
This is a collection of blood on the surface of the brain that lies beneath the outer covering of the brain (the dura) and the brain's surface. Acute SDH are often as the result of a head injury, although they can occur spontaneously. Chronic SDH occur most often in the elderly and in infancy with trauma being the likely cause.

Secondary benefits Benefits resulting from a treatment in addition to the primary, intended outcome.

Secondary osteoarthritis The type of osteoarthritis (OA) where there is another predisposing cause rather than a problem with the cartilage itself for example a fracture of the tibial plateau may result in secondary OA in later life.
See *Osteoarthritis*

Selective movement This is a term used by physiotherapists to describe a movement that is precise, co-ordinated, purposeful and is based on the appropriate background of stability.

Self-advocacy Most often applied to people with learning difficulties. It concerns people speaking up for themselves, defending their rights and organizing themselves to promote their interests as a group. As a political movement, it is the struggle over whose demands, concerns, choices and perspectives should prevail.
See *Advocacy*

Self-awareness The reflective ability of people to take themselves as the objects of their own thoughts. It can include self-conception and self-monitoring, which involves the observation and control of self-presentation.

Self-directed learning/study A student-centred learning strategy where the student determines: their learning needs, strategies to fulfil these needs, learning resources required and how to evaluate and reflect on the process.

Self-efficacy The belief that a person can successfully undertake a particular behaviour.

Self-esteem The degree to which a person values him or herself.

Self-fulfilling prophecy A process whereby people may become what others think they are or expect them to be. For example a child who is labelled 'very bright' by important people in his or her life, is likely to live up to that expectation.

Self-help The collective activities of groups of people who are experiencing similar problems. Self-help groups may remain small but can expand into social movements, for example, the Disabled People's Movement and Gay Pride.

Self-image An image of the self we suppose ourselves to be. Self-image may be discrepant with what we achieve or how others see us.

Semester A period of academic time – usually 15 weeks.

Semi-circular canals These are a series of canals containing endolymph and are part of the vestibular apparatus found within the inner ear. Different movements of the head lead to information being transmitted to the vestibular component of the VIII cranial nerve (auditory nerve) and hence the semi-circular canals are important in the maintenance of balance.

Seminar A learning session where students make a presentation (usually on something they have read) to a small group of peers and a tutor as a basis for further discussion by the group.

Senate The committee in a university with ultimate responsibility for academic matters.

Sensation Sensation is the term used to describe the afferent input from the world around us or from the body itself. It allows us to function safely and adapt in ever-changing circumstances. Sensory receptors convert information into electrical activity that is then processed by the CNS. Sensation requires the peripheral and central nervous system to be intact.

● Clinical note Movement is possible without sensation but it is clumsy and slow and is heavily reliant on visual information.

Sensitivity (of a test) The proportion of individuals classified as positive by the gold (or reference) standard, who are correctly identified by the study test. The proportion of people with disease who have a positive test.

Sensitizing concept Research term – a term used to describe how certain concepts may guide the researcher towards a certain behaviour.

Sensorimotor feedback This involves the integration and interaction of afferent (sensory) information during motor activity, which may then alter the movement or lead to adaptation of the motor response. Feedback allows errors to be corrected.

Sensorimotor feed forward This involves the integration and interaction of afferent (sensory) information prior to a motor activity and thus allows adaptation to be made before the execution of a movement.

Sensory ataxia See *Ataxia*
   This results from lesions affecting the peripheral sensory nerves, conditions affecting the dorsal columns, such as tabes dorsalis, or lesions affecting the primary sensory cortex.

● Clinical note Patients often have a wide based high-stepping gait pattern.

Sensory integration This is the meaningful organization of sensory information received by the body in order to maximally function in the world at large.

SEP Common medical abbreviation – Sensory evoked potentials.
This is a response that is recorded over the parietal region in the brain in response to the stimulation of a peripheral nerve.

○ Clinical note It allows the conduction time of a nerve to be calculated and so can help detect lesions in the sensory pathways.

Septicemia A serious, rapidly progressive, life-threatening infection that can arise from infections, including infections in the lungs, abdomen and urinary tract.

Sequestrated disc A term describing the complete detachment of a portion of prolapsed intervertebral disc, with migration, often into the spinal canal.

Sesamoid Bone Small bone shaped like a sesame seed lying within a tendon at points of great pressure.

○ Clinical point Some people have more sesamoid bones that others. The patella is the largest sesamoid bone in the body.

Sesamoiditis Inflammatory condition affecting the sesamoid bones usually in the flexor tendon of the great toe. It is usually precipitated by trauma. Stress fractures of the sesamoid bone are quite common with overuse.

Severe acute respiratory syndrome (SARS) A serious form of pneumonia, resulting in acute respiratory distress and sometimes death.

Severity See *SIN factors*

Sever's disease Traction apophysitis of the separate ossification centre on the calcaneum for the insertion of the Achilles tendon. Can mimic Achilles tendinitis.

Sexism Stereotyped, negative beliefs, usually about women, which may lead to discrimination; for example, unequal pay and poor educational opportunities. Men may also be subject to sexism, for example, some colleges of physiotherapy were once closed to men.

SFL/SFR Common medical abbreviation – Side flex left/right.

SH Common medical abbreviation – Social history.

Shift The phenomenon where a person moves a part of the body, usually the spine, in an attempt to adopt the least painful posture.

Shin splints The term for a collection of common problems that affect both recreational and trained athletes. Runners are often affected. Periostitis occurs further toward the front of the leg than posterior tibial shin splints and the bone itself is tender. Anterior compartment syndrome affects the outer side of the front of the leg. Stress fractures of the tibia may occur, which usually produce localized, sharp pain with tenderness below the knee. Stress fractures commonly occur several weeks into a new training programme or after commencing a more strenuous training regimen.

Shock Medical context – a serious condition that occurs when the cardiovascular system is unable to supply enough blood flow to the body, usually associated with low blood pressure and cell or tissue damage.

Shock Electrotherapy context – electrical shock: macroshock (ampere level current, person in mains to earth circuit – see *Body protected areas*) or microshock (issued mainly in high-dependency units or intensive care units). There is a risk of a small shock with electrical stimulation: the machine should be turned on prior to testing its output and connecting the patient and turned off only after the intensity is fully down and the patient circuit disconnected. The reason for this is that a microprocessor circuit that is not fully powered is not totally predictable.

Short-term memory Short-term memory is the ability to retain and recall information and experiences from recent events.

  ◉ Clinical note If affected, for instance after stroke or head injury, it will make the re-learning of tasks more difficult and liaison with the occupational therapist or psychologist is essential for compensatory strategies.

Shortwave diathermy (SWD) Electrotherapy term – an electromagnetic radiation with a frequency of 27.12 MHz. Continuous (CSWD) or pulsed (PSWD) output. CSWD used for deep tissue heating and PSWD to promote healing. Types: capacitive or inductothermy. Dangers and contraindications include: indwelling pumps or stimulators within 3–5 m, indwelling metal within 30 cm and, if local circulation reduced, there is a risk of heat induced damage.
  See *PEME*

Shoulder-hand syndrome This may also be called complex regional pain syndrome and may occur for no apparent reason or following trauma. Signs and symptoms include pain and loss of movement in the shoulder and wrist joints, with swelling of the hand and the skin may become red and shiny. It usually develops 1–6 months after stroke. The syndrome is considered to develop in three consecutive phases: I – acute, II – dystrophic and III – atrophic.

  ◉ Clinical note It is important to maintain as much range as possible in the joints but pain relief may be necessary. Sometimes a sympathetic nerve block is carried out (Zyluk & Zyluk 1999).

Sickle-cell anemia An inherited disease in which the red blood cells, normally disc-shaped, become crescent shaped. As a result, they function abnormally and cause small blood clots. These clots give rise to recurrent painful episodes called 'sickle cell pain crises'.

Sick role The role a person is expected to assume when ill. This will depend on historical and cultural factors. In Britain, at the present time, the obligations of this role are to obtain competent medical help and to comply with medical treatment. In return, the individual is relieved of everyday responsibilities and is not blamed for his or her illness. The concept is more applicable to acute illness than chronic illness or impairment. This conceptualization of the sick role was first formulated by Parsons in 1951.

SIDS Common medical abbreviation – Sudden infant death syndrome, also known as cot death syndrome.

Sigmoidoscopy Flexible sigmoidoscopy is a procedure that enables examination of the rectum and the lower colon. The instrument is a flexible tube.

Sign Objective evidence of disease or abnormality that is perceptible to the examiner, e.g. there is a positive patellar tap – this is a sign, 'my knee aches all the time' – this is a symptom.

Significance level Research term – the probability of incorrectly rejecting the null hypothesis, i.e. saying that there is a difference between two groups when actually there is no difference. Otherwise known as the probability of Type I error. By convention, the level of significance is often set to a P value of 0.01 (99% significance level) or 0.05 (95% significance level).

SIJ Common medical abbreviation – Sacro iliac joint.

Simultaneous oppression The way in which social divisions of gender, age, class, race, sexual orientation and disability combine in important and varying ways to exacerbate the experience of oppression.

SIN (Severity, irritability and nature) factors

Severity
A symptom is defined as severe if the activity that causes the pain needs to be interrupted and stopped because of the intensity of the pain. In many cases this is an indication that caution is needed in examination and treatment procedures.

Indications to severity:
- High number of pain killers.
- Disturbed sleep.
- Off work due to severity of pain.
- High visual analogue scale (VAS).

Irritability
This means that a little activity causes a lot of pain that takes a relatively long time to settle. In many cases this is an indication that caution is required regarding examination and treatment procedures.

Indicators for irritability:
- Susceptibility to become painful.
- How painful it becomes.
- The length of time this pain takes to recover.

Nature of the disorder
This refers to the aspects of problems that require consideration in examination and treatment procedures. It may include the pathobiological processes underlying the disorder, contributing factors such as osteoporosis, stage of healing, stage and stability of the disorder and certain personal features, such as fear of moving.

Sinding–Larsen–Johansson's disease Traction osteochondrosis at the patella's inferior pole.

Sinuvertebral nerve From the spinal nerve, after its formation from the joining of the ventral and dorsal nerves, comes a small filament of nerve, which is joined by a branch from the sympathetic trunk.

Skeletal traction The insertion of a wire or pin through a bone and a weight system attached to allow localized, effective traction.

The picture below shows skeletal traction. The pin shown is a Steinman pin. Common sites for this are the tibial plateau or the calcaneum. Pin sites must be kept clean and infection free.

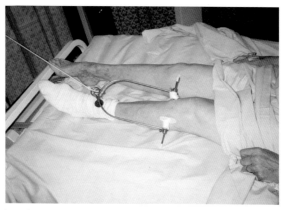

Skeletal traction

Skyline X-ray A type of X-ray view that portrays the patella sitting in the groove between the femoral condyles, it is useful in highlighting mal-tracking of the patella.

This X-ray shows a mal-tracking patella.

SL Common medical abbreviation – Sub lingual (under the tongue), usually refers to method of drug administration.

Slap lesion A shoulder joint pathology, it stands for superior glenoid labral tear in an anterior to posterior direction.

SLE Common medical abbreviation – Systemic lupus erythematosus.

Sleep apnoea The cessation of breathing during sleep.

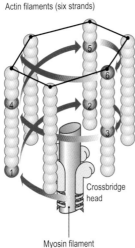

Actin filaments (six strands)

Crossbridge head

Myosin filament

Sliding filament theory

Sliding filament theory See *Actin and Myosin*

The concept that within the myofibrils, actin and myosin filaments slide across each other, thus inducing shortening. This is the fundamental mechanism underlying contraction of muscle.

Slow-twitch muscle fibres One of three skeletal muscle fibre subclasses; characterized by abundant mitochondria, fatigue resistance and myosin with low ATP sensitivity.

Slump Test See *Neurodynamics*

Smart See *Goal setting*

The term used to assist in the formation of treatment goals, it stands for:

- **S**pecific
- **M**easurable
- **A**chievable
- **R**ealistic
- **T**imely.

Typical examples of orthopaedic goals (these possess all the SMART characteristics shown above).

Good goals
- Mr X will be able to safely negotiate stairs, partial weight bearing with two elbow crutches in 4 days' time.
- Mrs Y will have attained 50° of active knee flexion by 1 week from today.
- Mrs Z will be able to transfer safely from bed to chair within 2 days' time.

Bad goals
Test yourself. Each of these goals fails to achieve one or more of the SMART criteria:

1. Mr X will be totally pain free within 1 day of sustaining his fractured femur, tibia and humerus.
2. Mr X will be able to walk in 8 months' time.
3. Mr X will be much better in 1 week.
4. Mr X will mobilize full weight bearing on the unstable fracture within 1 week.
5. Mr X will have more knee flexion within 1 week.

Why each goal is unacceptable:

1. Not realistic – it is extremely unlikely that Mr X will be totally pain free 1 day after three such major fractures.
2. Not timely – the end point of this goal is too far in the future.

3. Not specific – what does much better mean?
4. Not achievable – the orthopaedic protocol does not permit this.
5. Not measurable and not specific – what does 'more' mean?

Smiths fracture This is similar to a Colles fracture but with volar (towards the palm) as opposed to dorsal displacement of the distal fragment.

SNAG Common medical abbreviation – Sustained natural apophyseal glide.

Snowball sampling Research term – in which selection of additional respondents is based on referrals from the initial respondents, continuing until no new respondents are identified.

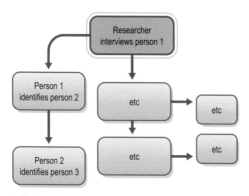

Snowball sampling

SOB (OE) Common medical abbreviation – Short of breath (on exertion).

Social class The structural position in society of an individual or a group compared to other individuals and groups. It is a central term within the social sciences and the subject of significant controversy and disagreement. In official statistics people are generally classified on the basis of occupation and income.

Social inclusion Refers to the full incorporation and participation of people in society as a result of fundamental changes within attitudes, behaviour and societal structures.

Social movement The organized efforts of significant numbers of oppressed people (including women, black people and disabled people) to change a major aspect of society. A social movement is a politically generated and committed force that is opposed to the status quo. Social movement usually operate outside regular political channels.

Social policy The process of developing measures to reduce social problems and implementing these measures. Social policy is also an academic field of study where these processes are analyzed.

Social role valorization This concept evolved from the concept of 'normalization' and was first formulated by Wolfensberger in 1998. This was partly due to mounting criticisms of the concept of 'normalization'. Social role valorization refers to the process of improving the lives and social standing of devalued groups, particularly people with learning difficulties, so that their social value in the eyes of others is enhanced. Such measures include de-institutionalization and allowing people to participate and contribute to society.

See *Normalization*

Socio-economic status A measure for classifying individuals, families and households. Indicators include occupation, income, education and housing.

See *Social class*

Sociology The study of human societies.

Sodium pump See *Calcium pump*

Sonophoresis Electrotherapy term – the use of therapeutic ultrasound to drive an active compound across the skin barrier, e.g. analgesics, anti-inflammatory creams are used as a contact medium between the applicator and skin.

Spasm This term describes a transient increase in tone in a muscle or group of muscles in the presence of neurological pathology.

✚ Clinical note The cause of spasms should be explored as it may indicate, for instance, a urinary-tract infection or the start of a pressure sore in a spinal injury patient.

Spasmodic torticollis See *Torticollis*

Spastic dystonia This is a term to describe the sustained chronic contraction of muscle that continues in the absence of movement. It is thought to be caused by sustained efferent muscular hyperactivity, dependent upon continuous supraspinal drive to the alpha motor neurones (Burke 1988).

Spasticity This term is often interchanged with increased tone, hypertonicity and hyper-reflexia.

In its true sense it describes a motor disorder that is characterized by a velocity-dependent increase in tonic stretch reflexes. It can be seen in a variety of neurological conditions such as stroke, multiple sclerosis and head injury.

✚ Clinical note The presence of spasticity in some patients is essential for function; therefore, a full and careful assessment must be carried out.

Spatial awareness For people to be able to function effectively within their environment they must know where each part of their body is in relation to the immediate environment.

✚ Clinical note This may be affected following brain injury and has major implications for safety, i.e. judging the depth of stairs or how far away a car is whilst crossing the road.

Special needs The concept of needs is widely used in the social sciences and in service policy, practice and provision. It can denote the lack of something required by or necessary for a person, particularly for survival. Though basic human needs can be agreed, such as for food, sleep and shelter, broader social and psychological needs are contested. When applied to specific groups, particularly disabled people, the notion of needs is often qualified by the term 'special' within an individual or medical model of disability. With regard to the need for provision of services, 'special' has meant separate or segregated and is seen by many disabled people as an expression and justification of oppression. It can be argued that the needs of disabled people should be mainstream rather than 'special'.

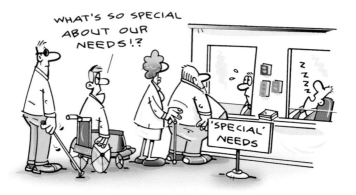

Specificity (of a test)   The proportion of individuals classified as negative by the gold (or reference) standard, who are correctly identified by the study test. The proportion of people free of a disease who have a negative test.

Spina bifida   A congenital defect of the spinal column, characterized by the absence of the vertebral arch through which the spinal cord may protrude.

Spina bifida occulta   Non-union of the laminae. It may be simply due to a failure of ossification of a neural arch, or else it may be associated with quite severe abnormalities of the dural sac, cauda equina and spinal cord.

Spinal anaesthesia   See *Epidural anaesthesia*
   This is a form of anaesthesia that is useful in operations that are undertaken below the level of the umbilicus, such as total hip or knee replacement. It is useful particularly in people who would not tolerate a general anaesthetic such as the frail or those with lung or cardiac problems.

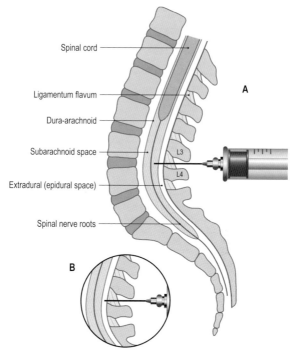

Spinal cord

Ligamentum flavum

Dura-arachnoid

Subarachnoid space

Extradural (epidural space)

Spinal nerve roots

A

L3

L4

B

Spinal and epidermal anaesthesia

Spinal canal stenosis – also known as spinal stenosis Reduction of the anterior-posterior and lateral diameters of the spinal canal. May be due to congenital factors, developmental factors or degenerative disease. Features include: pain or numbness in the buttocks, thighs or calves that worsens on walking or exercise. Back pain that radiates to the legs and leg weakness.

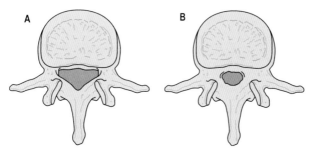

A   B

Spinal canal (shaded below) to indicate **(A)** normal size; **(B)** spinal stenosis.

Spinal-cord injury Damage to the spinal cord that results in neurological deficits.

Spirometry The measurement of airflow and lung volumes over time. Measurements include the forced expiratory volume in 1 s (or other time specified) (FEV_1), forced vital capacity (FVC) and forced expiratory ratio (FER), i.e. the FEV_1/FVC. Such measurements can be used for both diagnostic and monitoring purposes, but are effort dependent so correct technique is required for accurate results:

- FEV_1: the volume of air exhaled in the first second.
- FVC: the total volume of air exhaled from a maximal inspiration.
- FER: this is the ratio of FEV_1 to FVC, i.e. FEV_1/FVC $\times$ 100. This should normally be around 80%. Where the ratio is <70% airflow obstruction is detected, e.g. chronic obstructive pulmonary disease (COPD) and asthma; while a normal or raised ratio (with reduced values for both FEV_1 and FVC) is indicative of restrictive disorders such as fibrosis; oedema; chest wall deformity and neuromuscular disorders.

When more detailed analysis of lung function is required, other volumes may be measured.

These include:

- FRC: functional residual capacity (approximately 2500 ml). This is the amount of air residual in the lungs after a normal tidal exhalation. (Plethysmography is required to measure this lung volume.)
- TLC: total lung capacity (approximately 6 l). This is the total volume of air in the lungs after a maximal inhalation.
- RV: residual volume (approximately 1200 ml). This is the amount of air left in the lungs after a maximal exhalation. This volume cannot be measured using normal spirometric techniques. Body plethysmography (the body box) or gas dilution techniques are required to obtain this value.
- Vt: tidal volume (approximately 500 ml). This is the volume of air exchanged during normal resting breathing.

Splinting Splinting is an adjunct to physiotherapy treatment that can be used in a number of ways:

- Preventative – to help maintain a joint position and thus prevent loss of range of movement
- Corrective – to correct a loss of range or mal-alignment, e.g. serial casting
- For functional – a wrist splint to maintain extension to maximize finger extension, or an **AFO** to enable safe walking.

Spondylolisthesis Forward displacement of one vertebra on the bone below it. Most commonly seen at L5/S1. The degree of spondylolisthesis is determined by the distance the slipped vertebra travels on its lower counterpart – Grades 1–4.

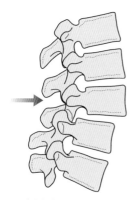

Spondylolisthesis

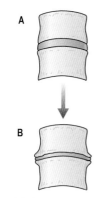

A

B

Spondylosis

Spondylosis See *Cervical spondylosis* and *Lumbar spondylosis*

Caused by a defect in the pars inter-articularis, a narrow strip of bone lying between the lamina and the inferior articular process below and the pedicle and the superior articular process above. May be congenital, traumatic or caused by overuse. In oblique X-ray views, which have the appearance of a Scotty dog, a spondylosis through the pars interarticularis showing will show up a 'collar' around the dog's neck.

The main characteristic of spondylosis is the loss of water from the disc. Tears also occur in the nucleus, annulus and endplates. The nourishment of the adult disc is more precarious than that of an immature disc and the first signs of spondylosis usually present clinically at about the age of 30 and is most common around the age of 45. The pathological changes that occur are the same regardless of site, but the differences in functional anatomy gives rise to different clinical signs and symptoms. Pathology involves a coarsening of the annulus fibrosis, collagen fibres separate and cracks appear in the annulus. The nucleus pulposus dehydrates and becomes more fibrous with the disc losing height overall. These changes can be present without causing any signs or symptoms. 'Lipping' of the vertebral bodies occurs, due to altered disc biomechanics, which causes traction of the periosteum by the attachments of the annulus fibrosis. There can also be decalcification within the vertebral body. The intervertebral ligaments may become contracted and thickened especially at the sites where there are gross changes. The dura mater of the spinal cord, which forms a sleeve round the nerve root, may undergo low-grade, chronic inflammatory changes. This can result in nerve-root adhesions with associated neural symptoms.

Most commonly, the major change is that of osteophytosis, the formation of bony spurs along the junction of the vertebral bodies and the corresponding intervertebral discs.

Sprain A sprain occurs when there is tearing of the ligament or capsular structures. A joint that is forced beyond its range of motion can stretch, tear and sometimes avulse the connective tissues that stabilize the joint. There are three categories.

First-degree sprain

Definition
A few fibres are torn.

Second-degree sprain

Definition
Approximately half of fibres are torn.

Third-degree sprain

Definition
Complete tear.

Squeeze test   See *Thompsons test*

Standard   Statement that describes the range of acceptable conduct or care. An agreed statement against which others are judged or measured.

Standard deviation   Research term – a measure of variability or spread of data. The standard deviation quantifies how much the values vary from each other. It is a measure of the spread of individual observations around the mean value of the sample. A normal, unskewed curve will have 34% of the cases between the mean and 1 standard deviation above or below the mean; 68% of cases between 1 standard deviation above and 1 below the mean; 95.5% of cases will be within two standard deviations of the mean.

Standard error of the mean   Research term – a measure of variability. The standard error of the mean quantifies how accurately the true population mean is known.

Statistical significance   Probability of the observed degree of association between variables, from this the statistical significance can be expressed, commonly in terms of the P value. For example: $P < 0.05$ means that for the results obtained there is a 95% chance that they have not occurred by chance alone; $P < 0.01$ means that for the results obtained there is a 99% chance that they have not occurred by chance alone.

For most physiotherapy research a P value of 0.05 is sufficient, but for research where an error in interpretation would have potentially disastrous consequences, e.g. for research into a new cancer therapy, a P value of 0.01 would be more appropriate.

Status epilepticus   This can be a life-threatening state, where a person is suffering from seizures (fits) and between seizures they remain unconscious. It is a medical emergency. This condition may be caused by a variety of reasons; head injury in the frontal region of the brain, infections and drug-induced being a few examples.

Steinman pin   See *Skeletal traction*

Stereognosis   This term relates to the ability to be able to recognize an object when placed or manipulated by the hand. It allows the detection of texture, weight, size and shape without the use of vision.

Stereotype An overgeneralized, oversimplified, biased and inflexible conception of a social group. Stereotypes are frequently associated with oppressed groups and provide justifications for and a means of maintaining oppression.

Sternotomy The incision used in thoracic surgery that splits the sternum vertically.

Stethoscope The instrument used for auscultation.

Stigma A term associated with the work of the sociologist Ervin Goffman. Its use generally denotes shame and disgrace attributed to the person (for example, the stigma of being a prisoner) though in more formal theory it denotes a relationship of devaluation (for example, the stigma of being disabled).

Stirrups Technique of ankle strapping using rigid tape (usually zinc oxide). The tape is placed on the ankle, medial to lateral adhering to the undersurface of the heel, mimicking a 'stirrup'.

Strabismus Deviation of the alignment of one eye in relation to the other.

Straight leg raise (SLR) See *Neurodynamics*

Strain Non-specific term given to excessive or abnormal loading of tissues. Can be used interchangeably to describe the sensation felt during exercise or activity. A strain occurs when there is a tear in the muscle or tendon. There are three classifications of strains.

First-degree strain

Definition
Few fibres of muscle stretched or torn.

Symptoms
Local pain, which is increased with stretch, slight loss of strength and stability.

Second-degree strain

Definition
Approximately half of muscle and/or tendon fibres are torn.

Symptoms
Significant pain with muscle on stretch, moderate loss of strength and stability.

Third-degree strain

Definition
Complete tear of muscle or tendon.

Symptoms
Significant loss of strength and joint stability, major loss of function.

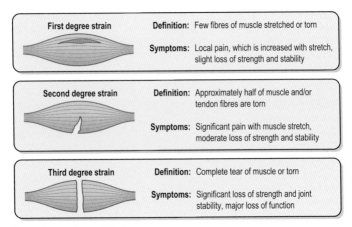

First degree strain — **Definition:** Few fibres of muscle stretched or torn

Symptoms: Local pain, which is increased with stretch, slight loss of strength and stability

Second degree strain — **Definition:** Approximately half of muscle and/or tendon fibres are torn

Symptoms: Significant pain with muscle stretch, moderate loss of strength and stability

Third degree strain — **Definition:** Complete tear of muscle or torn

Symptoms: Significant loss of strength and joint stability, major loss of function

Three classifications of strains

Strength–duration testing Electrotherapy term – a quick method (in conjunction with clinical assessment of sensory and motor deficits and functional changes) of obtaining information about a damaged peripheral nerve. Used to establish integrity and serial testing (7–14 days later) can indicate direction of change. Largely replaced by modern electrophysiological testing that is more accurate and able to provide more reliable differential diagnoses. Equipment required: monophasic pulses, frequency 1 Hz, range of 6–8 pulse durations between 10 μs and approximately 300 ms.

See *Rheobase* and *Chronaxie*

Stress Psychological strain, which can have physical manifestations, associated with events, experiences or circumstances that are difficult to tolerate and manage.

See *Anxiety*

Stress fracture Fracture caused by cumulative bone overload. Can be caused by a number of factors, including: overstraining, incorrect biomechanics, fatigue, hormonal imbalance, poor nutrition or osteoporosis.

Stretching Stretching exercises are normally used to mobilize neural and muscle tissue to the limits of the available range. Stretches may be applied in one of two ways: either dynamic or static.

Dynamic stretching

This involves gaining range by an active movement and should not be confused with ballistic stretching, which involves the use of repetitive, bouncing, dynamic, rhythmic movements performed at higher velocities. Dynamic stretching involves progressively increasing the range through successive movements until the end of range is reached. These exercises are especially useful when dealing with more advanced sports-related rehabilitation problems, they enhance dynamic function and neuromuscular control due to repetition and practice, thereby enhancing the movement memory.

Static stretching

As the name suggests, this involves maintaining a position for a sustained period to gain the desired effect. It is widely suggested that an effective time to hold a static stretch for is duration of 30 s. Static stretching is a controlled, slow movement with emphasis on correct bodily alignment. An element of fine motor control and postural awareness is important during static stretching exercises and this can be enhanced by use of feedback and correction from the physiotherapist, as well as use of equipment such as mirrors.

Stretching exercises: a practical guide

Before performing the stretch

- Before commencing a stretching programme, ensure that your assessment has not identified any contraindication to stretching
- Ensure that there is a logical, reasoned basis for your stretching programme, e.g. if there is a bony block to movement caused by osteophytes
- Consider how you will get your client to assist in his or her own stretching programme at home
- Explain how and why you are performing the stretch to ensure maximum compliance and minimal resistance
- Consider how the stretch might be made more comfortable prior to stretching, e.g. use a hot pack or hydrotherapy

During the stretch

- Make you handling firm, but maintain patient comfort, reassure the patient that you will stop the stretch at their command
- Stabilize the joints as necessary
- Stretch across one joint at a time for two joint muscles
- Make the stretch slow and sustained, do not bounce
- The patient should experience a pulling sensation, not pain
- Hold the position for 30 s (Bandy 1997)
- If tension releases, take the movement a little further
- Release slowly

After the stretch

- Warn the patient what feeling to expect following the stretch
- Remember that once movement has been regained, active muscle control throughout that range will be needed as well as some form of maintaining the stretch in the long term

Stretch reflex This consists of monosynaptic and polysynaptic pathways that conduct sensory information (afferent) from muscle spindles and can lead to a resultant contraction of a muscle fibre/muscle. The role of this reflex remains unclear, but it is thought to play a part in everyday activity.

Stridor A whistling sound usually heard on inspiration, it indicates obstruction of the trachea or larynx.

Stroke A stroke is defined as a sudden neurological deficit lasting more than 24 h of presumed vascular origin. Damage to the brain is caused by an interruption of the blood supply, most commonly caused by an infarct (85%) and is less often due to a haemorrhage (15%). Both may result in damaged brain tissue. Stroke is the leading cause of disability in the world.

Stroke unit This is a usually a geographically defined space that is dedicated to the treatment and management of stroke patients. It is characterized by organized specialist care delivered by a multidisciplinary team, who receive ongoing training and education in stroke, meet regularly (minimum weekly) and involve the carers and relatives in the rehabilitation process. Stroke units have been found to lead to better outcome for strokes with less mortality and morbidity (Stroke Unit Trialists 2002).

Student counsellor A professional employed by a university who has the skills necessary to help students with a range of personal problems or study needs requiring special learning strategies.

Students union The term used to describe the funded organization formed by students who manage social and sporting activities for students whilst at university. Its head is usually termed the president of the student union.

Subacromial decompression Surgical decompression of the shoulder, often with excision of the lateral portion of the clavicle, it is performed to relieve impingement.

Subacromial space Region of the shoulder that is bordered by the so-called subacromial joint – a joint made up by the humerus and a superior arch, consisting of the acromion process and the coracoid process of the scapula, joined by the coraco-acromial ligament. This arch is lined by the synovium of the subacromial bursa. In the subacromial space runs the rotator cuff.

Subcostal Below the ribs.

Subcutaneous Positioned under [sub-] the skin (e.g. a pacemaker and its batteries, wires and electrodes are inserted fully subcutaneously, under the skin).

Subdiaphragmatic Underneath the diaphragm. The following chest X-ray depicts the presence of sub-diaphragmatic air, e.g. post laparotomy or in the presence of a bowel rupture.

Subdural hematoma A collection of blood on the surface of the brain. It lies beneath the outer covering (the dura) of the brain and the brain's surface. Often the result of a head injury, although they can occur spontaneously.

Subjective assessment The data that are gained from speaking with the patient or carer, it aims to: gather all relevant information about the site, nature and behaviour of a person's symptoms and gain insight into the past behaviour and treatment. The patient's general health, previous investigations, medication and social circumstances are also recorded or reviewed.

Subjectivity A state of mind which emanates from personal feelings, opinions and emotions.

Subluxation This is where there is a partial dislocation of a joint. The shoulder joint is particularly vulnerable due to its inherent mobility from its anatomical structure and support given by the rotator cuff muscles. In hemiplegia or other forms of neurological damage the shoulder can sublux due to a lack of tone in the muscles surrounding the joint or in some cases the presence of increased tonal activity can cause some muscles to pull harder than others and thus cause a subluxation.

✪ Clinical note   Great care must be taken when handling a hemiplegic shoulder in order to try to prevent trauma, but it is important to remember that subluxation does not necessarily lead to pain.

Subtalar joint – also known as talocalcaneal joint The joint formed by the articulation of the talus with the calcaneus. This is a complex joint with a cylindrical axis.

Suction Respiratory care context – a means of removing excess bronchial secretions in a person who is unable to expectorate themselves, nasopharyngeal suction means that the catheter is inserted via the nose or oropharyngeal suction through the mouth, suction may also be administered via an airway, in a person who is intubated or via a tracheostomy.

The hazards of suctioning include hypoxia as ventilation is interrupted, raised intracranial pressure, trauma to the bronchial mucosa and cardiac arrhythmia (Pryor & Prasad 2002).

Suction Electrotherapy context – suction is used to hold electrodes against the skin. Can be a constant or a varying level of suction. Current passes from the stimulator output through a fine wire in each suction lead to a metal electrode in the suction cup. A damp sponge in the patient side of each suction cup completes the circuit. There is a risk of bruising if excess pressure is used or in patients with risk of bleeding, such as those taking anticoagulant medication.

Sudeck's atrophy A condition presenting as spontaneous pain. The underlying pathophysiology is still unknown. It is characterized by severe pain, swelling and disability, hyperalgesia (over sensitivity) that is not limited to a single nerve territory and is often out of proportion to the inciting event. It probably represents a neurovascular disorder leading to an intense hyperaemia and osteoporosis. Has been considered part of the reflex sympathetic dystrophy 'family' of conditions.

SUF(c)E Common medical abbreviation – Slipped upper femoral (capital) epiphysis.

A condition common in adolescents where the head of the femur slips on its growth plate like the ice cream slipping off an ice cream cone, it can cause pain, stiffness, loss of function and a limp.

Sulcus test See *Inferior draw test*

Supination Movement of the forearm so that the hand faces upwards.

Suppository A method of delivering a drug or medication via the rectum or vagina.

Supraspinatus impingement If the subacromial space is narrowed, impingement of the supraspinatus tendon may occur, characterized by pain, into shoulder abduction, and positive impingement tests. The person will often attempt to deviate away from the impingement, attempting to gain the necessary movement by using a trick movement.

Supraspinatus tendonitis Inflammation of the supraspinatus tendon. Commonly seen when there is a degree of supraspinatus tendon degeneration or degradation. Active contraction of the supraspinatus will cause pain and there is usually an arc of pain on abduction – described as 60–120° in most textbooks.

See *Painful arc*

Supraspinatus test – also known as empty can test The person sits or stands 90° with the shoulders in abduction full available medial rotation and 30° horizontal flexion. The physiotherapist resists abduction of the shoulder.

Abnormal finding Supraspinatus is the main support for the suspended arm in this position. Pain on resistance suggests a lesion of the supraspinatus muscle or tendon.

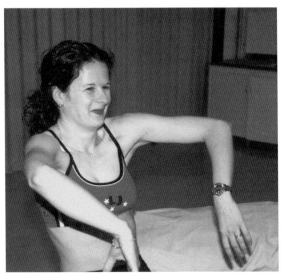

Empty can test

Surgical emphysema A collection of air in the tissues under the skin usually around the chest or neck, this makes a cracking sensation when compressed. It occurs when air from the mediastinum has tracked upwards.

Surfactant This is a substance secreted by Type II pneumocytes within the alveolus that forms a thin fluid layer on the alveolar surface. It reduces surface tension thus maintaining alveolar wall stability and preventing collapse.

Sustentaculum tali The talus sits on top of the calcaneus but not completely, so the calcaneus needs a scaffold to sustain or hold the talus up. This is called the sustentaculum tali.

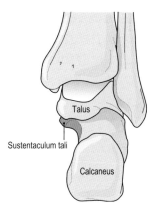

Sustentaculum tali

SVT Common medical abbreviation – Supra ventricular tachycardia.

Sway-back posture The posture typified by cervical spine extension, increased upper trunk flexion, lumbar flexion, posterior pelvic tilt, hyperextended hips and knees.

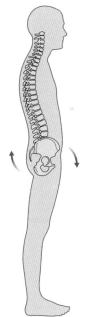

Sway back posture

Swan-neck deformity A common finger deformity seen in rheumatoid arthritis.

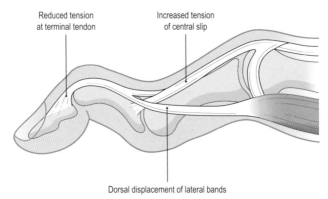

Reduced tension
at terminal tendon

Increased tension
of central slip

Dorsal displacement of lateral bands

Swan neck deformity

Sweat chloride test The sweat chloride test is a common and simple test used to evaluate a patient who is suspected of having cystic fibrosis (CF).

Sympathetic nervous system See *Autonomic nervous system*

Symphysis pubis See *Pubic symphysis*

Symptom Any perceptible, subjective change in the body or its functions that indicates disease or phases of disease, as reported by the patient, e.g. my knee aches all the time – this is a symptom. There is a positive patellar tap – this is a sign.

Syndesmophyte See *Bamboo spine*
   The bony outgrowth seen in ankylosing spondylitis, different in appearance and direction to osteophytes.

Syndrome A group of symptoms and diseases that is characteristic of a specific condition.

Synergist A muscle teams up with another muscle in the production of a movement that neither could perform alone.

Synovial fluid This is produced by the synovial membrane and is present in small amounts in all synovial joints.
   An increase in volume of synovial fluid often occurs after trauma, presence of infection, loose bodies or as a response to other pathology. Too much synovial fluid in a joint is known as an effusion. Synovial fluid is a clear or straw-coloured fluid, which is thixotropic. This unusual quality means that the more quickly a joint moves, the less viscous its synovial fluid becomes. Synovial fluid contains nutrients and the glycoprotein hyaluronate. It bathes and nourishes the joint, it also plays an important role in absorbing joint stresses. When moving from sitting to standing, stresses on the hip joint have been calculated to be in excess of 2610 pounds per square inch.

Studies show that 90% of this load may be borne by hydrostatic pressure within the synovial fluid between the articulating surfaces. This protects the cartilage matrix from otherwise catastrophic pressures (Makirowski et al. 1994).

Synovial sweep The term for the phenomenon whereby articular hyaline cartilage gains its source of nutrition (synovial fluid) by the process of joint movement and compression which facilitated the spread of synovial fluid across the surface of a joint, clinical point, for this reason many intra-articular fractures are now managed by early movement or CPM.

Synovitis Inflammation of the synovial membrane.

Syringomyelia A disease of the spinal cord in which cavities form in the grey matter. It is characterized by loss of pain and temperature sensation.

Systematic review A research process that summarizes the evidence on a clearly formulated question according to a pre-defined protocol and using a thorough approach. The report should make explicit the methods used to identify, select and appraise relevant studies and to extract, collate and report their findings. It may or may not use meta analysis.

T

TA Common medical abbreviation – Tendo Achilles.

Tachycardia A rapid heart rate (in excess of 100 beats per minute).

Tachypnoea An increased respiratory rate.

TACI Common medical abbreviation – Total arterial cerebral infarction.
This is a stroke caused by an infarct involving the total anterior circulation.

Tailor's muscle The old name for the sartorius muscle (tailors used to sit cross legged hence sartorial: the combined actions of sartorius hip flexion, abduction and lateral rotation).

Talar tilt test A musculoskeletal test this assesses integrity of the calcaneofibular ligament. The subject is supine or in side lying with a relaxed foot. The talus is tilted into abduction and adduction.
Excessive tilting means excessive laxity or rupture of this ligament.

Talipes equinovarus – also known as clubfoot A common congenital abnormality of the foot. Clubfoot may occur in several forms, but talipes equinovarus is the most common. In this case the foot turns downward and inward.

Tamponade See *Cardiac tamponade*

TAR Common medical abbreviation – Total ankle replacement.

TATT Common medical abbreviation – Tired all the time.

TB Common medical abbreviation – Tuberculosis.
An infectious pulmonary disease caused by tubercle bacilli (previously known as consumption). Fear and stigma are still high concerning the diagnosis of pulmonary TB, but reassurance should be given as to the curable nature of the illness with appropriate anti-tuberculous therapy. Open TB is the only form of TB considered to be an infection risk for staff and other patients (DoH 1998).

TBI Common medical abbreviation – Traumatic brain (head) injury.
See *Traumatic brain (head) injury*

T-cell A class of lymphocytes, derived from the thymus. Involved primarily in controlling cell-mediated immune reactions and in the control of B-cell development. They coordinate the immune system by secreting lymphokine hormones.

TDS Common medical abbreviation – Three times a day.

Teamwork Teamwork refers to working in collaboration with others. Most healthcare professionals work in teams and there is a widespread belief that they achieve more when working collaboratively than when working alone. Teams work by pooling skills, knowledge and resources. Each individual has his or her specific role but the team has common interests and objectives. Each member shares responsibility for the decisions made within the team, its overall functioning and the quality of its output. Teamwork allows for a broader base of skills, attitudes and values to be brought into practice and the decision-making process. Patients and clients should be central to any team involved in their care.

See *Inter-disciplinary team, Intra-disciplinary team* and *Multidisciplinary team*

Technetium bone scan A sensitive radiological investigation, utilizing a radio-isotope, used in the detection of stress fractures, as well as other bony pathology.

Telangiectasia A permanent dilation of blood vessels that creates small red lesions, in the skin or mucous membranes.

Temperomandibular joint (TMJ) Joint between the condyle of the mandible and the mandibular fossa and the temporal bone. There are separate joints on each side of the face, but these function together as one unit. It is lined by fibrous cartilage and not hyaline cartilage. It contains an intra-articular meniscus that divides the joint into two separate synovial cavities.

Tendonitis Inflammatory condition of the tendon. Pain is reproduced with resisted movements and tendon stretching, with active range of motion often normal, but with pain experienced at the end of range.

Tennis elbow See *Lateral epicondylitis*

Tenosynovitis Inflammation of a tendon sheath. May follow trauma, overuse or inflammatory conditions. There is a complaint of pain, swelling and/or restricted movements. The swelling has a characteristically linear appearance, along the tendons.

Tenotomy The division of a tendon or the act of dividing a tendon.

Tenovaginitis Thickening of the fibrous tendon sheath.

Tension A measure of force developed within a muscle during contraction when it is not allowed to shorten, i.e. isometric contraction.

Tests Electrotherapy context – three specific tests are used on the relevant cutaneous area prior to applying a specific electrophysical agent:

1. Thermal discrimination if risk of thermal burns – test patient's ability to accurately distinguish heated from cooled objects applied cutaneously in treatment area.

2. Sharp/blunt discrimination if risk of skin irritation, pain or electrolytic skin burns – test patient's ability to accurately differentiate sharp and blunt objects applied cutaneously in treatment area.

3. Ice reaction test if risk of adverse skin reaction to ice – test response of skin to local application of ice for 30 s or check under an icepack after 5 min.

Testing machine output

Prior to using many electrotherapeutic machines the therapist should test the output to ensure the machine is working and to obviate any risks to the patient. For example:

- Ultrasound output: applicator in small metal bowl with face covered by water, rapidly increase and decrease output, bulk streaming visible as beam reflects from side of bowl (using other methods can damage applicator crystal).
- Electrical stimulation: turn on and set output parameters, connect leads and place damp fingers on electrodes or end of leads, gradually increase output until you feel it. Turn back to zero and connect to patient if operating satisfactorily.
- Laser: needs specialized equipment (photodiode).
- PSWD: needs specialized equipment.

Other specific tests
- Erythema: the grade of reddening caused in response to a dose of ultraviolet rays (UVR).
    See *Erythema* and *UVR*
- S-D test: a test of the normality of the response of a nerve to electrical stimulation.
    See *Strength–duration testing, Rheobase* and *Chronaxie*

Tetanus Sustained contraction of skeletal muscle in response to high-frequency stimulation.

Tetralogy of Fallot A heart condition.
    See *Fallots tetralogy*

Tetraplegia This term relates to loss or impairment of motor and/or sensory function from damage to the cord in the cervical spine area. This may also be described as quadraparesis.

TFCC Common medical abbreviation – Triangular fibrocartilaginous complex (at the wrist).

TFT Common medical abbreviation – Thyroid function tests.

Thalamic pain This is pain that arises in the central nervous system (CNS) caused by injury to the thalamic region. The pain can feel like intense burning pain, which is often made worse by touch and is on the side contralateral (opposite) to the lesion.

Thalassaemia A genetic form of anaemia in which there is abnormality of the globin portion of haemoglobin. Affected individuals cannot synthesize haemoglobin properly.

Thematic analysis Research term – in qualitative research, the researcher attempts to categorize and analyze the themes that are produced from interviews.

Theoretical saturation (Data saturation) Research term – used in qualitative research, the point where no new themes or concepts emerge from the data being collected.

Theory of reasoned action This theory is underpinned by the belief that human beings usually behave in a rational way. Behavioural intentions, for example, to give up smoking, are influenced by the person's belief that a desired outcome will occur and that the outcome will be beneficial. Beliefs about what other people think the individual ought to do, the individual's motivation to comply with the wishes of others and how much control the individual believes he or she has are also important.

Therapeutic environment A therapeutic environment is one that is arranged and designed to allow patients to achieve their best performance. Environment has been shown to be a very important factor in rehabilitation, both physically and mentally.

Therapeutic play Professional-led play with specific goals to achieve.
See *Normative play*

Thermoplastics Materials that can be made soft by the application of heat and which harden when they become cool. Many braces and splints are now made from this material.
See *Functional brace/cast brace*

Third heart sound Occurs in early diastole and corresponds with the end of the first phase of rapid ventricular filling.

Thixotropy This term, which originates in engineering, relates to the inherent stiffness or viscosity in a muscle. It has been likened to the property of paint before and after stirring. Synovial fluid is also thoxotropic.

Thomas test Determines the presence of a fixed flexion deformity at the hip. The patient is supine, the hip is fully passively flexed and the lumbar lordosis is obliterated.

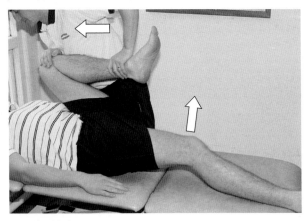

Thomas test (positive)

Abnormal finding If the opposite hip rises off the bed, this indicates a fixed flexion deformity of that hip. This may be due to tightness or restriction in the capsule, iliopsoas or rectus femoris. To differentiate between the iliopsoas and rectus femoris as the source of restriction, the patient's knee is passively extended. If this results in the patient's hip dropping down into less flexion, then the restriction is in the rectus femoris muscle, since, by extending the knee, an element of stretch has been removed. If the hip is unaffected and remains in the same degree of flexion, independently of the knee extension, then the restriction is in the iliopsoas muscle.

Thompsons test – also known as squeeze test This tests the integrity of the gastrocnemius/soleus Achilles tendon complex. The patient lies prone. The physiotherapist squeezes the calf firmly just distal to its maximum circumference. If the tendon is intact, the foot will plantarflex. A positive test will occur if the tendon or muscle is ruptured and the ankle will not plantarflex.

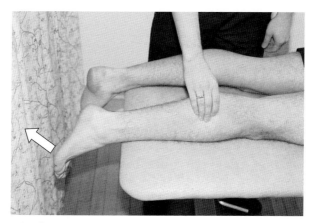

A negative Thompson test

Abnormal finding A palpable gap in the tendon or muscle belly may sometimes be observed if the tendon is ruptured.

Thoracic Pertaining to the chest.

Thoracic outlet syndrome Compression of the neurovascular bundle, comprising the brachial plexus and the subclavian artery, it produces a mix of symptoms, ranging from shoulder and arm pain, to neurological or vascular symptoms. The compression usually occurs in the thoracic outlet of the neck.

Thoracic spine Comprising 12 vertebrae, sitting between the cervical and lumbar spines. Provide attachments for the ribs.

Thoracolumbar fascia The fascia that covers the deep muscles of the back.

Thoracotomy Surgery to resect part or all of a lung. It involves rib resection and transection of major chest wall muscles.

THR Common medical abbreviation – Total hip replacement.

Thrombin time Test of the conversion of fibrinogen to fibrin by thrombin in which clotting time of plasma mixed with a thrombin solution is measured.

Thrombocytopenia A decrease in the number of blood platelets, it results in the potential for increased bleeding and decreased clotting ability.

Thromboembolism The obstruction of a blood vessel by material carried in the blood stream from the site of origin to plug another vessel.

Thymus gland A bilaterally symmetric lymphoid organ situated in the anterior superior mediastinum. It is the site of the production of T-lymphocytes. The thymus reaches its maximal development at about puberty.

TIA Common medical abbreviation – Transient ischaemic attack.
These are episodes of focal neurological symptoms that last less than 24 h and caused by insufficient blood supply to the brain. They can be an impending warning of a stroke and should be treated as an urgent medical condition.

Tibia The shin bone, articulates with the femur superiorly and the talus inferiorly, also joins the fibula at the superior and inferior tibiofibular joints.

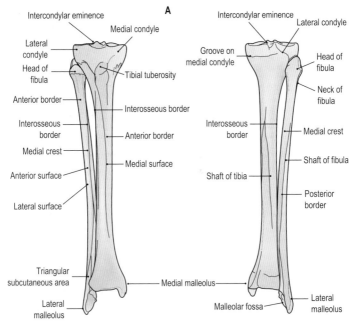

(**A**) Right tibia and fibula, anterior view and posterior view

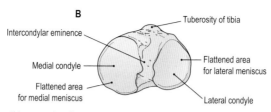

B

Tuberosity of tibia

Intercondylar eminence

Medial condyle

Flattened area for lateral meniscus

Flattened area for medial meniscus

Lateral condyle

(**B**) Right tibia, superior view

Tibial nerve See *Sciatic nerve*

TIC Involuntary movements that may be found in cases of obsessive compulsive disorder or other diseases.

Tilt table This is a mechanical standing device that enables patients who are unable to stand to be stood. Patients, even ventilated unconscious patients, can be stood using one of these as it is externally controlled through a range from horizontal to almost vertical and can be stopped at any angle in between.

Tinel's sign A test for damage or inflammation of the ulnar nerve, the examiner taps the nerve in the ulnar groove, a positive test occurs when there is tingling.

Tinnitus This is a condition that causes a sensation of noise in the ear. Patients describe the noise such as high or low pitched, buzzing, ringing or hissing. If it is accompanied by deafness it is called Meniere's disease.

TKR Common medical abbreviation – Total knee replacement.

T Lymphocyte Thymus-formed lymphocytes.

TMS Common medical abbreviation – Transcranial magnetic stimulation. This is a neuropsychological test whereby magnets are placed on the skull and stimulation can be applied to the brain to cause muscle movement dependent on the site of the stimulus. TMS can be more easily used in a clinical setting to provide a measurement tool of cerebral activity.

Tonsil One of the two glandular organs situated in the throat.

Torticollis, spasmodic – also known as wry neck or Cervical dystonia In torticollis, the muscles in the neck are affected, causing the head to twist and turn to one side. In addition, the head may be pulled forward or backward.

Total burn surface area (TBSA) A formula for gauging outcome in people who have sustained burns:

$$100 - (age + TBSA) = percentage\ chance\ of\ survival$$

For example:

$$100 - (60\ years + 30\%\ TBSA) = 10\ (10\%\ chance\ of\ survival)$$
$$100 - (20\ years + 30\%\ TBSA) = 50\ (50\%\ chance\ of\ survival)$$

It is interesting to note that if both legs are burnt, 36% TBSA is affected. Therefore, a 50-year-old patient with such extensive burns has $100 - (50 + 36) = 14\%$ chance of recovery.

The greater the TBSA, the poorer the prognosis.

A method for gauging the TBSA is 'the rule of nines'. This rule divides the body surface into 11 separate areas, each constituting 9%. The perineum is counted as 1%. An experienced doctor should carry out the assessment of the TBSA, as the correct percentage area will determine the correct volume of fluid replacement required for the resuscitation process.

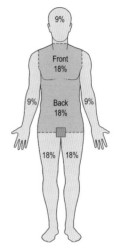

Illustrating the 'rule of nines'

Tourniquet An apparatus designed for the compression of the vessels of the limb. A loosely applied tourniquet will restrict venous blood flow out of the extremity. A tightly applied tourniquet will impede arterial blood flow into the extremity.

Trachea The major airway marking the commencement of the upper respiratory tract. The trachea is constructed of C-shaped rings of cartilage (to maintain airway patency), smooth muscle (to accommodate necessary changes in airway diameter) and ciliated columnar epithelium (to facilitate the mucociliary escalator).

Tracheostomy A surgically created opening in the neck that allows direct access to the trachea (the breathing tube). It is maintained open with a hollow tube called a tracheostomy tube.

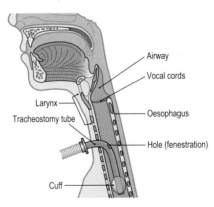

Tracheostomy

Tracheitis Inflammation of the trachea.

Traction Therapy to provide a distraction force, whether it is to the spine, or to the peripheral joints.

Tragus The prominence that is situated at the front of the external opening of the ear.

Physiotherapists sometimes use this as an objective marker when measuring spinal movements against a wall for example.

Transcutaneous Externally applied energy passes through the skin to the underlying tissues (e.g. electrical stimulation using surface electrodes passes through [trans] the skin to affect underlying tissues). Transcutaneous electrical nerve stimulation (TENS) is often used to mean electrical stimulation for pain control, but really describes any use of current that is passed through the skin.

Transcutaneous electrical nerve stimulation (TENS) TENS involves the delivery of short duration (50–250 µs) electrical pulses which target sensory nerves and can thereby achieve effective symptomatic pain relief. It is a widely used modality and one that is well supported by the evidence. TENS devices are usually small, battery-powered and well suited to patient self-management. Some of the larger, clinic-based electrical stimulators offer a TENS option that will achieve the same effects. TENS is a generally well tolerated form of electrical stimulation. With traditional or high TENS (@ 80–150 Hz) the target nerves are the sensory (Aß) fibres. Once stimulated, they will serve to close the pain gate and thus reduce the awareness of pain. Stimulation at lower frequencies (2–5 Hz) using acupuncture like AL-TENS aims to stimulate the Aδ sensory fibres and stimulate opioid production at spinal cord level by means of descending extra-segmental modulation.

Burst-mode TENS employs an interrupted output with machines commonly pre-set to burst at 2–3 times a s. Modulated output is also a standard feature and can be achieved by varying the amplitude, frequency or duration of the stimulating pulses.

Electrodes are commonly placed either side of the painful site, providing segmental stimulation. Alternative (and evidenced) electrode placements include stimulation of spinal nerve roots, peripheral nerves, motor points, dermatome, myotome or sclerotome, acupuncture and trigger points.

Transferable skills Academic or practical skills that can be used in another (different) situation (e.g. problem solving).

Transfer of care The term to describe the process of transferring the responsibility of care from one service to another.

Transfers This is a term to describe the assisted or independent movement of a patient from one position to another, i.e. from bed to wheelchair.

Transfusion The transfer of blood or blood products from one person (donor) into another person's bloodstream (recipient).

Transitional epithelium A highly distensible epithelium with large cuboidal cells in the relaxed state, but broad and squamous in the distended state occurs in the kidney, ureter and bladder.

Transpulmonary pressure The difference between the alveolar and pleural pressures.

Transverse frictions See *Deep transverse frictions (DTF)*

Transverse myelitus This is a rare condition that is associated with infections such as measles, mumps, herpes zoster/simplex. Paralysis with sensory loss and incontinence may be preceded by fever, back and/or limb pain.

Transverse plane The plane that divides the body into superior and inferior portions.

Traumatic head injury This is caused by an insult to the brain from an external force, which may lead to altered consciousness and loss of movement, speech and altered cognition amongst other impairments. Head injury is the commonest cause of accidental death.

Tread-mill training This is a form of therapy intervention that focuses on gait re-training following a neurological insult. It usually involves a specialist treadmill with a body de-weighting support system.

Treatment allocation Assigning a participant to a particular arm of the trial.

Trendelenburg gait Intrinsic disorder of the abductors of the hip due to either a weakness or an inhibition to function. As a result, the hip abductors are unable to stabilize the hip, as body weight is transferred to the affected side, resulting in a pelvic drop or tilt towards the opposite side.

Trendelenburg test/sign Tests the ability of the hip abductor mechanism to stabilize the hip, while the patient stands on one leg. The Trendelenburg test is positive when the patient stands on one leg and the opposite side of the pelvis then drops.

This is quite a difficult concept to grasp, the following figures help you to understand the concept.

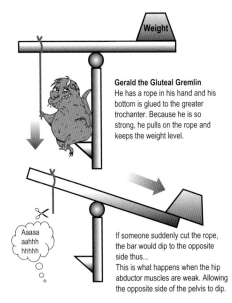

Weight

Gerald the Gluteal Gremlin
He has a rope in his hand and his bottom is glued to the greater trochanter. Because he is so strong, he pulls on the rope and keeps the weight level.

Aaaaa aahhh hhhhh

If someone suddenly cut the rope, the bar would dip to the opposite side thus...
This is what happens when the hip abductor muscles are weak. Allowing the opposite side of the pelvis to dip.

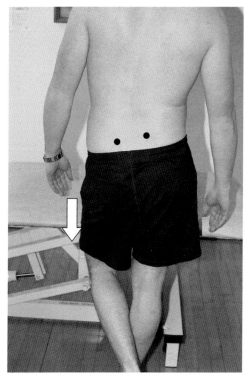

Positive Trendelenberg sign, note the different levels of the PSIS (indicated by black dots)

Triage The name for a system of sorting patients according to their illness or severity of injury so that patients can be steered to the most appropriate health worker.

Triangulation Research term – the process whereby the same data are obtained from various means as an attempt to improve its validity. Determining the consistency of evidence gathered from different sources of data and/or different research methods about a particular research question of interest. For example, one may wish to interview a group of students and then bring them together for a focus group as a means of data triangulation.

Trigeminal neuralgia A very painful disorder of the fifth cranial nerve. It causes episodes of intense electric-shock-like pain in the lips, eyes, nose, scalp and forehead.

Trigger finger Occurs when there is nodule formation within the flexor tendon of the hand. It usually occurs secondary to tenosynovitis (usually due to overuse) or to rheumatoid arthritis. Most commonly, the nodule is trapped under the metacarpophalangeal ligament, as the tendon flexes. Corticosteroid injection may relieve the symptoms, but sometimes surgery is indicated.

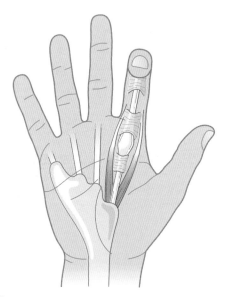

Trigger finger

Trigger point See *Myofascial trigger point*

Tri-malleolar fracture A fracture that involves both malleoli and the posterior part of the tibial articular surface.

Trochanteric bursitis Often associated with tendinitis of gluteus medius, it is characterized by an inflammation of the bursae overlying the greater trochanter of the femur. It is usually an overuse injury, seen in runners. Pain is often reproduced on stretch (hip flexion to 90° with full lateral rotation of hip) or contraction of the gluteus medius as in resisted hip abduction.

Trochlea Anatomical term for a pulley or a structure resembling a pulley, e.g. the trochlea or pulley-like end of the humerus that articulates with the ulna.

Troponin Muscle protein binding actin and tropomyosin; when calcium is present, it 'pulls' tropomyosin to uncover binding sites for myosin.

Tropomyosin The protein that winds along the actin 'thin filament' and covers the myosin-binding sites in the absence of calcium.

'T' Roll This is a 'T'-shaped piece of equipment that is used to help position patients by breaking up established patterns of tone and distributing weight more equally in patients with soft tissue shortening.

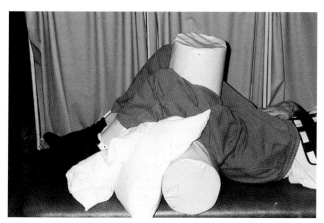

Supine lying with a T-roll

True leg length See *Leg length*

Truncal ataxia Uncoordinated movement of the trunk.

T4 syndrome Symptoms associated with a hypomobility lesion at T4 ($\pm$1–2 levels). The person complains of vague arm pain or discomfort, accompanied by paresthesia, which does not follow any dermatomal patterns. Hand symptoms are also considered to be an integral part of T4 syndrome. The pathology is unknown, but autonomic nerve control may be compromised.

TTO Common medical abbreviation – To take out (medication).

Tubercle The anatomical term for a circumscribed bony projection.

Tuberosity An anatomical term for roughened bony projections for the attachment of ligaments or muscles.

Tuberosity of fifth metatarsal A tubercle at the base of this bone to the posterior part to which the tendon of the peroneus brevis muscle attaches.

Tumour necrosis factor (TNF) A macrophage-produced cytokine that helps activate T-cells. Anti-TNF medications are currently revolutionizing management in rheumatology.

Turp Common medical abbreviation – Trans-urethral resection of prostate.

Two-tailed hypothesis Research term – it implies a difference but no direction to the change, e.g. physiotherapy students in group A will have a different score than physiotherapy students in group B.

Whereas a one-tailed hypothesis, implies a direction to a predicted change, e.g. physiotherapy students in group A will score higher physiotherapy students in group B.

See *One-tailed hypothesis*

Twitch   Rapid contraction of muscle in response to single stimulus.

Type I error (Alpha error)   Deciding to reject the null hypothesis when the null hypothesis is in fact true. The investigator determines that there is something going on when in fact there is not.

Type II error (Beta error)   Failing to reject the null hypothesis when the alternative hypothesis is in fact true. The investigator determines that there is nothing going on when in fact there is.

U

. . . .

U&E Common medical abbreviation – Urea and electrolytes.

Ulna See *Radius*

Ulnar nerve

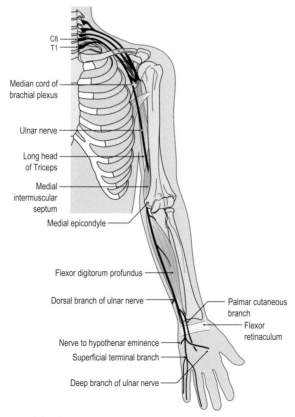

The course of the ulnar nerve

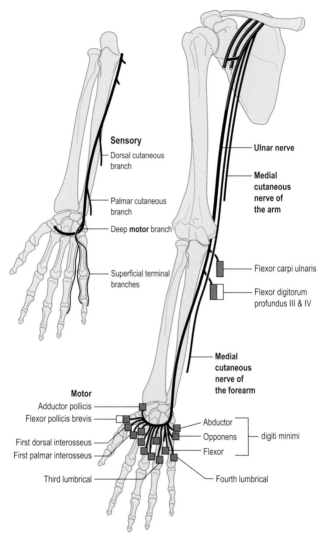

Sensory
- Dorsal cutaneous branch
- Palmar cutaneous branch
- Deep **motor** branch
- Superficial terminal branches

Ulnar nerve

Medial cutaneous nerve of the arm

Flexor carpi ulnaris

Flexor digitorum profundus III & IV

Medial cutaneous nerve of the forearm

Motor
- Adductor pollicis
- Flexor pollicis brevis
- First dorsal interosseus
- First palmar interosseus
- Third lumbrical

- Abductor ⎤
- Opponens ⎬ digiti minimi
- Flexor ⎦
- Fourth lumbrical

The muscles supplied by the ulnar nerve

Ultraviolet radiation (UVR) Electrotherapy term – an electromagnetic radiation. Three types (UVA, UVB and UVC) divided by wavelength because of differences in effects and hence clinical uses. UVA, wavelength 400–315 nm, also called long UV used with sensitizers (e.g. psoralen, PUVA method) to treat psoriasis, main component solar UVR. UVB, wavelength 315–280 nm, medium UV or erythemal UV main cause of skin damage from sun; UVC, wavelength 280–100 nm, also called short UV or abiotic UV, used to treat wounds. Main effect bactericidal, zero component solar UVR as absorbed in ozone layer.

Umbilical hernia Protrusion of soft tissues through the umbilicus.

Umbilicus The anatomical name for the navel or belly button.

Undergraduate The term used to describe work, levels or students prior to the award of an honours degree.

Underwater seal drainage A system of drainage that allows air or fluid to be removed from the thorax and transported to a drain. The underwater component ensures that only one way flow occurs.

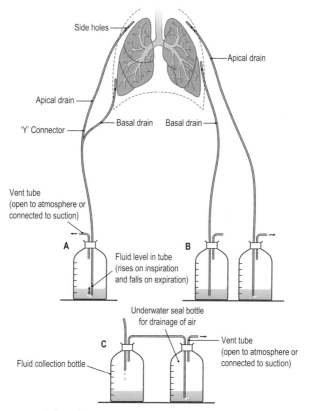

Underwater seal chest drainage

Unilateral neglect Unilateral neglect is a syndrome that can be seen in patients with brain injury and is characterized as a failure to respond, report to or orientate to meaningful stimuli presented to the side contralateral to the cerebral lesion (Heilman et al. 1993).

➕ Clinical note This may present as the patient ignoring their own arm, eating half their food on the plate and bumping into objects on their affected side.

Unipolar Electrotherapy term – an electrode arrangement in which one electrode (indifferent electrode) is larger than the other (stimulating or active electrode). The higher current density under the active electrode means stimulation of nearby nerve or muscle is more likely than if under the larger indifferent electrode with its lower current density. The outcome depends on the relative sizes of the electrodes. To stimulate quadriceps femoris: unipolar – use a small electrode over the femoral nerve, as it exits with the femoral artery under the inguinal ligament, place the larger indifferent electrode on the lateral aspect of the contralateral thigh or the abdomen or lower back.
    See *Bipolar*

Units of measurement Pulse duration (e.g. pulses of electrical current):

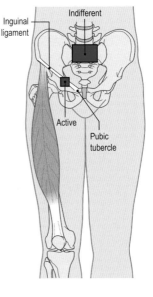

    1 s = 1000 ms

    1 ms = 1000 μs

    600 μs = 0.6 ms = 0.0006 s.

    Frequency (e.g. ultrasound):

    1 MHz = 1000 000 Hz (10^6 Hz)

    1 MHz = 1000 kHz

    0.78 MHz = 780 kHz = 780 000 Hz

    20 kHz = 20 200 Hz.

    Power output (e.g. laser, ultrasound):

    1 W = 1000 mW

    0.5 W = 500 mW.

    Wavelength (e.g. laser, infrared, SWD, MW):

    904 nm = 0.904 μm = 0.000904 mm.

Unmyelinated fibres This refers to nerve fibres that are not covered by myelin.
    Type C fibres are very small in diameter and carry sensory information about pain and temperature.

Unstable cavitation See *Cavitation*

Upper-limb tension test (ULTT) See *Neurodynamics*

Upper motor neurone syndrome This is a term used to describe a collection of positive and negative signs that are associated with cerebral lesions.

Positive features include spasticity, increased tendon reflexes, clonus and resistance to passive movement.

Negative features include muscle weakness, loss of dexterity and coordination, slowness of movement.

Urea A by product of protein metabolism.

Urge incontinence The complaint of involuntary leakage accompanied by, or immediately preceded by, urgency, i.e. a sudden compelling desire to pass urine (ICS 2002). This form of leakage occurs when the detrusor contracts inappropriately as the bladder fills.

Urinalysis An analysis of the urine.

Urinary retention In hypotonic ('floppy') bladders, the normal response to the increase in pressure, which occurs during filling, may be absent and the detrusor fails to contract. Retention is associated with outflow obstruction (e.g. in men with prostate disease), neuropathy, low spinal cord lesions, radical pelvic surgery and multiple sclerosis, or it may be secondary to drug (especially psychotropic) therapy. Incontinence sometimes, but not always, occurs with retention (Brook et al. 2003).

URTI Common medical abbreviation – Upper respiratory tract infection.

UTI Common medical abbreviation – Urinary-tract infection.

U/S or US Common medical abbreviation – Ultrasound.
See *Longwave ultrasound*

Ultrasound: general points
Sound waves with a frequency of >20 kHz are called 'ultrasound'. Used to promote healing (frequency 0.8–3 MHz), for diagnosis (frequency 1–10 MHz and applicator has receiver) and for tissue destruction (varies). Requires 'coupling' of applicator to skin with gel or water or similar as not transmitted in air at MHz frequency. Penetration inversely proportional to frequency (i.e. 3 Hz absorbed more rapidly in superficial tissue depth than 1 MHz frequency). Absorption rate higher in collagen-based tissues than, for example, fat. Properties of kHz frequency ultrasound very different from MHz. Used for teeth and jewellery cleaning and car alarms (i.e. travels in air). Beam divergence very wide and most energy penetrates through bodies with little effective absorption.

Ultrasound: mechanism of effect
Ultrasound energy heats tissue (thermal effects) and has mechanical pressure effects (non-thermal) at the same time to different degrees depending on intensity and frequency and underlying tissue properties. Mechanical pressure effects: acoustic streaming, either bulk streaming (i.e. movement of fluid in a direction in response to the ultrasound) or microstreaming (i.e. fluid eddies adjacent to a source of ultrasound). Contribution of streaming to treatment outcomes not clear. Cavitation, the formation of bubbles from gas previously in solution, does not occur in human body at usual frequency or intensity range of therapeutic ultrasound, though is a risk near gas-filled cavities such as lungs and gut.

Ultrasound: output

Output can be continuous (CUS) or pulsed (PUS). Operator sets intensity. The average intensity in the beam at a defined point is called the 'spatial average' (SA). For spatial peak (SP), see below. The peak intensity set is the 'temporal peak' (TP). If pulsed, the intensity is described as the 'temporal average' (TA) – the equivalent intensity if it were continuous and not pulsed (i.e. $TA = TP \times$ pulsing rate; if $2\,W.cm^2$ output [TP] pulsed at 20% duty cycle the TA is $0.4\,W/cm^2$).

Ultrasound: beam

Is complex, changing with distance from applicator according to frequency of ultrasound and diameter of applicator. For 1 MHz frequency, near zone (Fresnel) extends 10–15 cm from applicator, very uneven energy distribution, beam remains collimated ($\sim$4 divergence). Far zone (Fraunhofer) beam less intense and has more even energy distribution. Variations in energy distribution reported as beam non-uniformity ratio (BNR):

$$= \text{spatial peak intensity (SP)/spatial average intensity (SA)}$$

Usual BNR for therapeutic equipment is 5–6, for fracture healing is 2.16. Implication: energy distribution in higher BNR beam very irregular and applicator must be moved (even if pulsed output) during treatment to avoid effects of localized high-intensity beam energy.

Ultrasound: applicator

Energy applied with applicator for therapeutic US. Applicator is site of production of ultrasound – contains crystal, stimulated by high-frequency alternating current (reverse piezoelectric effect). Applicator sizes usually 1, 2, 5 or $10\,cm^2$ depending on area being treated. Actual radiating area usually less than applicator face size – effective radiating area (ERA). Couple energy produced in applicator to skin with gel or water or other transmissive substance as US not transmitted through air at MHz frequencies.

Ultrasound: clinical effectiveness

Effectiveness of MHz frequency ultrasound for acute soft-tissue injuries is still debated. One reason is that it is very difficult to identify a reduction in healing time over 5–7 days healing time. Another reason is unreliable equipment output – intensity is often not accurate. There is clear evidence of the effectiveness of MHz frequency ultrasound in fracture healing of delayed and non-uniting fractures. In chronic conditions, each application is for longer and there are more of them.

Ultrasound: dosage

These include frequency, size of applicator and ERA, intensity (SATA and SATP), location and size of area treated, duration of treatment, which machine, etc.

User involvement An approach to health and social care where the users of services are involved in the planning and evaluation of services. Government policy, such as the NHS and Community Care Act (1990), has encouraged and made mandatory some degree of user involvement.

Utilitarianism An ethical approach that advocates actions that provide the greatest good for the greatest number.

Utility measure A means of determining the strength of an individual's preference for a specific health state in relation to alternative health states. A utility measure assigns numerical values on a scale from 0 (death) to 1 (optimal or 'perfect' health). As health states can be considered worse than death, negative values can be recorded.

Uvulopalatopharyngoplasty (UVPPP) A surgical method of treatment for obstructive sleep apnoea in carefully selected patients (OSA SIGN Guidelines 2003).

V

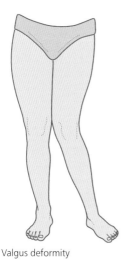

Valgus deformity

Valgus deformity Refers to a lateral inclination of a distal bone, of a joint, from the midline.

Valgus stress test (medial collateral ligament of the knee) The patient lies supine. The therapist applies a valgus strain to the knee joint.

Abnormal finding Excessive opening up on the medial side of the joint or pain.

The test is normally performed with the knee in 20–30° of flexion. If the test is done with the knee held in full extension, a positive sign would suggest major ligamentous injury involving the medial collateral, posterior cruciate and potentially the anterior cruciate injury.

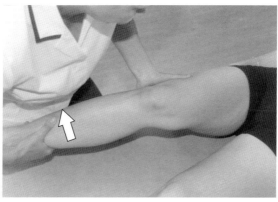

Valgus stress test

Validation The process of assessing an academic course and determining whether it meets the criteria for recognition. Often this is done by the professional body, licensing agency and university at the same time.

Revalidation

After a period of time, usually 5 years, a course is reviewed for continuing approval.

Validity Research term – the 'truth' of the research. In simple terms, does a test record accurately what it is supposed to record? A clinical example would be that asking a person to perform a straight leg raise is not a particularly reliable test of quadriceps function, since it is isometric only and mainly works the hip flexors instead. There are many types of validity:

Internal validity

The extent to which results of the study are valid for the patient population studied.

External validity

This refers to whether or not the results are valid outside the population that has been studied. For example, are results from studies done on dogs also valid for cats?

Face validity

Is the subjective assessment of the measurement tool to ensure that it is relevant and clear, e.g. when designing a questionnaire, clarity is vital.

Content validity

Similar to the above, but this time examines the concepts and thinking behind a tool to ensure it has the potential to obtain the right information.

Criterion validity

Assessed on the ability of a test to correlate with other tools.

Predictive validity

The ability to predict outcomes.

Vancouver referencing A referencing system used in academic publications which uses numbers inserted into the text. The reference cited in the text is numbered 1 and it is listed as 1 in the reference list at the end. This system of referencing is used in some medical journals.

Van't Hoff's law Any chemical reaction capable of being accelerated is accelerated by a rise in temperature.

○ Clinical point The body initiates a fever to accelerate the physiological processes involved. This concept is also of key importance to physiotherapists, particularly when dealing with electrotherapy modalities.

Variable Research term – anything which is able to vary.
See *Independent*, *Dependent* and *Extraneous variables*

Varicose vein An abnormal swelling and tortuosity common in the superficial veins of the lower limb.

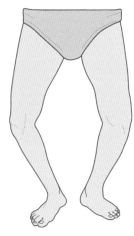

Varus deformity

Varus deformity Refers to medial inclination of a distal bone, of a joint, from the midline.

Varus stress test (lateral collateral ligament of the knee) The patient lies supine. The physiotherapist applies a varus force (i.e. the femur is pushed laterally and the leg pulled medially) to the knee joint. A positive sign is observed as excessive opening up or pain on the lateral side of the joint. The test is normally performed with the knee in 20–30° of flexion.

Abnormal finding With the knee held in extension a positive sign suggests major ligamentous injury involving the lateral collateral, posterior cruciate and potentially the anterior cruciate injury. The test is performed again with the knee in 20–30° of flexion.

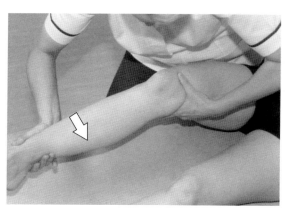

Varus stress test

Vasculitis Inflammation of a vessel.

Vasoconstriction Contraction of the smooth muscle encircling a blood vessel that results in a decrease in its diameter.

Vasodilation The opposite of vasoconstriction.

Vastus intermedius This forms part of the quadriceps muscle group. The fibres lie in a plane parallel with the anterior aspect of the shaft of the femur.

Vastus lateralis Forms the middle layer of the quadriceps group.

Vastus medialis – also known as vastus medialis obliquus (VMO) Part of the quadriceps femoris group. Located on the anteromedial aspect of the thigh. Recently investigated for its role in patellar stability, with particular reference to patellofemoral pain.

Vector A vector may be described as resultant force acting at a particular angle. They can be described in terms of vertical and horizontal directions.

Vegetative state See *PVS*

The vegetative state may result from severe brain injury or disease that irrevocably damages the central nervous system. The patient (person) is rendered dependent on others for all activities of daily living.

There are three prime features of the vegetative state:

1. The patient has sleep – wake cycles.
2. All responses can be identified as reflex patterns.
3. The patient makes no meaningful responses and has no awareness (Andrews 1999).

At the recommendation of the International Working Party (1996), the terms 'persistent' or 'permanent' should no longer be used as they confuse prognosis with diagnosis.

Ventilation The cyclical activity of breathing. Ventilation consists of inspiration (involving effort), expiration (usually a passive phase using the energy stored from inspiration) and rest (a time of no airflow) prior to the next inspiration. Ventilation occurs as a result of the pressure gradients generated by thoracic expansion and contraction. In healthy lungs, the distribution of ventilation is uneven, due to regional and local factors. In the upright position, ventilation is directed more to the bases and periphery of the lungs than to the apices and central zones. For ventilation to be efficient, it must exceed the body's requirements for oxygen uptake and carbon-dioxide removal.

Minute ventilation is calculated by multiplying the tidal volume (i.e. the amount of air expired with each breath) by the respiratory rate (number of breaths per minute).

Ventilation–perfusion (V/Q) ratio This is the ratio of alveolar ventilation to blood flow (perfusion). In the normal individual the ratio is approximately 80%, since V/Q varies throughout the lung. This is a major determining factor affecting the partial pressures of O_2 and CO_2 in the arterial blood.

In the normal upright lung, due to the effects of gravity, ventilation and perfusion gradients increase from apex to base. Ventilation increases toward the bases of the lungs since more volume is exchanged with each breath than that at the apex of lung (where a higher resting inflation volume exists); while the effect of gravity on the weight of the column of blood in the vessels increases perfusion at the bases. This of course alters with changes in body position; so positioning can be used to help improve V/Q mismatch, e.g. postural drainage to remove excessive secretions or positioning to facilitate the re-inflation of atelectatic segments/lobes.

Ventilators These are mechanical devices used to facilitate or perform breathing. These consist of invasive (requiring tracheal intubation) and non-invasive (being applied via a mask) systems. There are now numerous applications of ventilation with many combinations of control, phase and variables. These can broadly be explained in three categories:

1. CMV or controlled mandatory ventilation (infrequently used today), in which a precise minute ventilation can be delivered thus providing full ventilatory support.

2. IMV or intermittent mandatory ventilation, which combines both patient and machine triggered breaths.

3. Spontaneous breath modes, which are all patient initiated. Such modes include continuous positive airway pressure (CPAP), BiPAP and pressure supported ventilation (PSV).

Venous blood gas levels See *Blood gas*

Venous return The processes by which blood returns to the heart, it is achieved by means of:

• the respiratory pump
• the venous valves via the muscle pump
• venomotor tone.

➕ Clinical point Physiotherapists frequently encounter people who have a deficient muscle pump, for example, following lower limb surgery.

Verbal feedback Verbal or auditory feedback can be used by physiotherapists in reinforcing treatment goals in relation to performance. It is important to encourage appropriate effort, as accurate feedback is essential to the learning process. There should not be a mismatch between the action of the patient and the feedback of the therapist. However, negativity can also be non-motivational and so care should be taken to achieve a balance when treating patients.

Vertebral artery testing Vertebral arteries can be occluded by pathologies, such as atherosclerosis, arthritis and deformities of the spine. The vertebral arteries can also be occluded by certain movements of the cervical spine including rotation and extension. Subjective symptoms arising from vertebral artery insufficiency are known as the five 'Ds':

1. Diplopia
2. Dizziness
2. Dysphagia
4. Disarthria
5. Drop attacks.

Before performing any mobilization/manipulation or traction of the cervical spine, it is essential to ask the patient specifically for any of the above symptoms. If the patient has positive signs on subjective examination, it is necessary to conduct vertebral artery tests to support or negate vertebral artery insufficiency. Equally, if a patient is undergoing a technique that will compromise the vertebral artery, such as grade III/IV rotation of the cervical spine, vertebral artery insufficiency needs to be cleared objectively.

The following table shows vertebral artery tests for those who complain subjectively of symptoms and those who need vertebral artery clearance prior to treatment.

Vertebral artery test (Grant 1994)

Patient does not complain of symptoms related to VBI and manipulation is the choice of treatment	Patient complains of symptoms related to VBI
In sitting or lying:	**In sitting:**
Sustained extension	Sustained extension
Sustained L rotation	Sustained L rotation
Sustained R rotation	Sustained R rotation
Sustained L rotation/extension	Sustained L rotation/extension
Sustained R rotation/extension	Rapid movements
Pre-manipulation position	Sustained movements (more than 10 s)
	Any other movement

Vertebro basilar insufficiency (VBI) See *Vertebral artery testing*

Vertigo Vertigo can be caused from an infection or disease of the ear, or following damage to the vestibular nerve or its central connections. Vertigo gives the patient an illusion of rotatory movement due to disturbed orientation of the body in space, leaving the affected person with feeling that the environment around them is moving. It is often accompanied by nausea or vomiting, causes can include neurological damage, ear problems, sinusitis or medication.

Vestibular ataxia This may occur with peripheral vestibular disorders or central disorders that affect the vestibular nuclei and/or their afferent/efferent connections via the VIII cranial nerve. Peripheral lesions may be either bilateral or, more commonly, unilateral.
See *Acoustic neuroma*

⊕ Clinical point Patients with vestibular ataxia may demonstrate poor balance reactions, have a wide-based gait, with unilateral lesions leaning towards the side of the lesion and people with bilateral lesions have a tendency to lean backwards. Patients also tend to rely heavily on visual information and so may have increased problems with movement in reduced lighting or the dark.

Vestibular rehabilitation This is a type of rehabilitation for people suffering from vertigo (see *Vertigo*). Physiotherapists can help with vestibular rehabilitation by assessing the problems and prescribing specific exercises such as Cawthorne Cooksey and activities to increase independence.

⊕ Clinical point You must make a distinction when assessing these patients between positional triggers (see *BPPV*) and movement triggers. Peripheral problems respond better to these habituation exercises, central vertigo often only has limited success.

VF Common medical abbreviation – Ventricular fibrillation.

Vibration Vibration is sometimes used as a stimulation technique and can be applied to muscle or tendon. High-frequency vibration (100–300 Hz) will elicit a reflex called the tonic vibratory response. It can be used to facilitate activity in a hypotonic muscle or inhibit hypertonicity in a muscle belly.

Vice chancellor The chief executive and senior person in a university.

Victim blaming A tendency to blame the person who is experiencing ill-health or other difficulties. A heavy smoker, for example, may be blamed for contracting lung cancer. Victim-blaming denies the influence of wide social, economic and political factors on people's behaviour, over which they may have little control.

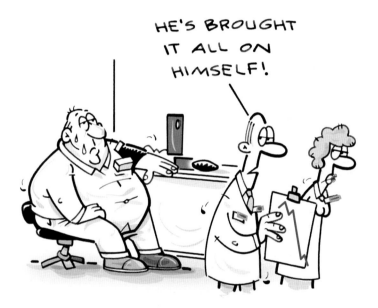

Virtue ethics An ethical approach that emphasizes the characteristics of people who make ethical decisions. It is deemed important for people to possess the personality traits of courage, wisdom, sensitivity, compassion and empathy in order to be capable of making sound ethical judgements. This approach may lead to the erroneous assumption that ethical decision making is simply about being the 'right' sort of person rather than having the ability to analyze ethical dilemmas skilfully and thoroughly.

Visio–spatial neglect See *Unilateral neglect*

Visual analogue scale (VAS) The visual analogue scale involves asking a person to make a mark on a line. The mark can then be measured and recorded for future comparisons using a ruler. Although these measures are not wholly objective, they do allow changes to be monitored as the treatment progresses.

Please mark on this line with a cross how you would rate your pain

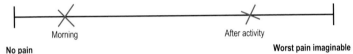

No pain   **Worst pain imaginable**

Example of visual analogue used in physiotherapy practice

Visual-evoked potentials (VEP) VEP is an electrical test that uses a stroboscopic flash to stimulate the retina of the eye or alternatively checkerboard pattern, can be used to stimulate the macula of the eye. The evoked visual signal is recorded over the occipital cortex. This test provides information about the conduction properties of the visual pathways.

✚ Clinical point The optic nerve is commonly one of the first signs in the development of multiple sclerosis and VEPs can be used to aid the diagnosis of this demyelinating disease.

Visual motor coordination This is the ability to co-ordinate vision with movement or parts of the body.

Vitalograph An instrument that tests lung function and is able to produce a trace that is very useful for diagnosis and assessment of treatment efficacy.

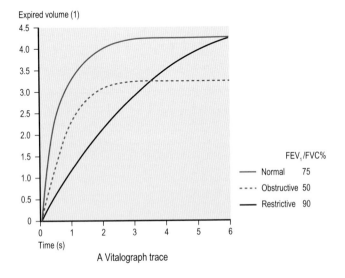

A Vitalograph trace

Vitalograph trace A useful diagnostic tool to identify normal, obstructive or restrictive airway disease states.

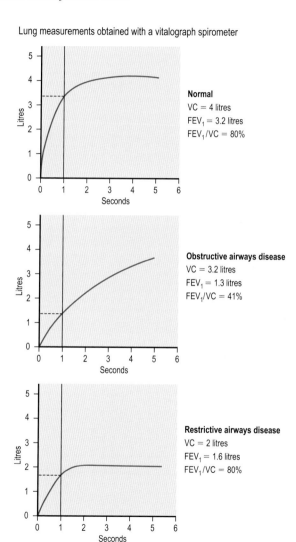

Lung measurements obtained with a vitalograph spirometer

Normal
VC = 4 litres
FEV_1 = 3.2 litres
FEV_1/VC = 80%

Obstructive airways disease
VC = 3.2 litres
FEV_1 = 1.3 litres
FEV_1/VC = 41%

Restrictive airways disease
VC = 2 litres
FEV_1 = 1.6 litres
FEV_1/VC = 80%

Viva (Voce) An examination where the candidate is asked questions directly by the examiner. This may be as the defence of a written piece of work, as in a PhD, or as an opportunity for a candidate to improve their mark following a written examination.

VMO Common medical abbreviation – Vastus medialis obliquus.

Volar On the same side of the hand as the palm.

Voltage Electrotherapy term – a measure (in volts [V]) of the electromotive force or potential difference between two points: the potential difference required between two points to move a coulomb of charge using a joule of energy.

Voluntary movement This is a commonly used term by physiotherapists to describe movement that is carried out by the patient under their own control.

von Recklinghausen disease (neurofibromatosis) An inherited disorder where multiple spots (known as café au lait spots) and neurofibromas appear. Joseph Merrick, the famous Elephant Man, was misdiagnosed as having this condition, it is now thought that he, in fact, had proteus syndrome (Tibbles & Cohen 1986).

VQ The ratio of alveolar ventilation to simultaneous alveolar capillary blood flow in any part of the lung:

Normal V (ventilation) = 4 l of air/min

Normal Q (perfusion) = 5 l of blood/min

A normal V/Q ratio is, therefore, 0.8. If the V/Q is higher than 0.8, it means ventilation exceeds perfusion. If the V/Q is <0.8, there is a VQ mismatch caused by poor ventilation.

VQ scan A scan that can be used to diagnose a pulmonary embolism.

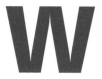

Wallerian degeneration This describes the physical and chemical process that occurs during changes to the axon following damage or trauma.

Warfarin A drug used as an inhibitor of prothrombin activation and, therefore, an inhibitor of blood clotting. Also used as a rat poison.

Warm up Warm up is used to improve circulation and increase body tissue temperature, therefore, physically and mentally preparing the participants for exercise. Warm-up exercise may also limit metabolite build up and subsequent acidosis during exercise. Proprioception may also be significantly more sensitive after warm up.

Warnings Following an explanation by the therapist of why they recommend using a particular therapy, the patient should be warned, prior to each treatment:

- what to expect to feel
- what they should not feel
- what to do if effect/feeling is not what was expected.

Then, obtain patient consent to use of the recommended procedure.

Wax A mixture of paraffin wax and mineral oil usually heated to 42–52°C in a purpose-designed container (wax bath). Used to provide superficial tissue heating, especially of hands to relieve chronic pain associated with various arthritic conditions or post fracture. Particular dangers are those associated with heating.

Wax bath Purpose-specific container, thermostat controlled and used to heat therapeutic wax clinically. Larger volumes usually require the container is within a surrounding water jacket to ensure even heating.

WBC Common medical abbreviation – White blood cell.

WCPT The World Confederation for Physical Therapy (WCPT) is a non-profit organization founded in 1951 supported by subscriptions from its 91 member organizations. The confederation represents over 225 000 physical therapists worldwide.

Wedges Wedges can come in a variety of sizes and can be used to help position patients and break up patterns of muscle activity, i.e. a wedge under the knees in supine lying can introduce flexion into an otherwise dominated extensor position. Alternatively, they can also be used to support areas of low tone, i.e. under the head and upper thorax to stop a low-tone shoulder 'dropping backwards'. Wedges are a useful adjunct to treatment.

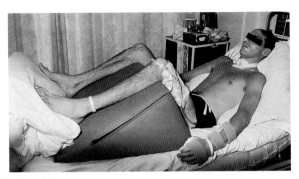

Supine lying with wedges

Weight distribution The distribution of body weight is a significant factor influencing postural stability. For instance, you are more stable on a wide base of support than when standing on tiptoes on one foot! For stability the centre of gravity of a body must fall within the base of support. A common problem with patients with hemiplegia (stroke) is their difficulty in moving the centre of gravity over the hemiplegic foot and hence problems with moving the so-called unaffected leg, but this is really due to their weight distribution still being proportionately more over the non-affected side.

Welfare state A system whereby government provides minimum, guaranteed services and income. In Britain the welfare state is linked to wide-ranging legislation, which was passed after the Second World War and which includes the National Health Service Act (1948) and the National Assistance Act (1948). The origins of the welfare state can, however, be traced back much further.

Wheeze A continuous high-pitched musical sound heard within the airways when obstruction is present.
See *Breath sounds*

Whiplash Injury to the cervical spine that results from rapid acceleration or deceleration pathology can be complex and prognosis varies remarkably. Medico legally, whiplash has become the subject of great debate.

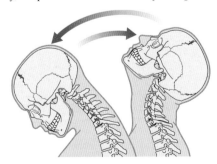

Whiplash

Whistle blowing A process whereby somebody employed by an organization makes known the incompetent or unethical practices or behaviour of colleagues. People who 'blow the whistle' are frequently victimized and, therefore, in 1998 the Public Interest and Disclosure Act was passed to provide them with some protection.

Winging scapula Elicited when the extended arm is pushed against resistance. The scapula 'wings' out when there is a weakening of the serratus anterior, usually caused by a long thoracic nerve lesion.

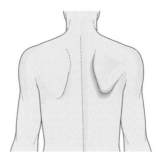

Winging Scapula

Wobble board An apparatus used for the re-education of proprioception and balance.

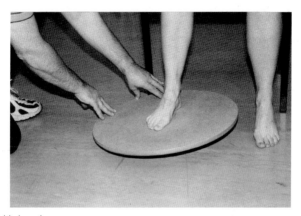

Wobble board

Wolf's law As bones are subjected to stress, they will change their internal architecture accordingly.

Put simply, bone is laid down when it is needed and absorbed when it is not.

✚ Clinical point This is of key importance to physiotherapists, since a person on prolonged bed rest will quickly start to lose bone mass, conversely a person who takes up jogging or weight lifting will begin to deposit extra bone – bone is alive.

Work of breathing (WOB) This is the amount of energy required to overcome the opposing forces of breathing (i.e. the elastic and resistive properties of the lung and chest wall). In order to move a given volume of air into the lung, a certain amount of effort is required.

Workshop A student-centred learning experience where the students and tutors work together using a range of materials/sources to achieve specified learning outcomes.

Wrist drop See *Radial nerve palsy*

Paralysis of the extensors of the wrist and fingers occurs following lesions of the radial nerve, these are particularly common following fractures of the shaft of the humerus (the radial nerve winds around the radial groove on the shaft of the humerus).

Wry neck See *Spasmodic torticollis*

X-rays Plain radiographs, usually taken when there is a history of trauma, to exclude fractures. Also used to confirm degenerative disease processes.

Y chromosome The chromosome that is male-determining in most mammals.

Yellow flag See *Flags*

Yergason's test A test for subluxation of the biceps tendon, at the shoulder. The physiotherapist resists shoulder flexion, elbow flexion and forearm supination. The biceps tendon is palpated to feel for any subluxation.

Yersinia pestis The bacterial cause of the bubonic plague that decimated Europe in the middle ages. It is transmitted to humans by the bite of fleas that have fed on infected rodents.

Z

Zimmer frame A four-point walking aid that can be used to assist patients who still require some extra support during the recovery process.

⊕ Clinical point Whilst assisting independence, be careful that the frame is at the right height so as to reduce the flexion influence, which may compound a balance problem. In some cases wheels may be used to replace the solid struts at the front of the frame in order to encourage a move-fluid pattern of walking. As with all walking aids, the Zimmer frame relies on upper-limb support and this needs to be taken into account when assessing the suitability of the patient.

Z-Line In muscle, these are the structures into which thin filaments are inserted. Z-lines define limits of the sarcomere.
See *Muscle structure*

Zona orbicularis Fibres of the articular capsule of the hip joint that encircle the neck of the femur.

Zygapophyseal joint – Also known as facet joint The pairs of spinal joints between the superior articular process, of the lower vertebra and the inferior articular process of vertebra above. These are plane synovial joints and they may be affected by degenerative changes in spondylosis. Their orientation serves to either allow or limit movement of the spine, e.g. in the thoracic spine they permit a great deal of rotation but block rotation in the lumbar spine.

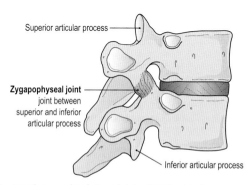

Facet joint – Rotation permitted; Facet joint – Rotation blocked

Zygoma The cheek bone.

Appendix: **Essay writing**

Sally French and John Swain

Northedge defines an essay as '... a short piece of writing on a specific subject' (1996: p. 110). You are frequently required to write essays as a means of demonstrating your mastery of a particular topic and your ability to express ideas coherently and in your own words. It is often the means by which you are assessed. Writing is demanding as it involves the development, shaping and expression of our thoughts and understandings. It is an active, dynamic process that takes considerable time, practice, patience and effort to perfect.

Constructing an essay does, however, demand skills other than the ability to write. It usually starts with note taking, where relevant material for the essay is gathered. At this stage it is crucial to read and select material that enables you to respond to the title precisely. A common mistake in essay writing is to pay insufficient attention to what is being asked. It is advisable, therefore, to highlight key words in the title to avoid the possibility of 'going off on a tangent'. The words you underline should be 'content' words (which indicate what you must write about) and 'command' or 'process' words (which indicate what you should do with the content you select). In the following examples the content words are underlined and the command words are in italics:

Evaluate the use of mobilizations in the treatment of capsulitis of the shoulder.

Justify the use of behaviour modification in the treatment of patients following brain injury.

The command word 'evaluate' is asking you to appraise the effectiveness or worth of mobilizations in the treatment of capsulitis of the shoulder. The content words are directing you to a particular medical condition (capsulitis) that is affecting a specific part of the body (the shoulder). You are not, therefore, being asked to consider capsulitis in any other joint or any other condition that might affect the shoulder. The command word 'justify' in the second example is asking you to provide grounds for the use of behaviour modification and to raise and allay any objections to it. The content words are directing you to a particular intervention (behaviour modification) in a particular circumstance (following brain injury). You are not being asked to consider behaviour modification for other patient groups or other interventions for people with brain injury.

Essay titles such as these also contain, implicitly, a controversy for you to consider. The first essay title implies that there are arguments both for and against the use of mobilizations in the treatment of capsulitis of the shoulder, with the likelihood of research articles supporting both opinions. The second essay title implies that there are objections to the use of behaviour modification following brain injury, on ethical grounds perhaps, as well as arguments that support it. Rather than coming down strongly on one side or the other, you are being asked to consider the evidence and to show that you have 'read round' the subject and understood it. It is always advisable to read carefully any guidance notes you are given on how to tackle the essay and what is expected of you. As you read around, keep careful notes about the literature and other sources you consult. It can be frustrating to have noted a quotation without the full information to reference the source (especially when you have returned the book to the library).

Before you start reading and selecting appropriate material it can be helpful to jot down all the ideas you have on the subject that you have accumulated from formal teaching, clinical education and your own experience. This will help you to get started and reassure you that you know something about the subject. Although it is likely that you will discard some of your jottings, other ideas and concepts will be important. You may organize them into 'mind maps' where the central idea is placed in the middle of the page with branches and arrows radiating outwards showing how the ideas and concepts are connected. This is an alternative to linear notes and may be more representative of our thought patterns in the early stages of formulating ideas.

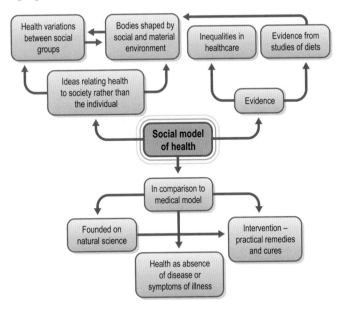

It is very important when writing essays to express the ideas in your own words. The ability to do this depends on your note taking skills and how well you understand the ideas. As Poole and Kelly state '... in order to develop the skill of writing in your own words you need to read actively processing meaning as you go' (2004: p. 43). Using somebody else's words and passing them off as your own is known as plagiarism. Although this is often done innocently, it usually indicates a weakness in note-taking skills and understanding and can also be regarded as a form of cheating; it must always be avoided as severe penalties can ensue. In order to avoid plagiarism, quotation marks must be placed around direct quotations and an indication made in the text of where important ideas have originated. This is usually done by placing the author's or researcher's name and date of the work in brackets. It is not acceptable to change the odd word or phase in somebody else's writing as this is still regarded as plagiarism. Most institutions have strict rules (often in course handbooks) and it is important to familiarize yourself with these.

As we have already discussed, your essay should demonstrate that you have grasped important ideas, that you have analyzed the evidence and that you have constructed a coherent argument. It will usually be necessary to draw upon material that you have covered in your course. It can be powerful to use examples from your own experience, but if this is done it is important to relate it to the theories or evidence that you are considering. You may, for example, recall a patient you treated with mobilizations for capsulitis of the shoulder and discuss the outcome of your treatment with reference to the research evidence. Similarly, you may have worked in a unit for people with brain injury where behaviour modification was used and relate this to various ethical considerations or to a particular theoretical perspective. Sweeping statements based on your own opinions or experience should generally be avoided.

A common question from students is, 'should I put in my own opinions?' What really matters is the quality of the argument, not what you personally believe one way or the another. For instance, if you personally take the position that there will always be a place for special schools in educational provision, it is your basis for your views (literature, argument, evidence, views of others, etc.) and also how you deal with counter-arguments that counts.

As we discussed above, it is important that your essay is your own work and not copied from the work of fellow students or published authors. It is wrong, however, to consider writing as necessarily a solitary activity. If you are experiencing problems in writing, or wish to improve your marks, support of various kinds can be helpful. This will depend both on the institution where you are studying and your own particular circumstances. The first source of support can be your tutor. If your tutor offers support in this way it can be useful to ask for a tutorial and to take along a plan of your essay and an introduction. Some students experience difficulties in expressing ideas in writing to such an extent that poor grammar, spelling and punctuation can be a barrier to the marker in understanding what the student is trying to say. This can be the case for people writing in a second language and for those who have dyslexia, for instance. Some universities and colleges offer specific support services that can be called upon. In general, you can seek out and use different sources of support while retaining the key principle that this is your piece of work, your ideas in your own words.

You may also experience difficulties with time management. This is especially true when the workload is high and a number of assignments need handing in around the same time. Time management is the key to ensuring that you organize your work to allow sufficient time for each of your writing tasks. A calendar can help in setting yourself personal deadlines for each aspect of your work.

STRUCTURING ESSAYS

It is important that your essay is structured so that your ideas flow and the people reading it (who are frequently assessing your work) can understand what you are saying. It is wise to plan your essay before you write it, although the plan may change and develop once you start. Most essays are structured in the following way:

- Title
- Introduction
- Main section
- Conclusion
- References.

However, Redman states that:

> ... an essay is always greater than its component parts, and it is how you put all those parts together that is often as important as the parts themselves.
>
> (2001: p. 18)

We have assumed that the title of the essay will be given to you, but you may, on occasions, be required to create a title of your own. In such circumstances it can help to check out your title with your tutor. As mentioned already, it is vitally important that you respond to the title of the essay precisely, whoever has constructed it. It is good practice always to include the full, exact title at the top of your essay. Some set titles provide a quotation followed by a process word such as 'discuss'. You should give the full quotation including, where possible, the reference for the source of the quotation.

The introduction

The introduction is more important than is generally recognized. It is not unusual to mark essays without an introduction or with a minimal couple of sentences to set the scene. For instance, we have marked essays that begin with a summary of the history of a topic with no explanation of where the discussion is going or why such a history is relevant to the particular issues being addressed. In the introduction you should show that you understand what is expected of you and briefly explain what you intend to do and how you are going to do it. Going back to the first of our two essay titles, you may indicate your understanding that there is a debate around the use of mobilizations in the treatment of capsulitis of the shoulder and that you are going to analyze the evidence from both sides. It may also be necessary to define key terms in the introduction, especially those that are contested. If you were writing an essay about disability, for example, it may be necessary to define the meaning of the word as it means different things to different people.

As the introduction should clearly state what you intend to do in the essay, it can be difficult to write it first (when the exact content of your essay is unclear). Redman points out that this is in no way necessary:

> The difficulty with introduction writing is that sometimes you only know what the core arguments are when you have finished your essay. So,

although writing the introduction can help to give you a clear idea of what you are doing, you may find it is a good idea to write it last.

(2001: p. 46)

As you progress through your course you may be encouraged to argue an issue from a particular position of your choice, rather than presenting both sides of an argument. If this is the case, you need to indicate in the introduction the line you intend to take. If, for example, you were presented with the following essay title, 'Physiotherapists play an important role in the ability of disabled people to become and remain independent. Discuss this claim with reference to one model of disability', you may decide to argue from the perspective of the social model rather than the medical model of disability. You can also state a particular focus for your essay. For instance, given this title you may wish to focus on people with learning difficulties. This can strengthen your essay if the focus is clearly defined in your introduction and you can justify it. You might argue that the issues have particular pertinence to physiotherapists working with people with learning difficulties or that you have personal experience of work in this area.

When the title includes a quotation, it is useful to consult and refer to the original source. It may be, for instance, that the quotation is from a paper based on research undertaken by the author(s). In this case, a sentence or two outlining the nature of the research can help put the quotation in context and set the scene for your discussion.

The main section

The main section of your essay is the longest part and is where you present the bulk of your material. It is here where you construct your argument being sure to engage with the title of the essay at all times and examining the issue from different points of view and theoretical perspectives. You will need to present and evaluate evidence and theory and may make use of your own experience if this is appropriate. You need to select the most important material to support your argument, which may include maps, numerical data and diagrams. As you will have a specific word count, your ability to précis material and write succinctly will be tested to the full.

The conclusion

The conclusion of your essay is usually no more than a paragraph or two in length. It is here that you need to summarize the main content of your essay and recap the core arguments. A good tactic in writing your conclusion is to return to your introduction and the title of the essay. This pulls the whole analysis and argument together and makes it clear that you have directly addressed the specific title. It is important not to raise new issues in your conclusion; that is, issues that have not been discussed in the body of the essay. You may, however, point out areas in the debate that need developing.

The references

At the end of your essay you should list in full the references that you have used and which appear in the text. There are various styles in which references are presented, the most common one being the Harvard style. The important thing is that all the information is present so that interested readers can look up the references if they wish. Some university and college libraries have booklets for students outlining the 'house style' for referencing for the institution. A list of references also indicates that you have engaged with the literature. The references you cite should always be relevant to what you are discussing and should generally be up to date. (For a full discussion of referencing styles see French & Sim [1993] and Northedge [1996].)

MAKING YOUR ESSAY FLOW

As well as attending to content, your essay should also be fluent and easy to read. This can be achieved in many ways, some of which have already been discussed. Outlining what you intend to do in the introduction, defining key terms and structuring your essay logically will all help the reader to follow your line of argument. Clear explanations and providing examples to illustrate the points you are making will help to give clarity and focus. Short sentences and simple language are also important in getting your meaning across. As Redman states:

> There is nothing to be gained from using complex language for its own sake. The real test lies in being able to communicate complex ideas in the form that is most easily understood. (2001: pp. 65–66)

Jargon and the excessive use of abbreviations should be avoided and paragraphs should be kept short and should generally contain just one major theme. Varying the length of sentences and paragraphs does, however, give your writing rhythm. The use of sub-heading can also help to structure your argument.

Keeping your readers on track is sometimes referred to as 'signposting'. You constantly need to tell discreetly or remind your readers of what you are doing, so that they do not lose the thread of your argument. A sound introduction and overall structure will assist with this, but you can also use 'linking' words and phrases to help your essay flow. Phrases such as 'as we have seen', 'on the other hand', 'to summarize', 'to conclude' and 'before we discuss x we need to consider y' all inform your readers of where you are going. Linking words, such as 'therefore', 'nevertheless', 'conversely' and 'however', also serve the purpose of linking together the ideas you are presenting. It is a good strategy to imagine that you are writing for the 'intelligent lay person' rather than your tutor. In that way points that may seem too obvious to mention will not be omitted. The overall presentation of your essay is also important. Handwriting should be clear, font size comfortable to read and margins wide enough to allow for the writing of comments. The correct level of formality or informality of your essay, for example, whether you write in the first person, varies across academic disciplines. Generally, the 'hard' sciences, such as physiology and physics, take a more formal stance than the social sciences.

It will usually be necessary to write at least two drafts before handing your essay in. In the first draft you need to concentrate on the content and overall structure of your essay and in the second draft you need to think about your reader and attend to the clarity of your writing including your spelling and punctuation. Considerable cutting and rearranging usually takes place at this stage. Both content and style are important in achieving a good grade.

CONCLUSION

As we mentioned at the beginning of this chapter, the skill of writing well is not easy and takes considerable time and effort. The rewards of writing are, however, great. Because you have engaged in a dynamic and challenging activity, your understanding of the topic, as well as your memory of the issues, will be enhanced. Furthermore, you will have practised a skill that is so important in the work of physiotherapists today.

References

French S, Sim J 1993 Writing: a Guide for Therapists. Butterworth Heinemann, Oxford

Northedge A 1996 The Good Study Guide. Open University. Milton Keynes

Poole L, Kelly B 2004 Preparing to Study DD100/DD121. Reading and Note Taking. Open University. Milton Keynes

Redman P 2001 Good Essay Writing: a Social Science Guide. Sage. London

References

AARC 1993 Clinical Practice Guideline- Directed Cough. Respir Care 38: 495–499

Altose MD 1989 Assessment and management of breathlessness. Chest (Suppl): 775–835

Alvarez DJ, Rockwell PG 2002 Trigger points: diagnosis and management. Am Fam Physician 65(4): 653–660

American Academy of Orthopaedic Surgeons 1987 A Glossary on Spinal Terminology. American Academy of Orthopaedic Surgeons, Chicago, pp. 34–35

Andrews K 1999 The vegetative state – clinical diagnosis. Postgraduate Medical Journal 75: 321–324

Barclay J 1994 In Good Hands: History of the Chartered Society of Physiotherapy, 1984–94. Butterworth Heinemann

Barlow JH and Williams B 1999 'I now feel that I'm not just a bit of left luggage': the experience of older women with arthritis attending a personal independence course. Disability and Society 14: 1, 53–64

Barnard G, Artiglas A, Bringham K et al. The Consensus Committee 1994 Report on the American-European consensus conference on ARDS: definitions, mechanisms, relevant outcomes and clinical trial co-ordination. Inten Care Med 20: 225–232

Bateman NT, Leach RM 1998 ABC of oxygen. Acute oxygen therapy. BMJ 317: 798–801

Birch A, Price A 2003 Joint arthroplasty. In: Porter S (ed.) Tidy's Physiotherapy, 13th edn. Butterworth Heinemann, Oxford

Bobath B 1985 Abnormal postural reflex activity caused by brain lesions, 3rd edn. Heinemann Physiotherapy, London

Bobath B 1990 Adult hemiplegia: evaluation and treatment, 3rd edn. Heinemann Medical Books, Oxford

Boissonnault JS, Blaschak MJ 1988 Incidence of diastasis recti abdominis during the childbearing year. Physical Therapy 7: 1082–1086

Borg G 1982 Psychophysical basis of perceived exertion. Med Sc Sports Ex 14: 377–381

Brook G, Brayshaw E, Coldron Y et al. 2003 Physiotherapy in women's health. In: Porter S (ed.) Tidy's Physiotherapy, 13th edn. Butterworth Heinemann, Oxford

Briemberg HR, Amato AA 2003 Dermatomyositis and polymyositis. Curr Treat Options Neurol 5(5): 349–356

BTS 1997 Current best practise for nebuliser treatment. Thorax 52; supplement 2

BTS 2001 Non-invasive ventilation in acute respiratory failure. Thorax 57(3): 192–211

BTS 2001 Guidelines for the Management of Community Acquired Pneumonia in Adults. 56; Suppl IV

BTS 2002 Guidelines for the Management of Community Acquired Pneumonia in Childhood. 57; Suppl I

BTS 2003 Guidelines on the Management of Asthma. Thorax 58: (suppl 1)

Burke D 1988 Spasticity as an adaptation to pyradimal tract injury. Advances in Neurology 47: 401–423

Byrnes WC, Clarkson PM 1986 Delayed onset muscle soreness and training. Clin Sports Med 5(3): 605–614

Calin A, Garrett S, Whitelock H, Kennedy L, O'Hea J, Mallorie P, Jenkinson T 1994 A new approach to defining functional ability in ankylosing spondylitis: the development of the Bath Ankylosing Spondylitis Functional Index. J Rheumatol 21(12): 2281–2285

Carne K 2003 Osteoporosis. In: Porter S (ed.) Tidy's Physiotherapy, 13th edn. Butterworth Heinemann, Oxford

Carr J, Shepherd R 1998 Neurological Rehabilitation: Optimizing Motor Performance. Butterworth Heinemann, Edinburgh

Chartered Society of Physiotherapy 2000 Rules of professional conduct, 3rd edn. CSP, London

Chartered Society of Physiotherapy 2002 Curriculum Framework for qualifying programmes in physiotherapy. CSP, London

Coggon D, Reading I, Barret D, McLaren M, Cooper C 2001 Knee osteoarthritis and obesity. Int J Obes Relat Metab Disord 25(5): 622–627

Concensus Conference 1999 Clinical indications for NIV in chronic respiratory failure due to restrictive lung disease, COPD and nocturnal hypoventilation – a Consensus conference report. Chest 116: 521–534

Court E, Lea R 2003 Tissue inflammation and repair. In: Porter S (ed.) Tidy's Physiotherapy, 13th edn. Butterworth Heinemann, Oxford

Cyriax J 1982 Illustrated manual of orthopaedic medicine. Butterworth Heinemann, Oxford

Davies A, Blackeley A, Kidd C 2001 Human physiology. Churchill Livingstone, Edinburgh

Department of Health 1990 NHS and Community Care Act. HMSO Stationery Office, London

Dyson M 1985 Therapeutic applications of ultrasound. In: Nyborg WL, Ziskin MC (eds) Biological effects of ultrasound (clinics in diagnostic ultrasound). Churchill Livingstone, New York

Edwards S (ed.) 2002 Neurological physiotherapy: a problem-solving approach. Churchill Livingstone, Edinburgh

European Respiratory Society Task Force 2001 ERS Guidelines on the use of nebulisers. Eur Respir J 18: 228–242

Falk M, Kelstrup M, Anderson JB, Pederson SS, Rossing I, Dirksen H 1984 Improving the ketchup bottle method with positive respiratory pressure, PEP, in cystic fibrosis. Eur J Resp Dis 65: 423–432

Fries JF, Spitz P, Kraines RG, Holman HR 1980. Measurement of patient outcome in arthritis. Arthritis Rheum 23: 137–145

Garay SM, Turino GM, Goldring RM 1981 Sustained reversal of chronic hypercapnia in patients with alveolar hypoventilation syndromes: long term maintenance with non-invasive nocturnal mechanical ventilation. Am J Med 70: 269–274

Giles LGF, Singer KP 1997 Clinical anatomy and management of low back pain, Butterworth Heinemann, London

Global Initiative for Chronic Obstructive Lung Disease Guidelines 2002 Guidelines for chronic obstructive pulmonary disease. Curr Opin Pulm Med 8(2): 81–86

Heilman KM, Watson R, Valenstein E 1993 Neglect and related disorders. In: Heilman KM, Valenstein E (eds) Clinical Neuropsychology, 3rd edn. Oxford University Press, Oxford

Hough A 2001 Physiotherapy in respiratory care: a problem-solving approach. Nelson Thornes, Cheltenham

Hunt SM, McKenna SP 1991 The Nottingham Health Profile: user's manual. Revised edn. Galen Research and Consultancy, Manchester

International Continence Society 2002 Standardisation of terminology in lower urinary tract function. International Continence Society Document

International Working Party 1996 Report on the Vegetative State. The Royal Hospital for Neuro-disability, London

Jaeschke R, Singer J, Guyatt G 1989 Controlled clinical trials 10: 407–415

Johnson LB, Bhan A, Pawlak J, Manzor O, Saravolatz LD 2003 Changing epidemiology of community-onset methicillin-resistant Staphylococcus aureus bacteremia. Infect Control Hosp Epidemiol 24(6): 431–435

Kearon C 2003 Natural history of venous thromboembolism. Circulation 107(23 Suppl 1): I22-I30

Kim SJ, Kim HK 1995 Reliability of the anterior drawer test, the pivot shift test, and the Lachman test. Clin Orthop 317: 237–242

Kramer N, Meyer TJ, Meharg J, Cece RD, Hill NS 1995 Randomised prospective trial of NIPPV in acute respiratory failure. Am J Resp Crit Care Med 151: 1799–1806

Laing RD 1983 The voice of experience. Penguin Books. Harmondsworth.

Lorig K, Chastain RL, Ung E, Shoor S, Holman HR 1989 Development and evaluation of a scale to measure perceived self-efficacy in people with arthritis. Arthritis Rheum 32: 37–44

Low J, Reed A 1999 Electrotherapy Explained. Butterworth Heinemann Publishers, Oxford

Kitchen S, Bazin S (eds) 1995 Clayton's electrotherapy. WB Saunders Co, London, pp. 3–30

Maitland GD 2001 Maitlands vertebral manipulation, 6th edn. Butterworth Heinemann, London

Macirowski T, Tepic S, Mann RW et al. 1994 Cartilage stresses in the human hip joint. Journal of Biomechanical Engineering 116: 106–107 Magnus 1926 as cited by Bobath B 1990 Adult hemiplegia: evaluation and treatment, 3rd edn. Heinemann Medical Books, Oxford

Mason D, Kilmurray S 2003 In: Porter S (ed.) Tidy's Physiotherapy, 13th edn. Butterworth Heinemann, Oxford

Meenan RF, Gertman PM, Mason JH, Dunaif R 1982 The Arthritis Impact Measurement Scales: further investigations of a health status measure. Arthritis Rheum 25: 1048–1053

Meenan RF, Mason JH, Anderson JJ, Guccione AA, Kazis LE. 1992 AIMS2: the content and properties of a revised and expanded Arthritis Impact Measurement Scales health status questionnaire. Arthritis Rheum 35: 1–10

Mehta S, Hill NS 2001 Non-invasive ventilation: state of the art. Am J Respir Crit Care Med 163: 540–77

Menkes H, Britt EJ 1980 Rationale for physical therapy. Am Rev Resp Dis 122 (2 part 2): 127–131

Morgan G, Wilbourn AJ 1998 Cervical radiculopathy and coexisting distal entrapment neuropathies: double-crush syndromes? Neurology 50(1): 78–83

National Institute for Clinical Excellence 2004 Chronic Obstructive Pulmonary Disease Guidelines. Thorax 59(Suppl 1)

National Institute for Clinical Excellence 2004 The guideline development process (current). Appendix K. NICE

North West Oxygen Group 2001 Emergency oxygen therapy for the breathless patient – guidelines. Emergency Med J 18(6): 421–423

Pryor JA, Prasad A 2002 Physiotherapy for respiratory and cardiac problems, 3rd edn. Churchill Livingstone, Edinburgh

Pongratz D, Spath M 2001 Fibromyalgia. Fortschr Neurol Psychiatr 69(4): 189–193

Porter S 2003 Tidy's Physiotherapy, 13th edn. Butterworth Heinemann, Oxford

Richards J 2003 Biomechanics In: Porter S (ed.) Tidy's Physiotherapy, 13th edn. Butterworth Heinemann, Oxford

Sackett DL, Rosenberg WMC, Muir Gray JA, Haynes G, Scott W 1996 Evidence based medicine: what it is and what it isn't. BMJ 312: 71–72

Schwartsman V, Choi SH, Schwartsman R 1990 Tibial nonunions. Treatment tactics with the Ilizarov method. Orthop Clin North Am 21(4): 639–653

Secretary of State for Health 1998 A First Class Service: Quality in the New NHS. Department of Health, London

Shakespeare T, Gillespie-Sells K, Davies D 1996 The Sexual Politics of Disability. Cassell. London

Shacklock M 1995 Neurodynamics. Physiotherapy 81(1): 9–16

Shapiro SH, Ernst P, Gray-Donals K et al 1992 Effect of negative pressure ventilation in severe COPD. Lancet 340: 1425–1429

Sharma LC, Lou C, Cahue S, Dunlop DD 2000 The mechanism of the effect of obesity in knee osteoarthritis: the mediating role of malalignment. Arthritis Rheum 43(3): 568–575

Shepherd JT, Rusch NJ, Vanhoutte PM 1983 Effect of cold on the blood vessel wall. Gen Pharmacol 14(1): 61–64

SIGN OSA Guidelines 2003 Available online at www.sign.ac.uk

Stephenson R, Edwards S, Freeman J 1998 Associated reactions: their value in clinical practice? Physiotherapy Research International 3: 69–78

Stokes 1998 Neurological physiotherapy. Mosby, London

Stroke Unit Trialists 2002 Organised Inpatient (Stroke Unit) Care for Stroke (Cochrane Review). In: The Cochrane Library Issue 1.Oxford: Update Software

Sturmer T, Gunther KP, Brenner H et al. 2000 Obesity, overweight and patterns of osteoarthritis: the Ulm Osteoarthritis Study. J Clin Epidemiol 53(3): 307–313

Sullivan CE, Issa FG, Berthan Jones M, Eves l 1981 Reversal of obstructive sleep apnoea by CPAP applied through the nares. Lancet 1: 862–865

Ter Haar G 1996 Electrophysical principles. In: Clayton's Electrotherapy, 10th edn. Bailliere Tindall, London

Tibbles JA, Cohen MM Jr 1986 The Proteus syndrome: the Elephant Man diagnosed. Br Med J (Clin Res Ed) 293(6548): 683–685

Tsong TY 1989 Deciphering the language of cells. TIBS 14: 89–92

Vickers AJ 2001 Time course of muscle soreness following different types of exercise BMC Musculoskelet Disord 2(1): 5

Wallston KA, Wallston BS, DeVellis R 1978 Development of the Multidimensional Health Locus of Control Scales. Health Educ Monogr 6: 161–170

Walshe F 1923 On certain tonic or postural reflexes in hemiplegia, with special reference to the so called associated movements. Brain 46: 1–37

Webber B 1988 The Brompton Hospital Guide to Chest Physiotherapy, 5th edn. Blackwell Scientific Publications, Oxford

Weilitz PB 1993 In: Ahrens T, Rutherford K (eds) Essentials of Oxygenation: Implication for Clinical Practice. Jones and Bartlett, Boston, Mass, pp. 132–141

Wendell S 1996 The Rejected Body: feminist philosophical perspectives on disability. Routledge. London

West JB 1977 Pulmonary gas exchange. Int Rev Physiol 14: 83–106

West JB 1982 Pulmonary pathophysiology, 2nd edn. Williams and Wilkins, Baltimore, p. 8–11

Woollam CHM 1976 The development of apparatus for intermittent negative pressure respiration 1832–1918. Anaesthesia 31: 537–547

World Health Organization 1991 Consensus Development Conference. Prophylaxis and treatment of osteoporosis. Am J Med 90: 107–110

Zyluk A, Zyluk B 1999 Shoulder-hand syndrome in patients after stroke. Neurol Neurochir Pol 33(1): 131–142